Role of Nutrition in Providing Pro-/Anti-Inflammatory Balance:

Emerging Research and Opportunities

Uğur Günşen
Bandırma Onyedi Eylül University, Turkey

Ramazan Mert Atan
Bandırma Onyedi Eylül University, Turkey

A volume in the Advances in Medical Diagnosis, Treatment, and Care (AMDTC) Book Series

IGI Global
DISSEMINATOR OF KNOWLEDGE

Published in the United States of America by
IGI Global
Medical Information Science Reference (an imprint of IGI Global)
701 E. Chocolate Avenue
Hershey PA, USA 17033
Tel: 717-533-8845
Fax: 717-533-8661
E-mail: cust@igi-global.com
Web site: http://www.igi-global.com

Library of Congress Cataloging-in-Publication Data

Names: Günşen, Uğur, 1965- editor. | Atan, Ramazan Mert, 1995- editor.
Title: Role of nutrition in providing pro-/anti-inflammatory balance : emerging research and opportunities / Uğur Günşen, Ramazan Mert Atan, editors.
Description: Hershey, PA : Medical Information Science Reference, [2020] | Includes bibliographical references and index. | Summary: "This book explores the role of nutrition in providing pro-/anti-inflammatory balance. It also examines the formation process of inflammation, biomarkers used for diagnosis, and diseases affected by inflammation"-- Provided by publisher.
Identifiers: LCCN 2019057184 (print) | LCCN 2019057185 (ebook) | ISBN 9781799835943 (hardcover) | ISBN 9781799835967 (ebook)
Subjects: MESH: Inflammation | Dietary Supplements | Inflammation Mediators | Biomarkers | Immune System Phenomena | Nutritional Physiological Phenomena
Classification: LCC RB131 (print) | LCC RB131 (ebook) | NLM QZ 150 | DDC 616/.0473--dc23
LC record available at https://lccn.loc.gov/2019057184
LC ebook record available at https://lccn.loc.gov/2019057185

This book is published in the IGI Global book series Advances in Medical Diagnosis, Treatment, and Care (AMDTC) (ISSN: 2475-6628; eISSN: 2475-6636)

British Cataloguing in Publication Data
A Cataloguing in Publication record for this book is available from the British Library.

For electronic access to this publication, please contact: eresources@igi-global.com.

Advances in Medical Diagnosis, Treatment, and Care (AMDTC) Book Series

ISSN:2475-6628
EISSN:2475-6636

MISSION

Advancements in medicine have prolonged the life expectancy of individuals all over the world. Once life-threatening conditions have become significantly easier to treat and even cure in many cases. Continued research in the medical field will further improve the quality of life, longevity, and wellbeing of individuals.

The **Advances in Medical Diagnosis, Treatment, and Care (AMDTC)** book series seeks to highlight publications on innovative treatment methodologies, diagnosis tools and techniques, and best practices for patient care. Comprised of comprehensive resources aimed to assist professionals in the medical field apply the latest innovations in the identification and management of medical conditions as well as patient care and interaction, the books within the AMDTC series are relevant to the research and practical needs of medical practitioners, researchers, students, and hospital administrators.

COVERAGE

- Experimental Medicine
- Alternative Medicine
- Patient Interaction
- Internal Medicine
- Cancer Treatment
- Diagnostic Medicine
- Disease Prevention
- Critical Care
- Medical Procedures
- Disease Management

IGI Global is currently accepting manuscripts for publication within this series. To submit a proposal for a volume in this series, please contact our Acquisition Editors at Acquisitions@igi-global.com or visit: http://www.igi-global.com/publish/.

The Advances in Medical Diagnosis, Treatment, and Care (AMDTC) Book Series (ISSN 2475-6628) is published by IGI Global, 701 E. Chocolate Avenue, Hershey, PA 17033-1240, USA, www.igi-global.com. This series is composed of titles available for purchase individually; each title is edited to be contextually exclusive from any other title within the series. For pricing and ordering information please visit http://www.igi-global.com/book-series/advances-medical-diagnosis-treatment-care/129618. Postmaster: Send all address changes to above address.

Titles in this Series

For a list of additional titles in this series, please visit:
http://www.igi-global.com/book-series/advances-medical-diagnosis-treatment-care/129618

Advanced Pharmacological Uses of Medicinal Plants and Natural Products
Ajeet Singh (National Dairy Research Institute, India) Padam Singh (Vaccine and Infectious Disease Research Centre, Translational Health Science and Technology Institute, India) and Navneet Bithel (Gurukul Kangri Universit, India)
Medical Information Science Reference • © 2020 • 540pp • H/C (ISBN: 9781799820949) • US $425.00

Quality Control of Cellular Protein in Neurodegenerative Disorders
Md. Sahab Uddin (Southeast University, Bangladesh) and Ghulam Md. Ashraf (King Abdulaziz University, Saud Arabia)
Medical Information Science Reference • © 2020 • 515pp • H/C (ISBN: 9781799813170) • US $295.00

Multidimensional Perspectives and Global Analysis of Universal Health Coverage
Yeter Demir Uslu (Istanbul Medipol University, Turkey) Hasan Dinçer (Istanbul Medipol University, Turkey) and Serhat Yüksel (İstanbul Medipol University, Turkey)
Medical Information Science Reference • © 2020 • 499pp • H/C (ISBN: 9781799823292) • US $265.00

Examining Biological Foundations of Human Behavior
Barre Vijaya Prasad (Dharwad Institute of Mental Health and Neurosciences, India)
Medical Information Science Reference • © 2020 • 266pp • H/C (ISBN: 9781799828600) • US $285.00

Handbook of Research on Medical Interpreting
Izabel E.T. de V. Souza (Osaka University, Japan) and Effrossyni (Effie) Fragkou (National and Kapodistrian University of Athens, Greece)
Medical Information Science Reference • © 2020 • 511pp • H/C (ISBN: 9781522593089) • US $345.00

For an entire list of titles in this series, please visit:
http://www.igi-global.com/book-series/advances-medical-diagnosis-treatment-care/129618

IGI Global
DISSEMINATOR OF KNOWLEDGE

701 East Chocolate Avenue, Hershey, PA 17033, USA
Tel: 717-533-8845 x100 • Fax: 717-533-8661
E-Mail: cust@igi-global.com • www.igi-global.com

Editorial Advisory Board

Table of Contents

Preface

Inflammation, which is one of the most important issues of health research in recent years, plays a role not only in a few diseases but also in the formation of many diseases that cause significant morbidity and contributes to early mortality (Couzin-Frankel, 2010).

Inflammation affects a wide range of diseases such as asthma, rheumatoid arthritis, cardiovascular diseases, obesity, diabetes, osteoporosis, certain types of cancer, depression, post-traumatic stress disorder, Alzheimer's and so on (Miller, Chen, & Parker, 2011; Slavich & Cole, 2013). Inflammation affects 8 of the top 10 causes of death in the US (Hoyert & Xu, 2012). However, there are many issues with a questionable link between inflammation and health. Furthermore, research on how and when to combat diseases associated with inflammation has been thought to reduce mortality and health care costs (Slavich, 2015).

Defining inflammation as good or bad is controversial. In addition, many issues related to inflammation are waiting to be elucidated. One of them is time. Time-dependent increases in inflammation are important to limit wound healing and the spread of infectious infections. Inflammation should therefore not always be described as bad and can be critical to survival, especially at times of injury and infection. However, to date, there is limited information about when elevated levels of inflammatory activity are protective against substances that may be harmful to our body (Irwin & Cole, 2011; Sternberg, 2006).

There is also some confusion regarding the mechanism of action of inflammation. Although classical theories have conceptualized inflammation as a localized process, new analyzes have created new ideas such as "systemic inflammation." It has also shown that inflammatory activity occurring at different locations such as peripheral tissues, different organs, oral fluids, and central nervous system is generally not correlated with a high degree of inflammation and possibly has different effects on health. Inflammation are thought to interact with some factors such as neural, cognitive, and emotional processes, diet, sleep and exercise, genetic factors and social-environmental problems. However, most human studies do not provide us with sufficient information about these factors that mitigate or increase the health effects of inflammation (Slavich, 2015).

Inflammation is the immune system's response to harmful stimuli, such as pathogens, damaged cells, toxic compounds (Medzhitov, 2010) and is effective in initiating the healing process by eliminating these harmful stimuli (Ferrero-Miliani, Nielsen, Andersen, & Girardin, 2007). Cellular, molecular events, and interactions usually occur during acute inflammatory responses, minimizes injury or inflammation. Thus, acute inflammation contributes to the restoration and healing of tissue homeostasis. This may contribute to various chronic inflammatory diseases (Zhou, Hong, & Huang, 2016). Chronic inflammatory diseases are one of the most important causes of death in the world. The World Health Organization (WHO) lists chronic diseases as the greatest threat to human health. Accordingly, the WHO expects the prevalence of chronic inflammation-related diseases to increase dramatically in the United States over the next 30 years. Worldwide, 3 out of 5 people die from chronic inflammatory diseases such as stroke, chronic respiratory diseases, heart disease, cancer, obesity, and diabetes (Chertov, Yang, Zack Howard, & Oppenheim, 2000; Takeuchi & Akira, 2010; Zhou et al., 2016).

Inflammation at the tissue level is characterized by redness, swelling, heat, pain and loss of tissue function as a result of vascular and inflammatory cell responses to local immunity due to infection or injury (Takeuchi & Akira, 2010). Important microcirculatory events that occur during the inflammatory process include changes in vascular permeability, leukocyte uptake, accumulation, and inflammatory mediator release (Chertov et al., 2000; Ferrero-Miliani et al., 2007). The etiology of inflammation can be divided into infectious or non-infectious (Table 1).

Table 1. Etiology of inflammation (Chen et al., 2018).

NON-INFECTIOUS FACTORS	INFECTIOUS FACTORS
Physical: Burn, frostbite, physical injury, foreign bodies, trauma, ionizing radiation **Chemical:** Glucose, fatty acids, toxins, alcohol, chemical irritants (including fluoride, nickel and other trace elements) **Biological:** Damaged cells **Psychological:** Excitement	Bacteria, viruses and other microorganisms

Although inflammatory response processes depend on the precise nature and position of the initial stimulus, they share a common mechanism, all of which can be summarized as follows:

1) Recognizes harmful stimuli from cell surface pattern receptors
2) Inflammatory pathways are activated
3) Inflammatory markers are released
4) Inflammatory cells are collected (Chen et al., 2018)

The discovery of cellular and molecular inflammatory mediators and the development of sensitive biomarkers has rapidly developed its role in the detection of inflammation and pathology (Brenner et al., 2014). Low-grade systemic inflammation is characterized by a two to three-fold increase in cytokine concentrations in the bloodstream, such as tumor necrosis factor alpha (TNF-α), interleukin-6 (IL-6) and high-sensitivity C-reactive protein (hsCRP) (Petersen & Pedersen, 2005; Ridker, 2007). In addition, other ILs (eg, IL-1β, IL-4, IL-8, and IL-10), adhesion molecules (e.g. vascular cell adhesion molecule 1 (VCAM1) and intracellular adhesion molecule 1 (ICAM1) are important biomarkers used to determine the inflammatory state of the individual (Demerath, Towne, Blangero, & Siervogel, 2001; Mozos et al., 2017).

According to many national and international health guidelines, a healthy and balanced diet pattern is one of the most important modifiable risk factors for the protection of individuals from chronic diseases. Adequate and balanced nutrition in terms of macro and micronutrients has a positive effect on the prevention, onset and prognosis of chronic diseases in the short and long term (WHO, 2019a; WHO, 2019b).

Unhealthy diets and negative behavioral patterns in lifestyle lead to the development of cardiovascular diseases, type 2 diabetes, cancer and other diseases, which are mainly due to inflammation. Consumption of foods containing natural antioxidants, fibers, refined carbohydrates, simple sugars, saturated fats, trans fats and omega-3 fatty acids stimulates innate immunity. Some of these foods increase the production of pro-inflammatory cytokines, while others increase the production of anti-inflammatory cytokines (Casas & Estruch, 2016).

Recent studies have emphasized the value of defining the relationship between diet and inflammation by evaluating dietary patterns (Ahluwalia, Andreeva, Kesse-Guyot, & Hercberg, 2013; Andersen, Murphy, & Fernandez, 2016; Calle, Vega-López, Segura-Pérez, Pérez-Escamilla, & Luz Fernandez, 2013). A dietary pattern can be described as a comprehensive dietary assessment, in which many types of nutrients are examined collectively (Jacobs & Steffen, 2003). Studying dietary patterns can be complex and challenging, in part due to the diversity of patterns within different cultures and populations, in addition to the inherent heterogeneity of physiological responses to diet due to variability in genetics, microbiome profiles, metabolic status, etc. (Reedy, Krebs-Smith, Hammond, & Hennessy, 2017).

The health impact of inflammation and the role of diet in inflammation have led to the development of dietary inflammatory index (DII). Accordingly, this index evaluates an individual's diet, the results of articles related to inflammatory biomarkers IL-1, IL-4, IL-6, IL-10, TNF-α, CRP, and with reference to, classifies the level of inflammation of the diet (Shivappa, Steck, Hurley, Hussey, & Hébert, 2014).

In addition to the fact that the whole diet is effective on inflammation, it appears that food groups in the diet affect inflammatory biomarkers separately. For example, higher consumption of both fruits and vegetables is associated with higher levels of antioxidant capacity indicators. This may result in lower levels of CRP, IL-6, and TNF-a, which are inflammatory biomarkers (Root at al., 2012).

Along with the modern society, there have been changes in the way individuals are fed. This diet, which changes with increasing consumption of packaged and processed carbohydrates, fast food, excessive sugary and carbonated beverages, is called "western type diet". Compared to other nutritional approaches, the Western diet is defined as malnutrition (Odermatt, 2011). The effect of chronic inflammation is remarkable in diseases that are rapidly increasing in society. Nutrition is one of the most important factors in the formation and treatment of inflammation. It is necessary to focus more on the effects of macro-micro nutrient selection, diet models, nutritional supplements, bioactive proteins and peptides on inflammation.

The main focus of this book is; pro- / anti-inflammatory balance is the effectiveness of nutrition and nutritional strategies. In this context, firstly information about the formation process of inflammation, biomarkers used for diagnosis, diseases affected by inflammation and their incidence in the society are given. Subsequently, affecting the balance of inflammation in individuals are discussed macro-micro nutrient consumption, nutritional supplements (probiotics and prebiotics), bioactive proteins and peptides, and dietary forms. This book is written at a level that can be used by students who are studying in medical faculties and health sciences, academicians working in this field and individuals who want to learn about this subject.

ORGANIZATION OF THE BOOK

The book is organized into eight chapters. A brief description of each of the chapters follows:

Chapter 1 provides a basic knowledge of inflammation. Distinctive features of acute and chronic inflammation and the factors causing this condition are mentioned. The methods used to reveal inflammation and newly added methods are included. In addition, the relationship between inflammation and other chronic diseases is explained.

Chapter 2 deals with the epidemiology of various diseases involving inflammation. Cardiovascular diseases, cancer, diabetes mellitus, asthma-chronic obstructive pulmonary disease, obesity, metabolic syndrome, inflammatory bowel disease and various diseases that cause premature death and morbidity are closely associated with inflammation. There is an increase in the rate of these diseases worldwide.

Chapter 3 discusses macro-nutrients that are effective in balancing inflammation in individuals. The individual's inflammatory response varies according to the daily intake levels, sources and types of carbohydrates, fats and proteins, which are macronutrients. Some macro nutrients disrupt this balance or vice versa. This section describes macronutrients with pro- or anti-inflammatory properties.

Chapter 4 discusses micronutrients that are effective in maintaining an individual's inflammatory balance. Accordingly, vitamins A, D, E, K, C, iron, selenium, and zinc are known to have anti-inflammatory properties. The intake of these nutrients in accordance with the requirements is an important step in the prevention and treatment of inflammation-related diseases. This section describes the effectiveness of these micronutrients in inflammation.

Chapter 5 describes the efficacy of bioactive peptides and proteins in inflammation, which have recently tended to be researched because of their effectiveness on human health. Bioactive peptides and proteins are considered as biologically active regulatory elements for individuals. It is thought to prevent oxidation and microbial deterioration in foods and may also be effective in the treatment of various diseases and disorders associated with inflammation.

Chapter 6 deals with probiotics and prebiotics, which have recently been the focus of health research. Probiotics can have many positive effects, such as enhancing the immune response, stabilizing the colony and increasing the endogenous defense capacity of cells. Prebiotics are indigestible carbohydrates that increase their effectiveness. This section discusses their effectiveness on inflammation.

Chapter 7 deals with diets that are effective on inflammation. Diet is one of the factors that play a role in the development of inflammation and prevents it from developing. Therefore, it is important to determine pro- and inflammatory properties of foods. Furthermore, the inflammatory index of the diet was developed to measure the inflammatory potential of a diet. In this context, the inflammatory index of the diet, diets thought to be effective in inflammation and recent studies on this subject are mentioned.

Uğur Günşen
University of Bandirma Onyedi Eylül, Turkey

Ramazan Mert Atan
University of Bandirma Onyedi Eylül, Turkey

REFERENCES

Ahluwalia, N., Andreeva, V. A., Kesse-Guyot, E., & Hercberg, S. (2013, April). Dietary patterns, inflammation and the metabolic syndrome. *Diabetes & Metabolism*, *39*(2), 99–110. doi:10.1016/j.diabet.2012.08.007 PMID:23062863

Andersen, C. J., Murphy, K. E., & Fernandez, M. L. (2016). Impact of Obesity and Metabolic Syndrome on Immunity. *Advances in Nutrition*, *7*(1), 66–75. doi:10.3945/an.115.010207 PMID:26773015

Brenner, D. R., Scherer, D., Muir, K., Schildkraut, J., Boffetta, P., Spitz, M. R., ... Hung, R. J. (2014). A review of the application of inflammatory biomarkers in epidemiologic cancer research. *Cancer Epidemiology, Biomarkers & Prevention*, *23*(9), 1729–1751. doi:10.1158/1055-9965.EPI-14-0064 PMID:24962838

Calle, M. C., Vega-López, S., Segura-Pérez, S., Pérez-Escamilla, R., & Luz Fernandez, M. (2013). Dietary Pattern Low in Fruits Explains Variations in Inflammation and in Biomarkers of Cardiovascular Disease in Latinos Diagnosed with Type-2 Diabetes. *British Journal of Medicine and Medical Research*, *3*(4), 1558–1573. doi:10.9734/BJMMR/2013/4248

Casas, R., & Estruch, R. (2016). Dietary Patterns, Foods, Nutrients and Chronic Inflammatory Disorders. *Immunologic Research*, *12*(2), 1–10.

Chen, L., Deng, H., Cui, H., Fang, J., Zuo, Z., Deng, J., ... Zhao, L. (2018). Inflammatory responses and inflammation-associated diseases in organs. *Oncotarget*, *9*(6), 7204–7218. doi:10.18632/oncotarget.23208 PMID:29467962

Chertov, O., Yang, D., Zack Howard, O. M., & Oppenheim, J. J. (2000). Leukocyte granule proteins mobilize innate host defenses and adaptive immune responses. *Immunological Reviews*, *177*(1), 68–78. doi:10.1034/j.1600-065X.2000.17702.x PMID:11138786

Couzin-Frankel, J. (2010). Inflammation bares a dark side. *Science*, *330*(6011), 1621. doi:10.1126cience.330.6011.1621 PMID:21163993

Demerath, E., Towne, B., Blangero, J., & Siervogel, R. M. (2001). The relationship of soluble ICAM-1, VCAM-1, P-selectin and E-selectin to cardiovascular disease risk factors in healthy men and women. *Annals of Human Biology*, *28*(6), 664–678. doi:10.1080/03014460110048530 PMID:11726042

Ferrero-Miliani, L., Nielsen, O. H., Andersen, P. S., & Girardin, S. E. (2007). Chronic inflammation: Importance of NOD2 and NALP3 in interleukin-1β generation. *Clinical and Experimental Immunology*, *147*(2), 227–235. PMID:17223962

Hoyert, D. L., & Xu, J. (2012). National Vital Statistics Reports Deaths: preliminary data for 2011. *National Vital Statistics System*, *61*(6), 1–51.

Irwin, M. R., & Cole, S. W. (2011). Reciprocal regulation of the neural and innate immune systems. *Nature Reviews. Immunology*, *11*(9), 625–632. doi:10.1038/nri3042 PMID:21818124

Jacobs, D.R. Jr, & Steffen, L. M. (2003). Nutrients, foods, and dietary patterns as exposures in research: A framework for food synergy. *The American Journal of Clinical Nutrition*, *78*(3 Suppl.), 508–513. doi:10.1093/ajcn/78.3.508S PMID:12936941

Medzhitov, R. (2010). Inflammation 2010: New Adventures of an Old Flame. *Cell*, *140*(6), 771–776. doi:10.1016/j.cell.2010.03.006 PMID:20303867

Miller, G. E., Chen, E., & Parker, K. J. (2011). Psychological Stress in Childhood and Susceptibility to the Chronic Diseases of Aging: Moving Toward a Model of Behavioral and Biological Mechanisms. *Psychological Bulletin*, *137*(6), 959–997. doi:10.1037/a0024768 PMID:21787044

Mozos, I., Malainer, C., Horbanczuk, J., Gug, C., Stoian, D., Luca, C. T., & Atanasov, A. G. (2017). Inflammatory markers for arterial stiffness in cardiovascular diseases. *Frontiers in Immunology*, 8. PMID:28912780

Odermatt, A. (2011). The western-style diet: A major risk factor for impaired kidney function and chronic kidney disease. *American Journal of Physiology. Renal Physiology*, *301*(5), 919–931. doi:10.1152/ajprenal.00068.2011 PMID:21880837

Petersen, A. M. W., & Pedersen, B. K. (2005). Taksonomi-Bloom-Revisi-New-9-638.

Reedy, J., Krebs-Smith, S. M., Hammond, R. A., & Hennessy, E. (2017). Advancing the Science of Dietary Patterns Research to Leverage a Complex Systems Approach. *Journal of the Academy of Nutrition and Dietetics*, *117*(7), 1019–1022. doi:10.1016/j.jand.2017.03.008 PMID:28465171

Ridker, P. M. (2007). C-Reactive Protein and the Prediction of Cardiovascular Events Among Those at Intermediate Risk. Moving an Inflammatory Hypothesis Toward Consensus. *Journal of the American College of Cardiology*, *49*(21), 2129–2138. doi:10.1016/j.jacc.2007.02.052 PMID:17531663

Root, M. M., McGinn, M. C., Nieman, D. C., Henson, D. A., Heinz, S. A., Shanely, R. A., ... Jin, F. (2012). Combined fruit and vegetable intake is correlated with improved inflammatory and oxidant status from a cross-sectional study in a community setting. *Nutrients*, *4*(1), 29–41. doi:10.3390/nu4010029 PMID:22347616

Shivappa, N., Steck, S. E., Hurley, T. G., Hussey, J. R., & Hébert, J. R. (2014). Designing and developing a literature-derived, population-based dietary inflammatory index. *Public Health Nutrition*, *17*(8), 1689–1696. doi:10.1017/S1368980013002115 PMID:23941862

Slavich, G. M. (2015). Understanding inflammation, its regulation, and relevance for health: A top scientific and public priority. *Brain, Behavior, and Immunity*, *45*, 13–14. doi:10.1016/j.bbi.2014.10.012 PMID:25449576

Slavich, G. M., & Cole, S. W. (2013). The emerging field of human social genomics. *Clinical Psychological Science*, *1*(3), 331–348. doi:10.1177/2167702613478594 PMID:23853742

Sternberg, E. M. (2006). Neural regulation of innate immunity: A coordinated nonspecific host response to pathogens. *Nature Reviews. Immunology*, *6*(4), 318–328. doi:10.1038/nri1810 PMID:16557263

Takeuchi, O., & Akira, S. (2010). Pattern Recognition Receptors and Inflammation. *Cell*, *140*(6), 805–820. doi:10.1016/j.cell.2010.01.022 PMID:20303872

WHO. (2019a). Diet, Nutrition and the Prevention of Chronic Diseases. Retrieved from https://www.who.int/dietphysicalactivity/publications/trs916/en/

WHO. (2019b). Healthy diet. Retrieved from http://www.who.int/news-room/fact-sheets/detail/healthy-diet

Zhou, Y., Hong, Y., & Huang, H. (2016). Triptolide Attenuates Inflammatory Response in Membranous Glomerulo-Nephritis Rat via Downregulation of NF-κB Signaling Pathway. *Kidney & Blood Pressure Research*, *41*(6), 901–910. doi:10.1159/000452591 PMID:27871079

Acknowledgment

We would like to thank the dear authors of this book, the scientific contributors as reviewers, and the staff at IGI Global Publishing.

Section 1
Knowledge of Basic Inflammation

Chapter 1
The Process of Acute and Chronic Inflammation:
Biomarkers and Their Relationship With Diseases

Sedat Demir
HC Clinic, Turkey

ABSTRACT

Inflammation is a physiopathological process that has been known for a long time but its relation with acute and chronic diseases and its role in the development of disease is becoming better understood. Diabetes, hypertension, ischemic heart disease, various organ cancers, rheumatologic diseases, the most common diseases of the liver, lungs and kidneys are either closely related to inflammatory processes or are caused by direct inflammatory processes. In one aspect, the aging process is a progressive inflammatory process. The understanding of what inflammation is and the mechanisms by which the inflammation occurs in the organism and by accurately identifying and following the clinical markers that show the course of inflammation. In this section, basic issues related to inflammation is examined.

BACKGROUND

Inflammation is one of the oldest medical conditions defined in history. It is the process of plasma proteins and leukocytes coming out of the vessel wall in tissues and destroying the antigenic structure or microorganism which is recognized as harmful due to their activation. During this process, there is a strong physiopathological

DOI: 10.4018/978-1-7998-3594-3.ch001

response to tissue damage in the organism at both cellular and humoral levels. Inflammation begins with the recognition of microorganisms or dead tissues. It can start with the natural immune system response and continue with the adaptive immune response. Inflammation can be defined as acute and chronic inflammation depending on time (Baştürk, 2017).

In all living things, a number of defensive mechanisms have been developed to protect the organism against living and inanimate harmful agents coming from outside for millions of years. In vertebrate and nonvertebrate organisms, it is aimed to defend the organism with acute and chronic responses to external factors through highly sophisticated, complex and detailed mechanisms. These defence mechanisms have been programmed to remove the alien from the organism in some way by the acute and chronic inflammatory responses of various cellular and chemical components through chain reactions.

The various components of the immune system protect the organism from outside and at the same time against a number of harmful substances and cells formed by a number of specific and nonspecific processes that are innate or acquired. Although acute and chronic inflammatory processes are mainly based on the logic of protection, they may also lead to undesirable consequences during these processes. Acute responses often result in symptoms of systemic disease and are often returned to normal physiological status.

Especially in the formation of chronic diseases and aging process, the main mechanism is usually chronic inflammatory processes. While these processes aim to defend the organism on the one hand, it also causes irreversible changes that lead to chronic tissue destruction and organ damage. Chronic inflammatory responses may lead to structural and functional changes in cells, resulting in diseases such as cancer, diabetes, and various chronic connective tissue diseases. In order to understand acute and chronic inflammation, cellular and chemical components of immune system and normal immune responses should be recognized (Barten at al. 2008)

IMMUNE SYSTEMS AND COMPONENTS

Human immunity is mainly created by two main elements.

1. Natural Immunity
2. Acquired Immunity
    - **Natural Immunity**: It is a naturally occurring immunity which occurs due to genetic factors during embryogenesis, carried from one generation to another.

- **Acquired immunity**: These are the answers that we do not bring with birth but that the organism develops as we face pathogens over the years. Both natural and acquired immunity are mainly accomplished by humoral and cellular components. In natural immunity, a variety of chemical mediators such as cells, complement and cytokines are present in the blood or tissues, such as macrophages, neutrophils and natural clays lymphocytes. Although the main cells of acquired immunity are t and b lymphocytes, the main humoral component is antibodies. Natural immunity consists of cellular and chemical defence mechanisms. It only responds to germs and damaged tissues.
- **Monocytes**: the form of tissue macrophages in the peripheral blood, and they produce specific and nonspecific responses in many bacterial and virus infections.
- **Eosinophils and Basophil Cells**: cells that are found mainly in the tissue in the peripheral blood.

  Eosinophil cells are primarily responsible for the control of parasitic infections and they are also responsible for the development of allergic responses.

  Basophil cells, also known as mast cells, regulate vascular permeability and provide eradication and immunization of allergic responses to bacterial, virus and parasitic infections.

  Eosinophil basophil and mast cells are often responsible for allergic reactions caused by exaggerated immune responses (Barten at al. 2008)

CHEMICAL COMPONENTS OF THE IMMUNE SYSTEM

Although both the natural and acquired immune system operate in part with different mechanisms, both systems have common pathways, common cells and chemical mediators. These structural elements have a common role in the formation of many diseases such as cancer and rheumatologic diseases, shaping of the aging process and long-term organ and tissue damage caused by acute and chronic inflammation. Determine the prognosis of the disease. In clinical practice, most of them are markers of inflammation that are used as laboratory tests.

Antigens: They are substances that can produce a reactive immune response in the organism. The antibodies and macromolecular substances which are specific to them are protein, polysaccharide, peptide, which may interact with the cell. They can be antigens. In some instances, nucleic acids may acquire antigenic properties.

Antibodies: Immune globulin mediators that are developed specifically for antigen and are composed of light or heavy chain proteins produced by B lymphocyte cells. When bacteria and other microorganisms are first encountered, the antigenic substances in their structures are perceived as foreign and specific antibodies are developed against each of them. The resulting antibodies combine with the antigen to form antigen antibody complexes. These complexes also provide the destruction of the cell to which they are attached. Unnecessary and excessive accumulation of antigen antibody complexes in tissues and vascular beds may cause tissue damage and cause many chronic organ diseases (White, 1999; Kuralay & Çavdar 2006; Wan, Haw, & Blackburn, 1989).

Complemantary System: These chemical mediators in the blood plasma, activated

Table 1. Chemical mediators of inflammation

Vasoactive amines	**Histamine** **Bradykinin**
Plasma Proteases	Quinines: Brachinin Kallikrein Complement system Coagulation and fibrinolytic system products
Arachidonic acid metabolites	Thromboxane Prostaglandins Endoperoxides Leukotrienes ...
Leukocyte products	Various lysosomal proteases Free oxygen radicals
Platelet activating factor	
Cytokines	
Growth factors	

by inflammatory processes and formed in various proteins, strengthen the inflammation process and destroy the foreign and harmful cells. During this process, they increase vascular permeability and provide vasodilatation. They also stimulate the secretion of vasoactive amines such as histamine from mast cells. They facilitate phagocytosis of macrophages. They attach to the foreign cell membrane and cause their sequence, allowing leukocytes to migrate to the inflammation site. The complement chain consists of a large number of sub-molecule structures and often performs their functions through chain reactions (Rus, Cudrici, & Niculescu, 2005).

Arachidonic Acid Metabolites: They are ansatured fatty acids formed from phospholipids in the cell membrane by various inflammatory stimuli. These metabolites follow two main pathways, leading to inflammatory processes. It is synthesized to prostoglandins (PG) by cyclooxygenase and to leukotrienes (LKT) by lipoxygenase. PG and leukotrienes are responsible for most of the systemic effects of tumor necrotizing factor-alpha (TNF-α) and interleukin (IL).

Cyclooxygenase Pathway: Arachidonic acid from the cyclooxygenase enzyme and arachidonic acid from PG G2 and then peroxidase effect PGH2 is formed. After several synthesis steps, they are converted to PGI2, Thromboxane A2, and other PG by the action of specific enzymes. While thromboxane A2 is a potent vasoconstrictor, some PG derivatives such as PGE2, PGD2, have vasodilatation and edema-enhancing effects.

Lipoxigenase Pathway: In this way, the enzyme lipoxygenase, which is abundantly found in neutrophil leukocytes, forms leukotrienes through arachidonic acid. They are chemical mediators that play an important role in inflammatory processes in leukotrienes. They increase the adhesion and aggregation of leukocytes to vascular endothelium. In many acute and chronic diseases (chronic obstructive pulmonary disease, various skin and kidney diseases) as intermediate mediators affect the course and prognosis of the disease (Donowitz, 1985; Kuralay & Çavdar,2006; Parkin, & Cohen, 2001).

Leucocyte Products: They are proteases and free oxygen radicals synthesized in leukocyte lysosomes. When stimulated by the immune stimulus, neutrophils and macrophages accompany the inflammation response by producing lysosomal enzymes and free oxygen radicals. In particular, free oxygen radicals have long-term adverse effects on the endothelial surface and vascular structure. They adversely affect vascular permeability and cause significant tissue damage. Free oxygen radicals are closely related to many chronic diseases and aging processes, especially atherosclerosis. Our tissue and organ systems have antioxidant defence systems that fight free oxygen radicals. When mediators such as elastase, collagenase, and leukocyte lysosomal proteolytic enzymes accumulate in the tissue, they break down other tissue proteins and cause tissue damage. For example, aging and skin elasticity are related to this process.

Thrombocyte Activing Factor: Platelet activating factor (PAF) is a phospholipid with strong physiological effects. 1-alkyl-2- (o) -acetyl-glycero-3-phosphocholine.

The source of basal PAF in plasma is the kidney. Other tissues in which PAF is synthesized are phagocytosis cells of the liver, spleen and blood. Many cells involved in inflammation or allergy, such as neutrophils, rnakrophages, lymphocytes, basophils and eosinophils, synthesize and release PAF when activated. Another source of PAF is human endothelial cells. Human endothelial cell cultures have been shown to synthesize PAF when stimulated with thrombin.

It causes activation of platelets, polymorphonuclear leukocytes, monocytes and rnakrophages. It also leads to increased vascular permeability, hypotension, decreased heart rate, glycogenolysis in the perfused liver, and stimulation of uterine contractions. It was found to function both in normal physiological events and to mediate some pathological events (Sarıahmetoglu & Çakıcı, 1996).

Cytokines: They are mediators formed in many cells such as CD4+ T lymphocytes and activated macrophrophages. CD4+ T lymphocytes are capable of evolving into T lymphocytes producing different cytokines. Cytokine secretion can be stimulated by bacterial products, immune complexes, various toxins, physical injuries and various inflammatory events. The most important of the polypeptide cytokines are IL and TNF-α. The three main effects are: triggering systemic acute phase reactants, leukocyte adhesion, procoagulant activity and Tenofovir alafenamide fumarate (TAF) activation from endothelial cells, increasing collagen synthesis and fibroblast production (Kishimoto, Taga, & Akira, 1994).

TNF-α and IL-8 are potent chemoattractive mediators and cause chemotaxis and activation of neutrophils. TNF-α plays an important role in acute inflammation and antitumoral activity and wound healing IL play a critical role in the etiopathogenesis and prognosis of many acute and chronic diseases such as rheumatologic diseases, septic shock, malignancy, and AIDS (Dinarello, 2002).

The soluble IL-1 receptor has been developed for anti-inflammatory and immunosuppressive therapy in the stimulation of haematopoiesis, protection against lethal doses of radiation and inhibition of growth of cancer cells (Leiva, Gardner, McKinnon, & Poretta, 2003).

Growth Factors: They are released from activated macrophages and act by binding to receptors in the cell membrane. Activated macrophages are capable of greater phagocytosis since cell volume and lysosomal enzyme levels are increased and secrete a variety of biologically active products that produce fibrosis, a characteristic of chronic inflammation. These are proinflammatory enzymes such as lysosomal proteases and plasminogen activator, coagulation and complement system fragments, reactive oxygen metabolites, AA metabolites, TAF and growth factors that affect proliferation of various cell types in addition to cytokines such as IL-1 and TNF (Sessle, 2001).

Nitric Oxide: Nitric oxide (NO) is synthesized in endothelial cells. It is one of the most important mediators of vascular resistance and inflammatory processes in circulation. It is found in many cells in the body that play a role in cardiovascular physiology with its various isomers.

Once synthesized in endothelial cells, the vessel enters into smooth muscle cells by diffusion. Relaxation occurs in vascular smooth muscle cells. It is also secreted in the vessel lumen, thereby inhibiting the adhesion of platelets and leukocytes. Slows down the growth of smooth muscle. The release of NO is regulated by physical and humoral stimuli. NO plays an important role in the pathogenesis of hypertension and complications. Inhibition of NOproduction leads to decreased vasodilatation, contraction of arteries and decreased blood flow. Chronic NO deficiency disrupts tissue circulation leading to target organ damage. With similar mechanisms, NO plays an important role, especially in the formation of diabetes and organ damage due to diabetes (Gültekin, Ersanlı, & Küçükateş, 1996; Radi, 2018).

Histamine: Histamine is common in the body, mast cells in connective tissue are the main source. Various physical stimuli such as trauma, cold, autoimmune events and antigen antibody complexes, complement fragments, and a number of neutrophil products cause histamine release. Histamine increases vascular permeability and provides vasodilatation. Histamine is also a chemotactic factor for eosinophils (Parsons, & Ganellin, 2006; Branco, Yoshikawa, Pietrobon, & Sato, 2018).

Serotonin: Serotonin is a biogenic amine similar to epinephrine and norepinephrine. Serotonin, also known as 5-hydroxytryptamine (5-HT), has an important role in the central nervous system as well as platelet aggregation, smooth muscle and vascular tone, pulmonary artery pressure and intestinal motility. It is also a mediator in acute and chronic inflammation. They are stored in the periphery in platelets and in the granules of mast cells (Shajib & Khan, 2015)

Plasma Proteases: They are peptide-mediated mediators with various biological activities in the inflammatory response and originating from plasma. In this chain, precallikrein is converted to prekallikrein, which is its active form with the stimulation of Hageman Factor (Factor 12). Kallikrein converts kininogen to bradykinin. Bradykinin is an important vasoactive mediator. It causes vasodilatation, natriuresis and diuresis, endothelial cell contraction and increased vascular permeability. It also provides neutrophil aggregation (Campbell, 2013).

Other Mediators: It has mainly examined mediators involved in chronic inflammation processes, substance P is involved in a number of mediators such as calpaines and hemigenigenase.

ACUTE AND CHRONIC INFLAMMATION FORMATION

As can be seen, acute and chronic inflammation processes are highly complex events with many cellular, humoral and chemical components. In fact, the main purpose of inflammation is to protect the organism from external and internal factors that cause cell damage, and to cleanse the necrotic tissues and cells and chemical substances of cell damage. However, this process may sometimes work against the organism in the chronic period and may cause some undesirable consequences and diseases. This condition takes place in the pathophysiology of many diseases seen in the clinic. In order to understand and define the pathological processes, it is necessary to examine how the physiological process works and how the mediators form chain reactions and how these reactions turn into pathological processes.

The inflammatory pathway consists of inducers, sensors, mediators, and target tissues. Inducers initiate the inflammatory response and are detected by sensors. Sensors, such as Toll-like receptors (TLRs), are expressed on specialized sentinel cells, such as tissue-resident macrophages, dendritic cells, and mast cells. They induce the production of mediators, including cytokines, chemokines, bioactive amines, eicosanoids, and products of proteolytic cascades, such as bradykinin. These inflammatory mediators act on various target tissues to elicit changes in their functional states that optimize adaptation to the noxious condition (e.g., infection or tissue injury) associated with the particular inducers that elicited the inflammatory response. The specific components shown represent only a small sample of the myriad different sensors, mediators, and target tissues involved in the inflammatory response (Medzhitov, 2010).

In acute inflammation, a series of events begins between the cellular and chemical components of the immune system, together with the factor that triggers inflammation. Acute inflammation develops in minutes and days, is characterized by extrapulmonary fluid and protein output and is characterized by more polymorphic neutrophils, while chronic inflammation is a process involving more lymphocytes and macrophages and mononuclear cells lasting for weeks and years. The role of chemical mediators in this process is more obvious and the determining factor of the process. Local temperature increase, redness, swelling, pain and loss of function in acute inflammation are the five main clinical symptoms; when the organ damage caused by chronic inflammation exceeds a certain level, symptoms start.

In general, inflammation has three periods: induction, regulation and resolution. Period of initiation, regulation of the process with inducing factor and finally cleaning and resolution of waste material caused by inflammation.

It is emphasized that many diseases, especially Type 2 diabetes, atherosclerosis, asthma, neurodegenerative diseases and cancer, may be related to chronic inflammation caused by some infections at an early age.

Several types of inflammation—differing by cause, mechanism, outcome, and intensity—can promote cancer development and progression. Persistent Helicobacter pylori infection is associated with gastric cancer and mucosa-associated lymphoid tissue (MALT) lymphoma. Infections with hepatitis B (HBV) or C (HCV) viruses increase the risk of hepatocellular carcinoma (HCC), and infections with Schistosoma or Bacteroides species are linked to bladder and colon cancer, respectively (Grivennikov, Greten, & Karin, 2010).

The relationship between chronic inflammation of non-infectious origin and these diseases and the course of the inflammation process in these diseases are known to determine the prognosis of the disease. Tissue damage during the inflammation process and a number of toxic substances occurring after injury are important causes of chronic inflammation (Hunter, 2012; Medzhitov, 2010).

CHRONIC INFLAMMATION AND ITS RELATIONSHIP WITH DISEASES:

Under this heading, both chronic inflammatory pathways on the basis of diseases and how this process has turned into disease will be examined.

Relationship Between Inflammation and Cancer: The transformation of inflammatory processes into cancer is a common occurrence and a number of mediators involved in inflammation and inflammation, and more importantly, tissue destruction products and toxic substances that result from inflammation can stimulate the emergence of tumor in a healthy tissue. Inflammation can induce every step of tumorogenesis. Reactive oxygen metabolites produced by immune cells in the initial process can lead to DNA damage. DNA damage is the earliest stage of tumor formation. There is a clear relationship between tumor cells and the immune system. One of the important tasks of the immune system is the destruction of cells that tend to become cancerous in various ways. In the area of inflammation, on the one hand, metabolites resulting from inflammation disrupt the DNA structure and stimulate the formation of new cancer cells, while at the same time disrupting the eradication process of formed cancer cells. This transformation, which often starts on a single cell basis (initation), then leads to the promotional phase and malignant transformation by uncontrolled proliferation of the cell. This new tissue, which invades the local area, then reaches the vessel bed or different channels and spreads to near and distant tissues and metastasizes (Hunter, 2012).

Recent data suggest that an additional mechanism involved in cancer-related inflammation (CRI) is induction of genetic instability by inflammatory mediators, leading to accumulation of random genetic alterations in cancer cells.

Oxidative stresses can activate a variety of transcription factors such as the nuclear factor (NF)-κB, AP-1, p53, HIF-1α, PPAR-γ, β-catenin / Wnt, and Nrf2. Activation of this transcription can affect around 500 different genes and alter the formation and effects of inflammatory growth cytokines, chemokines, molecular, and anti-inflammatory molecules that regulate cell cycle (Reuter, Gupta, Chaturvedi, & Aggarwal, 2010).

On the one hand, the inflammation process is the trigger for tumorigenesis, while on the other hand genetic tendencies, carcinogenic environmental factors such as smoking in lung cancer, and comorbid diseases such as obesity, the tendency to become cancerous increases significantly, and a small chronic inflammation can be an important cancer trigger. Low-grade chronic inflammation in diabetes and similar diseases increases the tendency to various organ cancers in the long term, combined with environmental factors (Smith & Missailidis, 2004).

Table 2. Chronic inflammation increases cancer risk (Grivennikov et al., 2010).

Subclinical, often undetectable inflammation may be as important in increasing cancer risk (for instance, obesity-induced inflammation).
Various types of immune and inflammatory cells are frequently present within tumors.
Immune cells affect malignant cells through production of cytokines, chemokines, growth factors, prostaglandins, and reactive oxygen and nitrogen species.
Inflammation impacts every single step of tumorigenesis, from initiation through tumor promotion, all the way to metastatic progression.
In developing tumors antitumorigenic and protumorigenic immune and inflammatory mechanisms coexist, but if the tumor is not rejected, the protumorigenic effect dominates.
Signaling pathways that mediate the protumorigenic effects of inflammation are often subject to a feed-forward loop (for example, activation of NF-kB in immune cells induces production of cytokines that activate NF-kB in cancer cells to induce chemokines that attract more inflammatory cells into the tumor).
Certain immune and inflammatory components may be dispensable during one stage of tumorigenesis but absolutely critical in another stage.

Inflammation, Obesity, Diabetes and Atherosclerosis: Type 1 Diabetes is a disease that usually occurs in childhood due to cellular mediated immune events and destruction of pancreatic Beta cells and loss of insulin production (Oever, Raterman, Nurmohamed, & Simsek, 2010).

Insulin resistance and Type II diabetes are not only metabolic components but also hyperuricemia, hyperleptinemia, obesity, microalbuminuria, more importantly endothelial dysfunction and inflammatory processes. There was a direct correlation between insulin resistance and CRP (C-reactive protein) elevation. CRP is an important inflammatory marker produced in the liver in response to IL-6 (Borazan, & Binici, 2010).

Hotamışlıgil and his friends with together Karasik and his friends Showed for the first time proinflammatory cytokines and TNFs that were formed in adipose tissue with potential systemic effects on increased metabolism (Hotamisligil, Shargill, & Spiegelman, 1993; Feinstein, Kanety, Papa, Lunenfeld, & Karasik, 1993).

Leptin, IL-6, resistin, monocyte chemoattractant protein-1 (MCP-1), Plasminogen activator inhibitor-1 (PAI-1), angiotensinogen, visfatin, retinol-binding protein-4, serum amyloid A (SAA) and others as stimulants and inducers of inflammatory events in adipose tissue determined. It has been understood that a number of inflammatory processes in adipose tissue increase the production of new adipose tissue and cause obesity. Increased adipocyte inflammatory in adipose tissue and liver.

MCP-1 and play a major role in the migration of other chemokinning macrophages into adipose tissue. These cytokines and chemokines activate the intracellular pathways, leading to the formation of insulin resistance and Type 2 diabetes.

Systemic products of oxidative stress play an important role in the formation of obesity and insulin resistance by increasing adipocyte (Wellen & Hotamisligil, 2005).

Lipids regulate and coordinate inflammation and metabolism. Increased plasma lipid levels are closely related to obesity infection and other inflammatory processes. When obesity and hyperlipidemia include peripheral insulin resistance, they produce acute phase responses that are proaterogenic in the long term, leading to atherosclerosis. There is a close relationship between macrophages, inflammation processes and metabolism. It is known that macrophages in adipose tissue are increased in obesity too. This helps us to understand the inflammatory changes in adipose tissue. Increased macrophages also play a role in the development of insulin resistance.

An important question is whether there are genetic differences between healthy individuals in terms of inflammation-induced insulin resistance. Genetic linkage and genetic predisposition have been demonstrated by different studies (Wellen & Hotamisligil, 2005).

Insulin resistance and inflammatory changes in the small vessel bed, which we will discuss in the next topic, are the most important causes and determinants of type 2 diabetes progression and end organ damage.

The local, portal and systemic effects of insulin resistance and atherogenesis, as well as diabetes and organ damage to diabetes occur (Shoelson, Lee, & Goldfine, 2006).

Other cell types in adipose tissue may also be involved in inflammatory processes. Multiple capialrization takes place by placing vascular cells in the adipose tissue. Thus, the adipose tissue is rapidly proliferating and increases the storage of nutrients. This increase in angiogenesis probably aggravates tumor development. Diabetes and obesity are among the reasons for the increase in the incidence of cancer.

Leukocytes, which cannot show adhesion on normal endothelium or show low adhesion, are more easily settled into vascular endothelium when high fat content is present.

IL-6 is a major inflammatory cytokine produced in many tissues, mainly activated leukocytes, adipocytes and endtelial cells. CRP is the most important indicator of inflammation among acute phase reactants. IL-6 is known to increase gluconeogenesis and compensate for hyperinsulinemia (Pradhan, Manson, Rifai, Buring, & Ridker, 2001).

Endothelial dysfunction is the most important factor in the pathogenesis of vascular disorders due to diabetes. Endothelium is a monolayer on the inner surface of the vessel, active tissue that forms a physical barrier between the circulating blood and the vessel lumen. In particular, it plays an important role in providing hemostasis and vascular tone. Regulates the balance between coagulation and fibrinolysis. An inflammatory activity in the endothelium also adversely affects cell proliferation and the function of other cell types such as smooth muscle cells, platelets, leukocytes, mesengial cells and macrophages through various chemical mediators. Endothelium is a tissue that is in continuous production and destruction, and disruption of this balance causes microvascular changes and microvascular apoptosis. This event is effective in the formation of early diabetic lesions (Oever, Raterman, Nurmohamed, & Simsek, 2010).

In physiological conditions, there is a balance between vascular expanding factors such as NO prostacyclin (PGI-2) released from the endothelium and contracting factors such as endothelin 1 (ET-1), prostaglandins, angiotensin2 (ANGT-II). Inflammatory processes, together with risk factors such as hypercholestrolemia, dyslipidemia, smoking and diabetes, lead to endothelial dysfunction and pave the way for atherosclerosis. Endothelial dysfunction, leukocytes lead to smooth muscle hypertrophy, vasoconstriction, impaired coagulation, vascular inflammation, thrombosis and lead to vascular complications. The most important mediator synthesized in endothelial cells is NO. The vasodilator plays an important role in preventing the adherence of NO leukocytes to the vascular endothelium, which reduces antithrombotic, anti-proliperative permeability and has antioxidant effects that reduce inflammation. Oxidative stresses are more effective because endothelial dysfunction brings with it the benefit of low NO. Oxidative stresses result in increased oxidant formation, decreased antioxidant production and inability to repair oxidative damage. Free radicals, on the other hand, activate oxygen atoms containing reactive anions. For example, hydroxyl radical, superoxide, hydrogen peroxide and peroxy nitrate increase in the endothelium. Many cardiovascular risk factors increase oxidative stress (Oever et al.,2010; Badawi, Klip, Haddad, Cole, Bailo, El-Sohemy, & Karmali, 2010).

Apoptosis is an important process in cell death and can be called cell suicide. Apoptosis can be controlled and regulated in healthy cells and is different from tissue necrosis. Necrosis is an uncontrolled condition that usually results from inflammatory processes resulting from tissue inflammation and cell destruction. Apoptosis or programmed cell death is a controlled process that continues throughout life. Provides healthy regeneration of cells. Throughout his adult life, apoptosis causes the destruction of old useless and damaged cells. Apoptosis and cell reproduction are in balance in a healthy organism. Many chronic diseases are caused by the deterioration of this balance. There are several factors that increase the speed of apoptosis in cells. Cytotoxic substances that bind to cell surfaces, also called death receptors, accelerate apoptosis (Oever et al.,2010; Badawi at al., 2010).

Endothelial dysfunction in diabetes; proliferation, low barrier function, adhesion of circulating cells and increased apoptosis sensitivity. NO has been shown to inhibit apoptosis in many cells, particularly endothelial cells. Insulin resistance is one of the most important triggers of endothelial dysfunction. Diabetes accompanying hypertension, obesity, such as the explanation of the presence of diseases mentioned above is the result of endothelial dysfunction and fat tissue problems (Navarro, & Mora, 2005).

Atherosclerosis is now described as an inflammatory disease. High lipid levels, smoking, hypertension, diabetes and possibly high serum homocysteine levels or microorganisms cause inflammatory responses in the endothelium. Increased vascular permeability, increased procoagulant activity, formation of vasoactive amines, various cytokines and growth factors cause persistent and slowly progressive inflammation and produce atheromatous changes (Borazan & Binici, 2010).

Although atherosclerosis is an aging process, it is caused by unhealthy diet and lifestyle and other facilitating factors. Endothelial cells that normally cover the inner surface of the arteries are resistant to adherence of leukocytes, but high saturated fat diet, smoking, hypertension, hyperglycemia, obesity or insulin resistance facilitate the adhesion of leukocytes. This adhesion binds lymphocytes and monocytes. Migration of leukocytes into the endothelium initiates a chronic inflammation, primarily with the release of cytokines and other inflammatory mediators, leading to accelerated atherosclerosis processes. The placement of monocytes in intima causes the migration of lipoproteins and the accumulation of cholesterol esters. Macrophages also secrete different growth factors. This transformation and proliferation leads to the formation of atherosclerotic plaques. The arterial lumen may become clogged due to rupture of the plaques or platelets on the plaques. Acute complications in atherosclerosis are related to this condition. T lymphocytes of the adaptive immune system play an important role in atherogenesis. However, the onset and development of atherosclerosis is determined by fat products (Libby, 2006).

The process of atherosclerosis may cause cardiovascular diseases as well as systemic vascular involvement, cerebral vascular diseases and peripheral vascular diseases. Reducing oxidative stresses or administering antioxidant drugs externally may slow down the process of atherosclerosis. During atherosclerosis, the early accumulation of proatherogenic oxidized LDL in the vascular bed is the earliest process. This cumulation stimulates the migration of vascular endothelium of macrophages. LDL elevation is an important marker in atherogenesis. HDL is another potential biomarker. HDL particles have antioxidant and anti-inflammatory effect.

Neopterin, produced in macrophages and dendritic cells and is an important marker of immune system activation, can be used to determine cardiovascular risk. Increased neopterin concentrations have been reported as an indicator of chronic immune activation from viral, bacterial, parasitic infections, autoimmune and malignant tumoral diseases. It is known that high neopterin concentrations in patients with atherosclerosis are accompanied by low levels of some antioxidant components and vitamins such as ascorbic acid (Mangge, Becker, Fuchs, & Gostner, 2014).

Many inflammation markers in plasma have been shown to be closely associated with heart disease and atherosclerosis. These include HS-CRP, serum amyloid A levels, IL-4, and intercellular allergy molecule type 1 (sICAM-1) (Ridker, Hennekens, Buring, & Rifai, 2000).

Oxidative stresses and free radicals in cardiac tissue play an important role in the prognosis of the disease. Oxidant and antioxidant balance in mitochondria (redox steate) adjust energy use by changing the permeability of pores in mitochondria. Increased NO production in mitochondria is associated with early atherosclerosis and hypercholestrolemia. Coronary circulation is easily affected by disruption of this balance and causes myocardial hypoxia (Elahi, Kong, & Matata, 2009).

Factor VIII, a coagulation factor that promotes inflammation rather than hypercoagulability, can be used as cardiac risk markers in elderly patients and D-dimer, a marker of plasmin activation in elderly patients (Tracy, 2003).

Aging and Inflamation: Aging is a complex phenomenon that is affected by environmental, stochastic, genetic and many factors throughout life. Human aging is associated with chronic, low-level inflammation, and this phenomenon is called inflamaging. Inflammation is a high predictor of morbidity and mortality in the elderly. CRP and IL levels in elderly patients are associated with morbidity and mortality. Under normal conditions, many toxic substances that arise as a result of immune system activities are easily eliminated and there is difficulty in eliminating residues in old age. Damaged cells and organelle components, oxidative stress-free radicals, metabolites such as extracellular ATP and many other tissue destruction products cannot be adequately eliminated. This means that a low-grade inflammation will persist. Low-level inflammation is a condition that significantly disrupts tissue dynamics during the aging process. This is the main mechanism underlying many chronic diseases such as type II diabetes, Alzheimer's, disease, cardiovascular disease, frailty, sarcopenia, osteoporosis, and cancer. There is overwhelming epidemiological evidence that a state of mild in ammation, revealed by elevated levels of in ammatory biomarkers such as CRP and IL-6 is associated and predictive of many aging phenotypes—for example, changes in body composition, energy production and utilization, metabolic homeostasis, immune senescence, and neuronal health.

Age-related changes to the immune system (immunosenescence) likely contribute to in_ammaging. Adaptive immunity declines with age, whereas innate immunity undergoes more subtle changes that could result in mild hyperactivity. These age-related changes most likely result from both lifelong exposure to pathogens and antigens, as well as intrinsic changes in immune cells and possibly genetic predisposition (Franceschi & Campisi, 2014; Fougère, Boulanger, Nourhashémi, Guyonnet, & Cesari, 2016; Ballou & Kushner, 1997).

Other Conditions Related to Inflammation: It is a known fact that many infections affect and direct the inflammation process. It has been shown that sytomegalovirus (CMV), hepatitis C virus, HIV virus and many other chronic infectious agents provoke inflammation by stimulating chronic inflammatory processes (Tracy, 2003).

Osteoporosis is a condition characterized by low bone mass and increased bone fragility, putting patients at risk of fractures, which are major causes of morbidity substantially in older people. Osteoporosis is currently attributed to various endocrine, metabolic and mechanical factors. However, emerging clinical and molecular evidence suggests that inflammation also exerts significant influence on bone turnover, inducing osteoporosis. Numerous proinflammatory cytokines have been implicated in the regulation of osteoblasts and osteoclasts, and a shift towards an activated immune profile has been hypothesized as important risk factor. Chronic inflammation and the immune system remodelling characteristic of ageing, as well as of other pathological conditions commonly associated with osteoporosis, may be determinant pathogenetic factors (Di Benedetto & De Martinis, 2005).

Bone loss occurs due to increased bone resorption, decreased bone formation, and often a combination of both. systemic bone loss is seen in inflammatory joint diseases, inflammatory bowel diseases and many inflammatory diseases. Many inflammatory diseases potentially lead to increased catabolism in the bone. In addition, malnutrition, general body weakness and corticosteroids often used in inflammatory diseases cause bone loss (Hardy & Cooper, 2009).

In many rheumatologic and autoimmune connective tissue diseases such as rheumatoid arthritis, SLE, Behçet's Disease systemic sclerosis (SSc), Sjögren's syndrome (SST), mixed connective tissue disease (MCTD), and various vasculitis, chronic inflammation processes play a role in the formation and progression of the disease. Chemotactic stochines play an important role in the development of both primary disease and complications by stimulating other mediators of inflammation.

Angiogenesis, the formation of new blood vessels, is a crucial process in a number of physiological processes, such as reproduction, development and tissue repair, as well as in disease states including, among others, rheumatoid arthritis (RA) and other inflammatory diseases (Bodolay, Koch, Kim Szegedi, & Szekanecz, 2002).

NO plays an important role in the pathogenesis of autoimmune diseases as it plays a role in the aging process and many other inflammatory processes. High amounts of NO, synthesized systemically and intra-articularly, play an important role in inflammatory joint diseases (Stichtenoth & Frölich, 1998).

Inflammatory processes play a role in many lung diseases, especially chronic obstructive pulmonary disease. Chronic obstructive pulmonary disease (COPD) is a major worldwide health problem with an increasing prevalence and incidence is characterized by chronic inflammation in the pulmonary tissue. The disease is associated with a switch from a self-limiting inflammatory response, mainly initiated by smoke inhalation, to a chronic persistent inflammatory response after prolonged interaction with cigarette smoke. The extent of the inflammatory reaction is correlated with the severity of the disease (Oudijk, Lammers, & Koenderman, 2003).

COPD is primarily characterised by the presence of airflow limitation resulting from airways inflammation and remodelling often associated with parenchymal destruction and the development of emphysema. However, in many patients the disease is associated with several systemic manifestations that can effectively result in impaired functional capacity, worsening dyspnoea, reduced health-related quality of life and increased mortality (Barnes & Celli, 2009).

Chronic inflammation is associated with a broad spectrum of neurodegenerative diseases of aging. Included are such disorders as Alzheimer's disease, Parkinson's disease, amyotrophic lateral sclerosis, the Parkinson-dementia complex of Guam, all of the tauopathies, and age-related macular degeneration (Mcgeer & Mcgeer, 2004).

Acute and chronic systemic inflammation are characterized by the systemic production of the proinflammatory cytokine TNF-α that plays a role in immune to brain communication. Previous preclinical research shows that acute systemic inflammation contributes to an exacerbation of neurodegeneration by activation of primed microglial cells (Holmes et al., 2009).

Ulcerative colitis (UC) and Crohn's disease (CD), the primary constituents of inflammatory bowel disease (IBD), are precipitated by a complex interaction of environmental, genetic, and immunoregulatory factors.

Inflammatory bowel diseases, which are very common in modern societies, are purely a chronic inflammation disease which is closely related to chronic inflammatory processes and even provoked by various other factors (Hanauer, 2006).

INFLAMMATION AND LABORATORY MARKERS

Acute and chronic inflammation, the occurrence, the course, to identify and monitor the damage caused by many different laboratory tests are used. Some of these may be cellular elements and various mediators directly involved in inflammation, and some are various chemical substances caused by tissue damage caused by inflammation. Theoretically, all cells and chemical mediators involved in the inflammation process are measurable and traceable. It is possible to identify and follow them with sensitive laboratory methods. However, many of these tests are not economically expensive, highly sensitive and specific. Laboratory markers used in the follow-up of inflammation processes should be easily identifiable, economically low-cost, highly sensitive to a disease or organ, that is, they should not be affected by other factors than inflammation.

Following years of clinical experience and numerous researches, the most widely used markers of inflammation in clinical practice are as follows.

CRP: CRP was first discovered in 1930 by Tillet and Francis in the serum of patients with S. pneumoniae pneumonia and is called an "C fraction protein akut. The infection was defined as a biomarker in the early periods as it was higher in the advanced infection periods than the baseline (Tillett & Francis, 1930).

CRP is a protein belonging to pentraxin family which is one of calcium dependent ligand binding plasma proteins and it is very low levels in healthy individuals (<1 mg / dl). Serum levels begin to rise 6-8 hours after the onset of inflammation, reach the highest value in about 48 hours and have a half-life of 4-9 hours.

Although CRP is considered as an acute phase reactant, it is used as a follow-up parameter to determine the severity and prognosis of the disease in many chronic diseases, especially cancer, diabetes and cardiovascular diseases.

Procalcitonin (PCT): Procalcitonin is a prohormone of 116 amino acids, the precursor of calcitonin, which is secreted from neuroendocrine cells in the lungs and small intestine, particularly in the C cells of the thyroid gland. Procalcitonin is an important marker of inflammation in the follow-up of acute inflammatory events, especially sepsis and septic shock (Becker, Snider, & Nylen, 2008).

Erythrocyte Sedimentation Rate (ESR): Erythrocyte sedimentation rate is a simple and inexpensive test that is often used to determine inflammatory activity. Blood erythrocytes with red cells that carry oxygen to the tissues through hemoglobin normally do not aggregate within the vessel due to the negative charges they carry in the vessel and collapse due to the fact that their densities are higher than plasma in vitro. However, since many plasma proteins are positively charged, the various proteins and chemical substances associated with inflammation reduce the repulsive forces of erythrocytes and increase aggregation and roll formation, thereby increasing the rate of collapse in plasma. This test, which is very simple, gives an important idea about the severity and progression of many chronic diseases.

In daily practice, total leukocyte count, neutrophil macrophages and monocytes, eosinophils, basophils, lymphocytes, such as the number and morphology of lower leukocyte cell groups are important tests that provide valuable information about inflammation.

Although most of the chemical mediators are used as markers, levels of IL-6, fibrinogen, angiotensin converting enzyme, complement levels, infection agents or antibodies against external and internal allergens are used in diagnosis and follow-up (Pradhan et al., 2001).

Measured values of various enzymes resulting from inflammation in tissues such as aspartate amino transferase, alanine amino transferase, amylase, lipase, creatine kinase take place in clinical practice as inflammatory markers.

CONCLUSION

Although it has examined the main examples here, it is known that many organ diseases, including liver and kidney diseases, are associated with chronic inflammatory processes and are actually a chronic inflammatory disease. Portal cirrhosis, alcoholic and nonalcoholic fatty liver, chronic hepatitis, acute and chronic nephritis, chronic renal failure can be considered in many clinical situations.

Diagnosis and follow-up of diseases in clinical practice is done by measuring inflammatory markers with various laboratory methods. Cellular and chemical mediators involved in chronic inflammatory process are used as markers of inflammation.

Good recognition and early diagnosis of signs and symptoms of ongoing inflammation, often at the subclinical level, will prevent the progression of many diseases and end-organ damage, save the patient in long and strenuous treatments, and provide significant economic savings. Knowledge of inflammation and its consequences is also very important in terms of preventive medicine and it can be prevented by some simple measures before many diseases occur. The most important factors preventing chronic inflammatory processes are; healthy environment, healthy eating and healthy living conditions.

REFERENCES

Abbas, A. K., Lichtman, A. H., & Pillai, S. (2009). *Cellular and molecular immunology*. England: Saunders.

Badawi, A., Klip, A., Haddad, P., Cole, D. E., Bailo, B. G., El-Sohemy, A., & Karmali, M. (2010). Type 2 diabetes mellitus and inflammation: Prospects for biomarkers of risk and nutritional intervention. *Diabetes, Metabolic Syndrome and Obesity*, *3*, 173–186. doi:10.2147/DMSO.S9089 PMID:21437087

Ballou, S. P., & Kushner, I. (1997). Chronic inflammation in older people: Recognition, consequences, and potential intervention. *Clinics in Geriatric Medicine*, *13*(4), 653–670. doi:10.1016/S0749-0690(18)30142-3 PMID:9354747

Barnes, P. J., & Celli, B. R. (2009). Systemic manifestations and comorbidities of COPD. *The European Respiratory Journal*, *33*(5), 1165–1185. doi:10.1183/09031936.00128008 PMID:19407051

Baştürk, B. (2017). Immune Response in Inflammation. *Turkiye Klinikleri Immunology Allergy-Special Topics*, *10*(3), 161–164.

Becker, K. L., Snider, R., & Nylen, E. S. (2008). Procalcitonin assay in systemic inflammation, infection, and sepsis: Clinical utility and limitations. *Critical Care Medicine*, *36*(3), 941–952. doi:10.1097/CCM.0B013E318165BABB PMID:18431284

Bodolay, E., Koch, A. E., Kim, J., Szegedi, G., & Szekanecz, Z. (2002). Angiogenesis and chemokines in rheumatoid arthritis and other systemic inflammatory rheumatic diseases. *Journal of Cellular and Molecular Medicine*, *6*(3), 357–376. doi:10.1111/j.1582-4934.2002.tb00514.x PMID:12417052

Borazan, A., & Binici, D. N. (2010). Relationship between insulin resistance and inflamation markers in hemodialysis patients. *Renal Failure*, *32*(2), 198–202. doi:10.3109/08860220903491232 PMID:20199182

Branco, A. C. C. C., Yoshikawa, F. S. Y., Pietrobon, A. J., & Sato, M. N. (2018). Role of histamine in modulating the immune response and inflammation. *Mediators of Inflammation*. PMID:30224900

Campbell, D. J. (2013). Bradykinin Peptides. In *Handbook of Biologically Active Peptides* (pp. 1386–1393). Academic Press. doi:10.1016/B978-0-12-385095-9.00188-3

Dinarello, C. A. (2002). The IL-1 family and inflammatory diseases. *Clinical and experimental rheumatology, 20*(5), 1-13.

Donowitz, M. (1985). Arachidonic acid metabolites and their role in inflammatory bowel disease: An update requiring addition of a pathway. *Gastroenterology*, *88*(2), 580–587. doi:10.1016/0016-5085(85)90525-6 PMID:2856909

Elahi, M. M., Kong, Y. X., & Matata, B. M. (2009). Oxidative stress as a mediator of cardiovascular disease. *Oxidative Medicine and Cellular Longevity*, *2*(5), 259–269. doi:10.4161/oxim.2.5.9441 PMID:20716913

Feinstein, R., Kanety, H., Papa, M. Z., Lunenfeld, B., & Karasik, A. (1993). Tumor necrosis factor-alpha suppresses insulin-induced tyrosine phosphorylation of insulin receptor and its substrates. *The Journal of Biological Chemistry*, *268*(35), 26055–26058. PMID:8253716

Fougère, B., Boulanger, E., Nourhashémi, F., Guyonnet, S., & Cesari, M. (2016). RETRACTED: Chronic Inflammation: Accelerator of Biological Aging. *The Journals of Gerontology: Series A*, *72*(9), 1218–1225. doi:10.1093/gerona/glw240

Franceschi, C., & Campisi, J. (2014). Chronic inflammation (inflammaging) and its potential contribution to age-associated diseases. *Journals of Gerontology Series A: Biomedical Sciences and Medical Sciences*, *69*(1), 4–9. doi:10.1093/gerona/glu057 PMID:24833586

Ginaldi, L., Di Benedetto, M. C., & De Martinis, M. (2005). Osteoporosis, inflammation and ageing. *Immunity & Ageing*, *2*(1), 14. doi:10.1186/1742-4933-2-14 PMID:16271143

Grivennikov, S. I., Greten, F. R., & Karin, M. (2010). Immunity, inflammation, and cancer. *Cell*, *140*(6), 883–899. doi:10.1016/j.cell.2010.01.025 PMID:20303878

Gültekin, N., Ersanlı, M., & Küçükateş, E. (1996). Güncel ve etkin bir transmitter: Nitrik oksit. *Türk Kardiyol Derneği Araştırmaları*, *24*, 311–320.

Hanauer, S. B. (2006). Inflammatory bowel disease: Epidemiology, pathogenesis, and therapeutic opportunities. *Inflammatory Bowel Diseases*, *12*(1), 3–9. doi:10.1097/01.MIB.0000195385.19268.68 PMID:16378007

Hardy, R., & Cooper, M. S. (2009). Bone loss in inflammatory disorders. *The Journal of Endocrinology*, *201*(3), 309–320. doi:10.1677/JOE-08-0568 PMID:19443863

Holmes, C., Cunningham, C., Zotova, E., Woolford, J., Dean, C., Kerr, S. U., ... Perry, V. H. (2009). Systemic inflammation and disease progression in Alzheimer disease. *Neurology*, *73*(10), 768–774. doi:10.1212/WNL.0b013e3181b6bb95 PMID:19738171

Hotamisligil, G. S., Shargill, N. S., & Spiegelman, B. M. (1993). Adipose expression of tumor necrosis factor-alpha: Direct role in obesity-linked insulin resistance. *Science*, *259*(5091), 87–91. doi:10.1126cience.7678183 PMID:7678183

Hunter, P. (2012). The inflammation theory of disease. *EMBO Reports*, *13*(11), 968–970. doi:10.1038/embor.2012.142 PMID:23044824

Kasper, D., Fauci, A., Hauser, S., Longo, D., Jameson, J., & Loscalzo, J. (2015). *Harrison's principles of internal medicine. McGraw-Hill Professional Publishing*. New York, NY: Blacklick.

Kishimoto, T., Taga, T., & Akira, S. (1994). Cytokine signal transduction. *Cell*, *76*(2), 253–262. doi:10.1016/0092-8674(94)90333-6 PMID:8293462

Kuralay, F., & Çavdar, Z. (2006). An overview of inflammatory mediators. *The Journal of Gene Medicine*, *16*(3), 143–152.

Leiva, L., Gardner, R. V., McKinnon, E., & Poretta, C. (2003). Hemopoietic Function After Use of IL-1 with. *Journal of Immunology*, *171*(3), 1202–1206. doi:10.4049/jimmunol.171.3.1202 PMID:12874206

Libby, P. (2006). Inflammation and cardiovascular disease mechanisms. *The American Journal of Clinical Nutrition*, *83*(2), 456–460. doi:10.1093/ajcn/83.2.456S PMID:16470012

Mangge, H., Becker, K., Fuchs, D., & Gostner, J. M. (2014). Antioxidants, inflammation and cardiovascular disease. *World Journal of Cardiology*, *6*(6), 462. doi:10.4330/wjc.v6.i6.462 PMID:24976919

Mcgeer, P. L., & Mcgeer, E. G. (2004). Inflammation and the degenerative diseases of aging. *Annals of the New York Academy of Sciences*, *1035*(1), 104–116. doi:10.1196/annals.1332.007 PMID:15681803

Medzhitov, R. (2010). Inflammation 2010: New adventures of an old flame. *Cell, 140*(6), 771–776. doi:10.1016/j.cell.2010.03.006 PMID:20303867

Navarro, J. F., & Mora, C. (2005). Role of inflammation in diabetic complications. *Nephrology, Dialysis, Transplantation, 20*(12), 2601–2604. doi:10.1093/ndt/gfi155 PMID:16188894

Oever, V. A. I. A., Raterman, H. G., Nurmohamed, M. T., & Simsek, S. (2010). Endothelial dysfunction, inflammation, and apoptosis in diabetes mellitus. *Mediators of Inflammation*. PMID:20634940

Oudijk, E. D., Lammers, J. J., & Koenderman, L. (2003). Systemic inflammation in chronic obstructive pulmonary disease. *The European Respiratory Journal, 22*(46), 5–13. doi:10.1183/09031936.03.00004603a PMID:14621102

Parkin, J., & Cohen, B. (2001). An overview of the immune system. *Lancet, 357*(9270), 1777–1789. doi:10.1016/S0140-6736(00)04904-7 PMID:11403834

Parsons, M. E., & Ganellin, C. R. (2006). Histamine and its receptors. *British Journal of Pharmacology, 147*(1), 127–135. PMID:16402096

Pradhan, A. D., Manson, J. E., Rifai, N., Buring, J. E., & Ridker, P. M. (2001). C-reactive protein, interleukin 6, and risk of developing type 2 diabetes mellitus. *Journal of the American Medical Association, 286*(3), 327–334. doi:10.1001/jama.286.3.327 PMID:11466099

Radi, R. (2018). Oxygen radicals, nitric oxide, and peroxynitrite: Redox pathways in molecular medicine. *Proceedings of the National Academy of Sciences of the United States of America, 115*(23), 5839–5848. doi:10.1073/pnas.1804932115 PMID:29802228

Reuter, S., Gupta, S. C., Chaturvedi, M. M., & Aggarwal, B. B. (2010). Oxidative stress, inflammation, and cancer: How are they linked? *Free Radical Biology & Medicine, 49*(11), 1603–1616. doi:10.1016/j.freeradbiomed.2010.09.006 PMID:20840865

Ridker, P. M., Hennekens, C. H., Buring, J. E., & Rifai, N. (2000). C-reactive protein and other markers of inflammation in the prediction of cardiovascular disease in women. *The New England Journal of Medicine, 342*(12), 836–843. doi:10.1056/NEJM200003233421202 PMID:10733371

Rus, H., Cudrici, C., & Niculescu, F. (2005). The role of the complement system in innate immunity. *Immunologic Research, 33*(2), 103–112. doi:10.1385/IR:33:2:103 PMID:16234578

Sarıahmetoglu, M., & Çakıcı, I. (1996). Platelet activating factor (paf): Cardiovascular effects and its role in ischemia-reperfusion meltem. *Journal of Pharmaceutical Sciences*, *22*, 119–124.

Sessle, B. J. (2001). New insights into peripheral chemical mediators of temporomandibular pain and inflammation. *Journal of Orofacial Pain*, *15*(1), 5. PMID:11889648

Shajib, M. S., & Khan, W. I. (2015). The role of serotonin and its receptors in activation of immune responses and inflammation. *Acta Physiologica*, *213*(3), 561–574. doi:10.1111/apha.12430 PMID:25439045

Shoelson, S. E., Lee, J., & Goldfine, A. B. (2006). Inflammation and insulin resistance. *The Journal of Clinical Investigation*, *116*(7), 1793–1801. doi:10.1172/JCI29069 PMID:16823477

Smith, G. R., & Missailidis, S. (2004). Cancer, inflammation and the AT1 and AT2 receptors. *Journal of Inflammation*, *1*(1), 3. doi:10.1186/1476-9255-1-3 PMID:15813980

Stichtenoth, D. O., & Frölich, J. C. (1998). Nitric oxide and inflammatory joint diseases. *British Journal of Rheumatology*, *37*(3), 246–257. doi:10.1093/rheumatology/37.3.246 PMID:9566663

Tillett, W. S., & Francis, T. Jr. (1930). Serological reactions in pneumonia with a non-protein somatic fraction of pneumococcus. *The Journal of Experimental Medicine*, *52*(4), 561–571. doi:10.1084/jem.52.4.561 PMID:19869788

Tracy, R. P. (2003). Emerging relationships of inflammation, cardiovascular disease and chronic diseases of aging. *International Journal of Obesity*, *27*(3), 29. doi:10.1038j.ijo.0802497 PMID:14704741

Wan, J. M. F., Haw, M. P., & Blackburn, G. L. (1989). Nutrition, immune function, and inflammation: An overview. *The Proceedings of the Nutrition Society*, *48*(3), 315–335. doi:10.1079/PNS19890048 PMID:2515541

Wellen, K. E., & Hotamisligil, G. S. (2005). Inflammation, stress, and diabetes. *The Journal of Clinical Investigation*, *115*(5), 1111–1119. doi:10.1172/JCI25102 PMID:15864338

White, M. (1999). Mediators of inflammation and the inflammatory process. *The Journal of Allergy and Clinical Immunology*, *103*(3), 378–381. doi:10.1016/S0091-6749(99)70215-0 PMID:10069896

Chapter 2
Epidemiology of Inflammation-Related Diseases

Kevser Tarı Selçuk
Bandırma Onyedi Eylül University, Turkey

ABSTRACT

Inflammation, a vital defense mechanism for health, is defined as the immune system's response to harmful stimuli such as pathogens, damaged cells, toxic compounds or irradiation. Inflammation is usually examined in two groups: acute and chronic. Chronic inflammation instigates various kinds of diseases that cause premature mortality and morbidity such us cardiovascular diseases, cancer, diabetes mellitus (DM), asthma-chronic obstructive pulmonary disease (COPD), obesity, metabolic syndrome (METs), inflammatory bowel disease (IBD), rheumatoid arthritis (RA), multiple sclerosis (MS), osteoporosis, and neurological diseases via dysregulation of various signaling pathways such as nuclear factor kappa-B (NF-κB), signal transducer, activator of transcription 3 (STAT3), etc. These inflammation-related diseases are among the major causes of mortality and morbidity in almost every region of the world. Studies have shown that these diseases associated with inflammation have tended to increase worldwide.

BACKGROUND

Inflammation, a vital defense mechanism for health, is defined as "the immune system's response to harmful stimuli such as pathogens, damaged cells, toxic compounds, or irradiation" (Chen et al., 2018). Inflammation is usually examined in two groups:

DOI: 10.4018/978-1-7998-3594-3.ch002

acute and chronic (Pahwa & Jialal, 2018). Acute inflammation is part of natural immunity initiated by immune cells that persist for a short time (Kunnumakkara et al., 2018). If acute inflammation persists for any reason (Chen et al., 2018), the second stage of infammation called "chronic infammation" lasts more than a few months (Pahwa & Jialal, 2018). Chronic inflammation commences which instigates various kinds of disease that cause premature mortality and morbidity such us cardiovascular diseases, cancer, diabetes mellitus (DM), asthma-Chronic Obstructive Pulmoner Disese (COPD), obesity, Metabolic Syndrome (METs), Inflammatory Bowel Disease (IBD), rheumatoid athritis, multiple sclerosis (MS), osteoporosis and neurological diseases via dysregulation of various signaling pathways such as nuclear factor kappa-B (NF-κB), signal transducer and activator of transcription 3 (STAT3) etc. (Kunnumakkara et al., 2018; Slavich, 2015; Elsayed & Norreddin, 2019; Calle & Andersen, 2019).

In this section, epidemiology of cardiovascular diseases, cancer, diabetes, obesity, METs, asthma, COPD, IBD, Rheumatoid arthritis, and MS will be evaluated.

CARDIOVASCULAR DISEASES

Cardiovascular diseases, which is one of the leading non-communicable diseases and also known as heart diseases, is defined as "a series of diseases affecting the heart and blood vessels such as coronary heart disease (heart attacks), cerebrovascular disease, raised blood pressure (hypertension), peripheral artery disease, rheumatic heart disease, congenital heart disease, and heart failure" (Joseph et al., 2017; Mishra & Monica, 2019). Cardiovascular diseases are the leading cause of mortality and morbidity worldwide. Physical inactivity, tobacco use, harmful use of alcohol and unhealthy dietary habits are identified as major risk factors for the development of cardiovascular diseases (Joseph et al., 2017; Meier et al., 2019). Studies have shown that these major risk factors play an important role in modulating the inflammatory response (Casas & Estruch, 2016). Inflammation triggers the early stages of the atherosclerotic process and increases in inflammatory cytokines may cause an increased risk of cardiovascular diseases and consequently, inflammation plays an important role in the development of cardiovascular diseases (Sorriento & Iaccarino, 2019; Yalçın & Rakıcıoğlu, 2018).

According to World Health Organization (WHO), in 2010, cardiovascular diseases account for 27.3% of all deaths globally and this ratio is 31.4% in 2016. Additionally in 2016 cardiovascular diseases account for 14.8%, 27.9%, 40.3% and 31.0% all deathts in low, lower middle, upper middle and high income countries according to World Bank income groups, respectively. The mortality rate due to cardiovascular diseases is 120 per thousand in low income countries, 205 per thousand lower middle income countries, 295 per thousand in upper middle income countries and 271 per hundred thousand in high income countries in 2016. It is reported that ischemic heart disease (16.6% of total deaths) is the first and stroke (10.2% of total deaths) is the second most common cause of death in 2000-2016 in the world. Ischemic heart diseases are the first and stroke is the second leading cause of death in lower middle, upper middle and high-income countries. In low-income countries, ischemic heart disease (6.5% of total deaths) is third and stroke (5.2% of total deaths) is the fifth cause of death. Ischemic heart disease and stroke are among the leading causes of death in all regions of the WHO except Africa (World Health Organization [WHO], 2016a).

Cardiovascular diseases are responsible for approximately 17.6 million deaths in 2016 globally and age-adjusted mortality due to these diseases has increased by 14.5% since 2006 (Benjamin et al., 2019). In a study examining the global, regional and national burden of cardiovascular diseases, it is reported that deaths due to these diseases are caused by 10 main causes such as ischemic heart disease, ischemic stroke, hemorrhagic and other stroke, atrial fibrillation, peripheral arterial disease, aortic aneurysm, cardiomyopathy and myocarditis, hypertensive heart disease, endocarditis, rheumatic heart disease, and a category for other cardiovascular diseases conditions and ischemic heart disease and stroke are responsible for 85.1% of deaths related to cardiovascular diseases (Roth et al., 2017; Zaidi et al., 2019). Cardiovascular diseases have been cited as the leading cause of deaths in the member states of the European Union (EU). It is reported that in 2015, 1.91 million deaths (36.7% of all deaths) occurred in 28 EU member states due to circulatory system diseases. The first three countries with the highest age-standardized mortality are Bulgaria, Romania and Lithuania, and the lowest is France, Spain, Denmark (European Union Statistical Office [Eurostat], 2015).

Globally, there were an estimated 422.7 million prevalent cases of cardiovascular diseases in 2015 and the age-standardized prevalence of cardiovascular diseases varied significantly by country. Countries with the lowest age standardized prevalence (<5,000/100,000) Singapore, Japan, South Korea, Chile, Argentina, Uruguay, Canada, Australia, New Zealand, Ireland, Cyprus, Malta, Italy, Greece, and Israel, countries with the highest age-standardized prevalence (>9,000/100,000) included most countries in West Africa, Morocco, Iran, Oman, Zambia, Mozambique, and Madagascar. In countries such as United States (US), Canada, Western Europe, Brazil, Australia, New Zealand, Japan, South Korea, Kenya, Cambodia, Laos, and India, a significant decline in the age-standardized prevalence of cardiovascular diseases (Roth et al., 2017). In US in 2016, the prevalence of cardiovascular diseases was reported to be 48.0% (121.5 million) in the age group 20 and over, and the prevalence is reported to increase with age (Benjamin et al., 2019).

Disability-adjusted life years (DALY) lost means loss of healthy years of life. Cardiovascular diseases is the leading cause of DALY (Joseph et al., 2017).

Cardiovascular disease accounts for 10% DALYs in low and middle-income countries and 18% in high income countries (Rehan, Qadeer, Bashir, & Jamshaid, 2016). In 2016, the share of ischemic heart disease and stroke in total DALY was 7.6% and 5.2%, respectively. Globally, ischemic heart disease has the largest share (10.4%) in the Years of Life Lost (YLL) (WHO, 2016a).

Increased risk factors such as tobacco use, unhealthy nutrition, obesity, physical inactivity and harmful use of alcohol increase the burden of chronic diseases, especially cardiovascular diseases (WHO, 2016b). The Global Action Plan, published by the WHO (WHO, 2013), aims to reduce premature mortality by 25% due to major noncommunicable diseases (cardiovascular diseases, cancer, diabetes mellitus, and chronic respiratory diseases) associated with these four risk factors, which contribute greatly to global mortality and morbidity by 2025. It is stated in the projections that if the risk factors continue with the current trend, the mortality rate related to these diseases will increase in some countries in Africa and there will be no detectable change in premature deaths in countries such as China, India, Russia, Mexico, and Ethiopia until 2025. In addition, in some countries, such as the US, Brazil, and South Africa, premature mortality will fall, but the 25% target will not be achieved (Roth et al., 2015).

CANCER

Cancer is a heterogeneous group of diseases that can affect any part of the body, each with many anatomical and molecular subtypes requiring specific diagnostic and management strategies (WHO, 2017). Cancer, one of the most important public health problems and it is one of the biggest obstacles to increasing life expectancy in the 21st century (Bray et al., 2018). Many studies have reported that chronic inflammation increases cancer risk, promotes tumor progression and metastatic spread (Multhoff, Molls, & Radons, 2012), and infection and inflammation are responsible for approximately 25% of cancer-related factors (Murata, 2018).

Cancer incidence and mortality are rapidly increasing worldwide due to aging, population growth, prevalence of major risk factors and changes in distribution (Bray et al., 2018). It is reported that by the International Agency for Research on Cancer (IARC) the number of new cancer cases worldwide was 18.1 million and the number of cancer-related deaths was 9.6 million in 2018 and it is estimated that the number of cancer cases will reach 29.5 million and the number of deaths will reach 16.4 million by 2040 (Ferlay et al., 2019; International Agency for Research on Cancer [IARC], 2018). According to GLOBOCAN 2018 data, the regions with the highest cancer incidence rates for both sexes were Asia (48.4%), Europe (23.4%), America (21.0%), Africa (5.8%), respectively and the regions with the highest mortality rates were Asia (57.3%), Europe (20.3%), America (14.4%), Africa (7.3%). The first four cancer types with the highest incidence rates for both sexes worldwide were lung (11.6%), breast (11.6%), colorectal (10.2%), prostate (7.1%) and the first four cancer types with the highest mortality rates for both sexes worldwide were lung (18.4%), colorectal (9.2%), stomach (8.2%) and liver (8.2%), respectively. Breast (24.2%), colorectal (9.5%), lung (8.4%), cervical uteri (6.6%) were the highest incidence of cancer in women. The highest incidence of cancer among men was lung (14.5%), prostate (13.5%), colorectal (10.9%) and stomach (7.2%), respectively. Breast (15.0%), lung (13.8%), colorectal (9.5%), cervical uteri (7.5%) were the highest mortality of cancer in women. The highest mortality of cancer among men was lung (22.0%), liver (10.2%), stomach (9.5%) and colorectal (9.0%), respectively (Bray et al., 2018).

According to World Bank income groups breast (12.9%), cervical uteri (12.6%), prostate (5.9%) and liver (5.4%) had the highest incidence rates for both sexes in low income countries. Cervical uteri (12.9%), breast (9.0%), liver (7.3%) and lung (6.8%) had the highest mortality rates for both sexes in low income countries. Breast (11.2%), colorectal (10.9%), lung (10.9%), prostate (10.3%) had the highest incidence rates for both sexes in high income countries. Lung (21.3%), colon (8.2%), pancreas (7.2%), breast (6.4%) had the highest mortality rates for both sexes in high income countries (IARC, 2018).

A study of cancer incidence and mortality patterns in 40 countries in Europe in 2018 revealed that there were more than 3.9 million (excluding nonmelanoma skin cancers) new cancer cases in Europe and 53% (2.05 million) occurring in men and 47% (1.85 million) in women. In Europe, the highest incidence rates for both sexes were breast (13.4%), colorectal (12.8%), lung (12.0), and prostate (11.5%), respectively and these four types of cancer account for 49.7% of the cancer burden in Europe. In Europe, breast cancer (28.2%), colorectal (12.3%), lung (8.5%) and corpus uteri (6.6%) had the highest incidence in women, and prostate (21.8%), lung (15.1%), colorectal (13.2%) and bladder (7.5%) had the highest incidence in men. It is reported that 1.93 million people (56% were in men, 44% were in women) died in Europe in 2018 due to cancer. Lung cancer (24.8%) is the leading cause of cancer-related death in men, followed by colorectal (12.0%) and prostate (10.0%) cancer. In women, breast cancer (16.2%) was the leading cause of cancer-related deaths, followed by lung (14.2%) colorectal (13.2%) cancer (Ferlay et al., 2018).

Cancer is responsible for 25% of all deaths in 2015 in a total of 36 countries, including 28 EU member states, 5 candidate countries and 3 European Free Trade Union countries and the second leading cause of death after cardiovascular diseases. In women, 29% of new cancer cases were breast, 12% colon and rectum, 10% lung and 8% uterine and cervical cancer. In men, 23% of new cancer cases were prostate, 14% lung, 13% colon and rectum cancer. The most common causes of cancer mortality in women were breast (16.0%), lung (15.0%), colorectal (12.0%)

and pancreas (7.0%). The most common causes of cancer mortality in men were lung (25.0%), colorectal (11.0%), prostate (10.0%) and pancreas (6.0%) and cancer mortality rates in all countries are reported to be higher in men than in women (The Organisation for Economic Co-operation and Development [OECD], 2018).

According to the American Cancer Society, the number of new cancer cases is expected to reach 27.5 million and cancer deaths will reach 16.3 million due to global growth and aging of the population in 2040. However, it is reported that the risk of future cancer burden may be higher than expected due to the increase in risk factors such as smoking, unhealthy diet habits and physical inactivity. In addition, the American Cancer Society suggests that cancer types such as lung, breast, colorectal cancers associated with these risk factors tend to increase in countries currently undergoing economic transition and if the necessary measures are not taken, this upward trend will continue (American Cancer Society, 2018).

DIABETES MELLITUS

DM is a chronic metabolic disease characterized by hyperglycemia caused by insulin secretion, insulin effect, or disorder in both of these factors (Yılmaz, 2019). DM is a serious public health problem that is increasing worldwide and with increasing treatment costs due to the frequent development of chronic complications (Guariguata et al., 2013). The causal and potentially primordial role of inflammation in the development of diabetes has been the subject of research for many years. Recent evidence has shown that cytokines and adipocytokines play an important role in the development of diabetes and diabetes-related complications (Saxena & Moodi, 2014).

The World Health Organization (WHO) reported that diabetes was 13th among the causes of death in 2000 (944 million deaths), while it rose to 7th place in 2016 (1,599 million deaths). In low-income countries, diabetes (1.7% of total deaths) is the 17th cause of death, while in high-income countries it ranks 8th (2.7% of total deaths). According to WHO regiions, diabetes is the 17th cause of death in Africa (2.7% of total deaths), 5th in America (5.0% of total deaths), 7th in Southeast Asia (3.6% of total deaths), 8th in Europe (2.0% of total deaths), 6th in Eastern Meditarrenean (3.2% of total deaths) and 12th in the Western Pacific (1.9% of total deaths) (WHO, 2016a).

Diabetes is responsible for 9.9% of deaths in the 20-99 age group worldwide in 2017. Diabetes-related deaths are highest in Western Pacific (1.7 million) and lowest in South and Central America (0.27 milyon). In addition, 36.5% of deaths attributed to diabetes occur under the age of 60 and Africa (%73.7) has the highest deaths caused by diabetes before the age of 60 years (Cho et al., 2018).

The prevalence of diabetes varies according to age groups, gender, World Bank income groups and geographical region. Worldwide, the prevalence of diabetes is 8.4% in women aged 18-99 years and 8.9% in men in 2017. Globally, 79% of people with diabetes live in low- and middle-income countries, and two-thirds live in urban areas. Western Pacific Region (37.0%) has the highest prevalence of diabetes in the 18-99 age group which is estimated to have 168.4 million people with diabetes. The region with the highest prevalence of age-adjusted diabetes is North American and Caribbean (10.8%) and the lowest prevalence of age-adjusted diabetes is Africa (4.2%). (Cho et al., 2018).

According to World Bank (World Bank, 2017) data, the prevalence of diabetes at the global level is 8.5% in 2017. The prevalence of diabetes by income groups is 5.5% in low-income countries, 8.9% in middle-income countries, and 7.9% in high-income countries. In Organisation for Economic Co-operation and Development (OECD) member countries, diabetes prevalence is 8.2% and the lowest prevalence is Zimbabwe (1.8%) and the highest prevalence is Marshall Island (30.5%).

OBESITY AND METABOLIC SYNDROME

Obesity adversely affects almost all physiological functions of the body and is considered one of the most important public health threats (Chooi, Ding, & Magkos, 2019). Obesity defined as "a condition of abnormal or excessive fat accumulation in adipose tissue, to the extent that health may be impaired" (WHO, 2000). Obesity increases the risk of developing cardiovascular disease, diabetes, many types of cancer, a range of musculoskeletal disorders and poor mental health, adversely affecting quality of life, work efficiency and health expenditure (Chooi, Ding, & Magkos, 2019).

Obesity prevelance have increased in all ages and both sexes regardless of geographic location, ethnicity or socioeconomic status. It is estimated that the prevalence of overweight and obesity has doubled compared to 1980 in the world. The prevalence of age-standardized overweight was 26.5% in 1980. In 2015, it increased by approximately 50% and reached 39.0%. Similarly, the prevalence of obesity was about 7% in 1980. In 2015, it reached 12.5% with an increase of approximately 80% (Chooi et al., 2019). In the last 30 years age-standardized obesity (BMI ³30 kg/m2) increased from 3.2% to 10.8% in men and from 6.4% to 14.9% in women. Current trends suggest that global adult obesity prevalence will reach 18% in men and 21% in women by 2025 (NCD Risk Factor Collaboration [NCD-RisC], 2016). Obesity ranks 6th among the causes of DALY around the world, and obesity-related DALYs have been increasing rapidly since 1990, especially in low- and middle-income countries (Ford, Patel, & Narayan, 2017).

The two regions with the highest overweight and obesity prevalence are the Americas and Europe. Overweight prevalence in the America increased from 45.3% in 1980 to 64.2% in 2015. On the other hands the prevalence of obesity was 12.9% in 1980, it reached 28.3% in the America in 2015. The prevalence of overweight in Europe was 48.0% in 1980 and 59.6% in 2015. The prevalence of obesity in the European region was reported to be 14.5% in 1980 and 22.9% in 2015. United States (US) and Turkey are two countries with the highest overweight and obesity prevelance in the American and European regions in 2015. France and Colombia are two countries with the lowest overweight and obesity prevelance in the American and European regions in 2015. The region with the lowest overweight and obesity prevalence at the global level is the Western Pacific. However, it is reported that the overweight prevalence has increased from 9.7% to 28.2% and the prevalence of obesity has increased from 0.8% to 4.9% between 1980 to 2015 (Chooi et al. 2019).

The prevalence of obesity in adults in OECD countries in 2015 is estimated to be 19.5%. The first three countries with the lowest prevalence are Japan (3.7%), Korea (5.3%), Italy (9.8%), the three countries with the highest rates are US (38.2%), Mexico (32.4%) and New Zealand (30.7%). It has been reported that overweight and obesity prevalence has increased significantly in Canada, France, Mexico, Switzerland and the US in the last 20 years and no significant change has been observed in England, Italy, Korea and Spain. According to OECD estimates, the prevalence of obesity is expected to reach approximately 47%, 39% and 35%, in the US, Mexico and the UK in 2030, respectively (OECD, 2017).

METs is also referred to as 'Insulin resistance syndrome', 'syndrome X', 'hypertriglyceridemic waist', and 'the deadly quartet'. METs is not considered as a single disease in the literature, but as a constellation of cardiovascular disease risk factors and it is defined in different ways by various organizations such as WHO, National Cholesterol Education Program (NCEP), International Diabetes Federation (IDF) (Rochlani, Pothineni, Kovelamudi, & Mehta, 2017; Saklayen, 2018). It is generally agreed that a a clustering of abdominal obesity, diabetes and prediabetes, high cholesterol and high blood pressure (De Silva et al., 2019).

The prevalence of metabolic syndrome varies according to age, sex, race / ethnicity and the criteria used for diagnosis and it is increasing with global obesity and diabetes outbreaks worldwide (Lee et al., 2018; Rochlani et al., 2017). Especially in developing countries, environmental and behavioral changes such as adaptation to westernized diet and sedentary lifestyle are considered as the main causes of METs pandemic (Lee et al., 2018). According to the IDF estimates, almost a quarter of adults worldwide have MetS (IDF, 2015). In addition, the mortality rate in people with METs is reported to be two times higher more than in those without METs (Sarebanhassanabadi et al., 2017).

ASTHMA AND CHRONIC OBSTRUCTIVE PULMONER DISEASE

Chronic respiratory diseases are among the leading causes of mortality and morbidity worldwide. Asthma and COPD are the most common chronic respiratory diseases (Şen et al., 2015; Chronic Respiratory Disease Collaborators, 2017). Asthma and COPD are two distinct diseases that are typically separated due to differences in their pathophysiological mechanisms as well as their epidemiological characteristics. For example, asthma is generally considered an allergic disease that begins in childhood. On the other hands COPD is a disease characterized by progressive and irreversible airway obstruction, typically associated with tobacco use, usually occurring after 40 years of age (Uchida, Sakaue, & Inoue, 2018).

The most comprehensive study evaluating the prevalence of asthma on a global scale is the World Health Survey conducted by the WHO in 2002-2003. This study was conducted with 178,215 adults aged 18-45 years in 70 countries. The prevalence of asthma was based on responses to questions relating to self-reported doctor diagnosed asthma, clinical/treated asthma, and wheezing in the last 12 months. According to this study, the global prevalence rates of asthma, clinical / treated asthma and wheezing in adults were 4.3%, 4.5%, and 8.6% respectively. It is reported that the prevalence of physician-based asthma in adults worldwide differs in the 70 countries included in the study and the lowest prevalence is China (0.2%) and the highest prevalence is Australia (21.0%). The prevalence of cured asthma (or treated asthma) varies from country to country, but is 4.5% globally. The country with the lowest prevalence is reported to be Vietnam with 1.0% and the country with the highest prevalence is Australia with 21.5%. In addition, the five countries with the highest prevalence of clinical asthma are reported to be Australia (21.5%), Sweden (20.2%), UK (18.2%), Netherlands (15.3%), and Brazil (13.0%). The region with the highest prevalence of clinical asthma is Western Pacifix (6.2%) The prevalence of clinical asthma in this region is similar in rural and urban areas, approximately one-fourth of those living with clinical asthma are smokers, one in two people reported wheezing in the last 12 months and one-fifth of these people were not receiving asthma treatment (WHO, 2018). The global prevalence of wheezing was estimated to be 8.6%. Countries with the highest prevalence of wheezing are reported as Australia (27.4%), the Netherlands (22.7%), the UK (22.6%), Brazil (22.6%), and Sweden (21.6%) (To et al., 2012).

In 2015, it was reported that approximately 0.40 million people died due to asthma on a global level, and asthma-related deaths were reduced by 26.7% and age-standardized death rates by 58.8% in all age groups compared to 1990 (Chronic Respiratory Disease Collaborators, 2017). In the Global Burden Disease (GBD) study, it is reported that asthma is 28th among the leading causes of disease burden and 16th among the causes of YLD (WHO, 2018).

COPD is a common, preventable and treatable disease that is characterized by persistent respiratory symptoms and airflow limitation that is due to airway and/or alveolar abnormalities usually caused by significant exposure to noxious particles or gases (Global Initiative for Chronic Obstructive Lung Disease [GOLD], 2017). It is reported that the prevalence of COPD was calculated as 10.7% in 1990 in the age group of 30 and over in the global scale and that it reached 11.7% in 2010. The highest prevalence in the WHO regions is America (13.3% in 1990 and 15.2% in 2010), and the lowest prevalence in South East Asia (7.9% in 1990 and 9.7% in 2010). The regions with the highest increase in COPD prevalence between 1990 and 2010 are Eastern Mediterranean (118.7%), African (102.1%) and the lowest increase is reported as European (22.5%). In addition, the study states that 13.6% of COPD cases live in urban areas, 9.7% live in rural areas, and COPD prevalence is higher in males (14.3%) compared to females (7.6%) (Adeloye et al., 2015).

According to the World Health Survey conducted by the WHO in 2002-2003, the prevalence of COPD increased by 44.2% compared to 1990 and reached 174.5 million in 2015. In addition, the decrease in age-standardized prevalence (14.7%) is reported to be lower than the age-standardized mortality rate. The greatest decrease in age standardised prevalence was seen in countries in the high-middle-SDI (SDI captures three different aspects of development: income, education, and fertility) quintile and the middle-SDI quintile. Also in this study it was reported that despite a 41% reduction in age-standardized mortality worldwide, the number of COPD-related deaths increased by 11.6% in 2015 to 3.2 million in 2015. Population growth and ageing of the global population outweighed the downward trend in age standardised mortality rates. The greatest reduction in age standardised mortality rates occurred in countries in the high-middle-SDI quintile and middle-SDI quintile (Chronic Respiratory Disease Collaborators, 2017).

In the GBD study, COPD was 11th in 1990 and 7th in 2017 among the causes of premature death. Among the causes of disability, it was fifth in 1990 and declined to 6th place in 2017. In the same study, the causes of premature death and disability are listed according to the development level of the countries and COPD is considered as the fifth cause of premature death and disability in countries with high SDI (Institute for Health Metrics and Evaluation [IHME], 2017).

INFLAMMATORY BOWEL DİSEASE

IBD is a term used for Crohn's disease (CD) and ulcerative colitis (UC), characterized by chronic inflammation of the gastrointestinal system (Crohn's and Colitis Foundation of America, 2014). In the past decade, IBD has emerged as a public health challenge worldwide (Kaplan, 2015).

In the literature stated that epidemiological differences between the Western world and newly industrialized countries in IBD are caused by the effects of genetic and environmental factors on disease development (Kaplan, 2015). Epidemiological studies show that the incidence of IBD has rapidly increased in the newly industrialized countries such as Middle East, Asia, and South America in the last 20 years, and that the incidence has stabilized in the 21st century despite the dramatic increase in the 20th century (Khalili, 2019).

IBD is described as a modern disease of modern times (Kaplan, 2015). In a recent systematic review, the regions with the highest prevalence of IBD are Europe (UC: 505 / 100,000 in Norway; CD: 322 / 100,000 in Germany) and North America (UC: 279 / 100,000 in USA; CD: 319 / 100,000 in Canada). It is predicted that prevelans will increase gradually in North America, many countries in Europe, Australia and New Zealand. It is also reported that the incidence is increasing in new industrialized countries such as Asia, the Middle East, South America, and Africa, particularly Brazil, Taiwan and Spain. IBD prevalence in newly industrialized countries is relatively low, but given the increase in incidence, it is estimated that prevalence in these countries will increased (Ng et al., 2018).

The incidence and prevalence of IBD varies according to geographic region (Ng et al., 2018). According to the Center for Disease Control and Prevention (CDC) data, while the rate of those diagnosed with IBD in the USA in 1999 was 0.9%, it was reported that it reached 1.3% in 2015 (Centers for Disease Control and Prevention [CDC], 2015). It is estimated that 267,983 people live in Canada with IBD in 2018. In the projections, it is estimated that the number of people living with IBD will reach 402,853 in 2030 and the prevalence will be higher than the rate in 2018 (Coward et al., 2019).

In a study conducted in Tavyan, it was reported that the crude incidence of CD was 0.17 / 100,000 in 2001, 0.47 / 100,000 in 2015, and UC incidence was 0.54 / 100,000 in 2001 and 0.95 / 100,000 in 2015. The prevalence of CD was reported 0.6 / 100.000 in 2001, 3.9 / 100.000 in 2015, and the prevelance of UC 2.1 / 100,000 in 2001 and 12.8 / 100,000 in 2015, respectively (Yen et al., 2019). Increasing evidence suggests that the incidence and prevalence of IBD in China remains lower than in developed countries, but that IBD is significantly increased. In a study conducted in China, the incidence of IBD, UC and CD was reported 1.80, 1.33 and 0.46 / 1.000.000 between 2010 and 2013 (Cui, & Yuan, 2018). In another study conducted in Portugal, in 2003, approximately 0.1% of the population was diagnosed with IBD and in 2019, this rate is 0.24-0.33%. It is estimated that this ratio will be 0.32-0.49% in 2030 (Santiago et al., 2019).

RHEUMATOID ARTHRITIS

Rheumatoid arthritis is a chronic autoimmune inflammatory disease associated with progressive joint damage and disability (Dargham et al., 2018). Rheumatoid arthritis is the most common inflammatory disease of the joints ve rheumatoid arthritis is associated with reduced mobility, disability, poor quality of life and death. Rheumatoid arthritis affects approximately 0.5–1.0% of the adult population in most developed countries (Kiadaliri, Felson, Neogi, & Englund, 2017).

In a study evaluating data from the GBD study, it was reported that the prevalence of rheumatoid arthritis worldwide was 0.24% (0.13% in males and 0.35% in females). Globally, of the 291 conditions studied, In 2010 RA was ranked as the 42nd highest contributor to global disability and represented 0.49% of total YLDs and it was ranked 74th in global DALYs, accounting for 0.19% of total DALYs (Cross et al., 2014). In addition, it is reported that approximately one quarter of rheumatoid arthritis patients are incapacitated for the first three years of diagnosis and 35% of them are incapacitated within 10 years. (Kiadaliri et al., 2017).

The prevalence of rheumatoid arthritis in low and middle income countries is reported to be 0.40% for Southeast Asia, 0.37% for Eastern Mediterranean, 0.62% for Europe, 1.25% for America and 0.42% for the Western Pacific. In the same study, the prevalence of rheumatoid arthritis in men and women in low- and middle-income countries was reported to be 0.16% and 0.75%, respectively, and the prevalence of rheumatoid arthritis was reported to be similar in rural and urban areas (Rudan et al., 2019).

When regional studies of the prevalence of rheumatoid arthritis are evaluated, it is reported that the prevalence of rheumatoid arthritis varies between 0.41% and 0.54% in the commercially insured adult US population between 2004 and 2014 (Hunter et al., 2017). In a study conducted in India in 2016, the rate of rheumatoid arthritis incidence was 18.5 / 100.000 person-yrs (25.2 in women, 8.8 in men), prevalence rates were 0.329 (0.464 for women, 0.123 for men) (Di et al., 2016). The prevalence of rheumatoid arthritis has been reported to be 0.84% in the age group 16 and over in the UK, 0.78% in adults 18 and over in Scotland and 0.94% in the age group 16 and over in Wales (Versus Arthritis, 2019). In a study conducted in Taiwan, the prevalence of rheumatoid arthritis in the 10-79 age group was reported to be 14.01 / 100.000 (22.25 / 100.000 in women and 5.37 / 100.000 in men) (Yang, Huang, Chiou, & Wei, 2018).

MULTİPLE SCLEROSİS

MS is the most common inflammatory neurological disease in young adults (Multiple Sclerosis International Federation, 2013). The cause of MS is unknown and the incidence and prevalance varies according to region, sex and ethnicity (Gilmour, Ramage-Morin, & Wong, 2018; Multiple Sclerosis Collaborators, 2019). Studies have shown that patients with MS are usually diagnosed in early adulthood and that patients have had to live with this progressive neurological disease for years (Multiple Sclerosis International Federation, 2013).

Globally, the number of cases was 2 012 000 in 2015 and MS is ranked 10th in the prevalence of neurological conditions (Multiple Sclerosis Collaborators, 2019). According to WHO data (WHO, 2016a), the number of MS cases is 24.065 in 2016 and this number is higher in women compared to men (F: 14.743, M: 9.322). Multiple Sclerosis Collaborators (2019) is estimated that the highest age-standardised MS prevalence were in high-income North America (164.6/100000), Western Europe (127.0/100000), and Australasia (91.1/100000), and the lowest were in eastern sub-Saharan Africa (3·3/100000), central sub-Saharan African (2·8/100000), and Oceania (2·0/100000). The prevelance of MS were significantly higher in women than in men (Multiple Sclerosis Collaborators, 2019).

Globally there were approximately 18 932 deaths due to MS and most deaths occurred in high SDI countries (10 021 deaths), and mortality in the USA was highest among all countries (3862 deaths) in 2016. It is reported that the age-standardized mortality rate for MS globally decreased by 11.5% in 2016 compared to 1990 (Multiple Sclerosis Collaborators, 2019) According to WHO data (WHO, 2016a) the regions with the highest deaths due to MS in 2016 are Europe, America and Southeast Asia respectively. According to the World Bank income groups, MS-related deaths were highest level in high-income countries and lowest level in low-income countries (WHO2016a).

Globally 1 151 478 DALYs due to MS in 2016. Countries in the highest SDI quintile accounted for half of the DALYs in 2016. According to the WHO, the three regions in which DALY was highest were Europe, America and Southeast Asia respectively, while Africa was the lowest in 2016 (WHO2016a). Overall, MS made up 0·04% of the overall DALYs from all neurological disorders (Multiple Sclerosis Collaborators, 2019).

REFERENCES

Adeloye, D., Chua, S., Lee, C., Basquill, C., Papana, A., Theodoratou, E., ... Rudan, I. (2015). Global and regional estimates of COPD prevalence: Systematic review and meta–analysis. *Journal of Global Health*, *5*(2), 020415. doi:10.7189/jogh.05.020415 PMID:26755942

American Cancer Society. (2018). *Global cancer facts & figures*. Atlanta: American Cancer Society.

Benjamin, E. J., Muntner, P., Alonso, A., Bittencourt, M. S., Callaway, C. W., Carson, A. P., ... Virani, S. S. (2019). Heart Disease and Stroke Statistics-2019 Update: A Report From the American Heart Association. *Circulation*, *139*(10), e56–e528. doi:10.1161/CIR.0000000000000659 PMID:30700139

Bray, F., Ferlay, J., Soerjomataram, I., Siegel, R. L., Torre, L. A., & Jemal, A. (2018). Global Cancer Statistics 2018: GLOBOCAN estimates of ıncidence and mortality worldwide for 36 cancers in 185 countries. *CA: a Cancer Journal for Clinicians*, *68*(6), 394–424. doi:10.3322/caac.21492 PMID:30207593

Calle, M. C., & Andersen, C. J. (2019). Assessment of Dietary Patterns Represents a Potential, Yet Variable, Measure of Inflammatory Status: A Review and Update. *Disease Markers*, *3102870*. doi:10.1155/2019/3102870

Casas, R., & Estruch, R. (2016). Dietary Patterns, Foods, Nutrients and Chronic Inflammatory Disorders. *Immunome Research*, *12*(2), 2. doi:10.4172/1745-7580.10000122

Centers for Disease Control and Prevention. (2019). Data and statics. Inflammatory bowel disease prevalence (IBD) in the United States. Retrieved from https://www.cdc.gov/ibd/data-statistics.htm

Chen, L., Deng, H., Cui, H., Fang, J., Zuo, Z., Deng, J., ... Zhao, L. (2018). Inflammatory responses and inflammation-associated diseases in organs. *Oncotarget*, *9*(6), 7204–7218. doi:10.18632/oncotarget.23208 PMID:29467962

Cho, N. H., Shaw, J. E., Karuranga, S., Huang, Y., da Rocha Fernandes, J. D., Ohlrogge, A. W., & Malanda, B. (2018). IDF diabetes atlas: Global estimates of diabetes prevalence for 2017 and projections for 2045. *Diabetes Research and Clinical Practice*, *138*, 271–281. doi:10.1016/j.diabres.2018.02.023 PMID:29496507

Chooi, Y. C., Ding, C., & Magkos, F. (2019). The epidemiology of obesity. *Metabolism: Clinical and Experimental*, *92*, 6–10. doi:10.1016/j.metabol.2018.09.005 PMID:30253139

Chronic Respiratory Disease Collaborators. (2017). Global, regional, and national deaths, prevalence, DALY, and YLD for chronic obstructive pulmonary disease and asthma, 1990–2015: A systematic analysis for the Global Burden of Disease Study. *The Lancet. Respiratory Medicine*, *5*(9), 691–706. PMID:28822787

Coward, S., Clement, F., Benchimol, E. I., Bernstein, C. N., Avina-Zubieta, J. A., Bitton, A., ... Kaplan, G. G. (2019). Past and future burden of inflammatory bowel diseases based on modeling of population-based data. *Gastroenterology*, *156*(5), 1345–1353. doi:10.1053/j.gastro.2019.01.002 PMID:30639677

Crohn's and Colitis Foundation of America. (2014). The facts about inflammatory bowel diseases. Retrived from http://www.crohnscolitisfoundation.org/assets/pdfs/updatedibdfactbook.pdf

Cross, M., Smith, E., Hoy, D., Carmona, L., Wolfe, F., Vos, T., ... March, L. (2014). The global burden of rheumatoid arthritis: Estimates from the global burden of disease 2010 study. *Annals of the Rheumatic Diseases*, *73*(7), 1316–1322. doi:10.1136/annrheumdis-2013-204627 PMID:24550173

Cui, G., & Yuan, A. A. (2018). Systematic review of epidemiology and risk factors associated with Chinese inflammatory bowel disease. *Frontiers in Medicine*, *5*, 183. doi:10.3389/fmed.2018.00183 PMID:29971235

Dargham, S.R., Zahirovic, S., Hammoudeh, M., Al Emadi, S., Masri, B.K., Halabi, H., … Arayssi, T. (2018). Epidemiology and treatment patterns of rheumatoid arthritis in a large cohort of Arab patients. *PLoS One*, *13*(12), 1-12.

De Silva, S. T., Niriella, M. A., Ediriweera, D. S., Kottahachchi, D., Kasturiratne, A., de Silva, A. P., ... de Silva, H. J. (2019). Incidence and risk factors for metabolic syndrome among urban, adult Sri Lankans: A prospective, 7-year community cohort, follow-up study. *Diabetology & Metabolic Syndrome*, *11*(1), 66. doi:10.118613098-019-0461-7 PMID:31428204

Di, W. T., Vergara, F., Bertiller, E., Gallardo, M. L., Gandino, I., Scolnik, M., ... Soriano, E. R. (2016). Incidence and prevalence of rheumatoid arthritis in a health management organization in Argentina: A 15-year study. *The Journal of Rheumatology*, *43*(7), 1306–1311. doi:10.3899/jrheum.151262 PMID:27084906

Elsayed, M. A., & Norredin, A. (2019). *The potential contribution of nanoparticles in the treatment of inflammatory diseases*. InTech Open. Retrieved from https://www.intechopen.com/online-first/the-potential-contribution-of-nanoparticles-in-the-treatment-of-inflammatory-diseases

Eurostat. (2015). Cardiovascular diseases statistics. Retrieved from https://ec.europa.eu/eurostat/statistics-explained/index.php/Cardiovascular_diseases_statistics

Ferlay, J., Colombet, M., Soerjomataram, I., Dyba, T., Randi, G., Bettio, M., ... Bray, F. (2018). Cancer incidence and mortality patterns in Europe: Estimates for 40 countries and 25 major cancers in 2018. *European Journal of Cancer*, *103*, 356–387. doi:10.1016/j.ejca.2018.07.005 PMID:30100160

Ferlay, J., Colombet, M., Soerjomataram, I., Mathers, C., Parkin, D. M., Piñeros, M., ... Bray, F. (2019). Estimating the global cancer incidence and mortality in 2018: GLOBOCAN sources and Methods. *International Journal of Cancer*, *144*(8), 1941–1953. doi:10.1002/ijc.31937 PMID:30350310

Ford, N. D., Patel, S. A., & Narayan, K. M. (2017). Obesity in low- and middle-income countries: Burden, drivers, and emerging challenges. *Annual Review of Public Health*, *38*(1), 145–164. doi:10.1146/annurev-publhealth-031816-044604 PMID:28068485

Gilmour, H., Ramage-Morin, P. L., & Wong, S. L. (2018). Multiple sclerosis: Prevalence and impact. *Health Reports*, *29*(1), 3–8. PMID:29341025

Global Initiative for Chronic Obstructive Lung Disease. (2018). Pocket guide To COPD diagnosıs, management, and preventıon a guide for health care professionals 2017 Report. Retrived from https://goldcopd.org/wp-content/uploads/2016/12/wms-GOLD-2017-Pocket-Guide.pdf

Guariguata, L., Whiting, D. R., Hambleton, I., Beagley, J., Linnenkamp, U., & Shaw, J. E. (2014). Global estimates of diabetes prevalence in adults for 2013 and projections for 2035 for the IDF Diabetes Atlas. *Diabetes Research and Clinical Practice*, *103*(2), 137–149. doi:10.1016/j.diabres.2013.11.002 PMID:24630390

Hunter, T. M., Boytsov, N. N., Zhang, X., Schroeder, K., Michaud, K., & Araujo, A. B. (2017). Prevalence of rheumatoid arthritis in the United States adult population in healthcare claims databases, 2004–2014. *Rheumatology International*, *37*(9), 1551–1557. doi:10.100700296-017-3726-1 PMID:28455559

Institute for Health Metrics and Evaluation (IHME). (2018). Findings from the global burden of disease study 2017. Retrived from http://www.healthdata.org/sites/default/files/files/policy_report/2019/GBD_2017_Booklet_Issuu_2.pdf

International Agency for Research on Cancer. (2018). Global cancer observatory. Retrieved from https://gco.iarc.fr/tomorrow/home

International Diabetes Federation. (2015). The IDF consensus worldwide defnition of the metabolic syndrome. Retrieved from http://www.idf.org/metabolic-syndrome

Joseph, P., Leong, D., McKee, M., Anand, S. S., Schwalm, J. D., Teo, K., ... Yusuf, S. (2017). Reducing the Global Burden of Cardiovascular Disease, Part 1: The Epidemiology and Risk Factors. *Circulation Research*, *121*(6), 677–694. doi:10.1161/CIRCRESAHA.117.308903 PMID:28860318

Kaplan, G. G. (2015). The global burden of IBD: from 2015 to 2025. *Nature Reviews. Gastroenterology & Hepatology*, *12*(12), 720–727. doi:10.1038/nrgastro.2015.150 PMID:26323879

Khalili, H. (2019). The changing epidemiology of inflammatory bowel disease: What goes up may come down. *Inflammatory Bowel Diseases*, izz186. doi:10.1093/ibd/izz186 PMID:31504537

Kiadaliri, A. A., Felson, D. T., Neogi, T., & Englund, M. (2017). Brief report: Rheumatoid arthritis as the underlying cause of death in thirty-one countries, 1987–2011: Trend Analysis of World Health Organization Mortality Database. *Arthritis & Rheumatology*, *69*(8), 1560–1565. doi:10.1002/art.40091 PMID:28425170

Kunnumakkara, A. B., Sailo, B. L., Banik, K., Choudhary, H., Prasad, S., Gupta, S. C., ... Aggarwal, B. B. (2018). Chronic diseases, infammation, and spices: How are they linked? *Journal of Translational Medicine*, *16*(1), 14. doi:10.118612967-018-1381-2 PMID:29370858

Lee, S. E., Han, K., Kang, Y. M., Kim, S. O., Cho, Y. K., Ko, K. S., ... Koh, E. H. (2018). Trends in the prevalence of metabolic syndrome and its components in South Korea: Findings from the Korean National Health Insurance Service Database (2009–2013). *PLoS One*, *13*(3), e0194490. doi:10.1371/journal.pone.0194490 PMID:29566051

Meier, T., Grafe, K., Senn, F., Sur, P., Stangl, G. I., Dawczynski, C., ... Lorkowski, S. (2019). Cardiovascular mortality attributable to dietary risk Factors in 51 countries in the WHO European Region from 1990 to 2016: A systematic analysis of the Global Burden of Disease Study. *European Journal of Epidemiology*, *34*(1), 37–55. doi:10.100710654-018-0473-x PMID:30547256

Mishra, M.R. (2019). Determinants of cardiovascular disease and sequential decision-making for treatment among women: A Heckman's approach. *SSM Population Health*, *7*, 100365. doi:10.1016/j.ssmph.2019.100365

Multhoff, G., Molls, M., & Radons, J. (2012). Chronic inflammation in cancer development. *Frontiers in Immunology*, *2*, 98. doi:10.3389/fimmu.2011.00098 PMID:22566887

Multiple Sclerosis International Federation. (2013). Mapping multiple sclerosis around the world. Retrieved from https://www.msif.org/wp-content/uploads/2014/09/Atlas-of-MS.pdf

Murata, M. (2018). Inflammation and cancer. *Environmental Health and Preventive Medicine*, *23*(1), 50. doi:10.118612199-018-0740-1 PMID:30340457

Ng, S. C., Shi, H. Y., Hamidi, N., Underwood, F. E., Tang, W., Benchimol, E. I., ... Kaplan, G. G. (2018). Worldwide incidence and prevalence of inflammatory bowel disease in the 21st century: A systematic review of population-based studies. *Lancet*, *23*(390), 2769–2778. PMID:29050646

OECD/EU. (2018). Health at a glance: Europe 2018: State of health in the EU cycle. Retrived from https://ec.europa.eu/health/sites/health/files/state/docs/2018_healthatglance_rep_en.pdf

Pahwa, R., & Jialal, I. (2019). *Chronic inflammation*. StatPearls. Retrieved from https://www.ncbi.nlm.nih.gov/books/NBK493173/

Rehan, F., Qadeer, A., Bashir, I., & Jamshaid, M. (2016). Risk factors of cardiovascular disease in developing countries. *International Current Pharmaceutical Journal*, *5*(8), 69–72. doi:10.3329/icpj.v5i8.28875

Risk Factor Collab, N. C. D. (2016). Trends in adult body-mass index in 200 countries from 1975 to 2014: A pooled analysis of 1698 population-based measurement studies with 19·2 million participants. *Lancet*, *387*(10026), 1377–1396. doi:10.1016/S0140-6736(16)30054-X PMID:27115820

Rochlani, Y., Pothineni, N. V., Kovelamudi, S., & Mehta, J. L. (2017). Metabolic syndrome: Pathophysiology, management, and modulation by natural compounds. *Therapeutic Advances in Cardiovascular Disease*, *11*(8), 215–225. doi:10.1177/1753944717711379 PMID:28639538

Roth, G. A., Johnson, C., Abajobir, A., Abd-Allah, F., Abera, S. F., Abyu, G., ... Murray, C. (2017). Global, regional, and national burden of cardiovascular diseases for 10 causes, 1990 to 2015. *Journal of the American College of Cardiology*, *70*(1), 1–25. doi:10.1016/j.jacc.2017.04.052 PMID:28527533

Roth, G. A., Nguyen, G., Forouzanfar, M. H., Mokdad, A. H., Naghavi, M., & Murray, C. J. (2015). Stimates of global and regional premature cardiovascular mortality in 2025. *Circulation, 132*(13), 1270–1282. doi:10.1161/CIRCULATIONAHA.115.016021 PMID:26408271

Rudan, I., Sidhu, S., Papana, A., Meng, S.J., Xin-Wei, Y., Wang, W. … Chan, K.Y. (2015). Prevalence of rheumatoid arthritis in low– and middle–income countries: A systematic review and analysis. *Journal of Global Health, 5*(1), 1-10.

Saklayen, M. G. (2018). The Global epidemic of the metabolic syndrome. *Current Hypertension Reports, 20*(2), 12. doi:10.100711906-018-0812-z PMID:29480368

Santiago, M., Magro, F., Correia, L., Portela, F., Ministro, P., Lago, P., & Dias, C. C. (2019). What forecasting the prevalence of inflammatory bowel disease may tell us about its evolution on a national scale. *Therapeutic Advances in Gastroenterology, 12*, 1–6. doi:10.1177/1756284819860044 PMID:31467592

Sarebanhassanabadi, M., Mirhosseini, S. J., Mirzaei, M., Namayandeh, S. M., Soltani, M. H., Pedarzadeh, A., ... Salehi-Abargouei, A. (2017). The incidence of metabolic syndrome and the most powerful components as predictors of metabolic syndrome in central Iran: A 10-Year Follow-Up in a Cohort Study. *Iranian Red Crescent Medical Journal, 19*(7), e14934. doi:10.5812/ircmj.14934

Saxena, M., & Modi, D. R. (2014). Inflammation and diabetes. *Interdisciplinary Journal of Microinflammation, 1 (110)*, 2.

Şen, E., Oğuzülgen, K., Bavbek, S., Günen, H., Kıyan, E., & Türktaş, H. … Yıldırım, N. (2015). Astım-KOAH overlap sendromu. *Tuberculozis and Throrax, 63*(4), 265–277. PMID:26963310

Slavich, G. M. (2015). Understanding inflammation, its regulation, and relevance for health: A top scientific and public priority. *Brain, Behavior, and Immunity, 45*, 13–14. doi:10.1016/j.bbi.2014.10.012 PMID:25449576

Sorriento, D., & Iaccarino, G. (2019). Inflammation and cardiovascular diseases: The most recent findings. *International Journal of Molecular Sciences, 20*(16), 3879. doi:10.3390/ijms20163879 PMID:31395800

The Organisation for Economic Co-operation and Development (OECD). (2017). Obesity update 2017. doi:10.100711428-017-0241-7

To, T., Stanojevic, S., Moores, G., Gershon, A. S., Bateman, E. D., Cruz, A. A., & Boulet, L. P. (2012). Global asthma prevalence in adults: Findings from the cross-sectional world health survey. *BMC Public Health, 12*(1), 204. doi:10.1186/1471-2458-12-204 PMID:22429515

Uchida, A., Sakaue, K., & Inoue, H. (2018). Epidemiology of asthma-chronic obstructive pulmonary disease overlap (ACO). *Allergology International, 67*(2), 165–171. doi:10.1016/j.alit.2018.02.002 PMID:29551279

Versus Arthritis. (2019). The State of Musculoskeletal Health 2019. Retrieved from https://www.versusarthritis.org/about-arthritis/data-and-statistics/state-of-musculoskeletal-health-2019/

Wallin, M. T., Culpepper, W. J., Nichols, E., Bhutta, Z. A., Gebrehiwot, T. T., Hay, S. I., ... Mokdad, A. H. (2019). Global, regional, and national burden of multiple sclerosis 1990–2016: A systematic analysis for the Global Burden of Disease Study 2016. *Lancet Neurology, 18*(3), 269–285.

World Bank. (2017). Diabetes prevalence. Retrieved from https://data.worldbank.org/indicator/SH.STA.DIAB.ZS

World Health Organization. (2000). Obesity: preventing and managing the global epidemic Report of a WHO Consultation. World Health Organization. doi:10.1007/BF00400469

World Health Organization. (2013). *Global NCD action plan 2013–2020*. Geneva, Switzerland: WHO Press.

World Health Organization. (2016a). Disease burden and mortality estimates. Cause spesific.

World Health Organization. (2016b). *HEARTS technical package for cardiovascular disease management in primary health care*. Geneva, Switzerland: WHO Press.

World Health Organization. (2017). *Guide to cancer early diagnosis*. Geneva, Switzerland: WHO Press.

World Health Organization. (2018). Global Asthma report, 2018. Retrieved from http://www.globalasthmareport.org/Global%20Asthma%20Report%202018.pdf

Yalçın, T., & Rakıcıoğlu, R. (2018). *Dietary factors, type 2 diabetes and inflammation*. Sakarya.

Yang, D. H., Huang, J. Y., Chiou, J. Y., & Wei, J. C. C. (2018). Analysis of socioeconomic status in the patients with rheumatoid arthritis. *International Journal of Environmental Research and Public Health*, *15*(6), 1–12. doi:10.3390/ijerph15061194 PMID:29875338

Yen, H. H., Weng, M. T., Tung, C. C., Wang, Y. T., Chang, Y. T., Chang, C. H., ... Wei, S. C. (2019). Epidemiological trend in inflammatory bowel disease in Taiwan from 2001 to 2015: A nationwide populationbased study. *Intestinal Research*, *17*(1), 54–62. doi:10.5217/ir.2018.00096 PMID:30449079

Yılmaz, C. (2019). Diabetes and diabetes education journey from past to present in Turkey. In N. Dinççağ (Ed.), *Turkish Diabetes Annual 2018-2019* (1st ed., pp. 33–46). Academic Press. Retrieved from http://www.diabetcemiyeti.org/var/cdn/0/0/diyabet-yilligi-2019.pdf

Zaidi, Z., Boussouf, K., Benkobbi, S., Bitat-Aouati, C., Boudiaf, S. B., Kaddour, F., & Djelaoudji, A. (2019). Burden of cardiovascular diseases in the maghrebian region, 1990-2017. *Health Science Journal*, *13*(1), 632. doi:10.21767/1791-809X.1000632

Section 2
Nutrition in Anti- and Pro-Inflammatory Balance

Chapter 3
Macronutrients Having Pro-/ Anti-Inflammatory Properties

Uğur Günşen
https://orcid.org/0000-0001-9858-6019
Bandırma Onyedi Eylül University, Turkey

Ramazan Mert Atan
https://orcid.org/0000-0003-4608-605X
University Bandırma Onyedi Eylül, Turkey

ABSTRACT

Inflammation is a physiological response to infectious agents and tissue damage. When the inflammatory process does not proceed appropriately, a low-grade chronic inflammatory response develops. Low-grade chronic inflammation is defined as a metabolic process characterized by the increase of the acute phase proteins such as CRP and the pro-inflammatory cytokines in plasma and by infiltration of macrophage and T cell and of chemotactic pro-inflammatory chemokines such as monocyte chemotactic protein-1 (MCP-1) in insulin-dependent tissues cells. Carbohydrates, fats, and proteins, which are among the most important macro nutrients are important for the individual's inflammatory response according to their daily intake levels, sources and types. Although their diet is rich in complex carbohydrates, pulp, MUFA, PUFA, the reduction of SFA, TFA, simple sugars, and processed carbohydrates can lead to positive effects on inflammatory pathways and prevent chronic diseases in the long term.

DOI: 10.4018/978-1-7998-3594-3.ch003

NUTRITION AND INFLAMMATION

According to many national and international health guidelines, a healthy and balanced diet pattern is one of the leading modifiable risk factors for the protection of individuals from chronic diseases. Adequate and balanced diet in terms of macro and micronutrients, has positive effects on prevention, onset and prognosis of chronic diseases in the short and long term (WHO, 2019a; WHO, 2019b).

In recent years, changing living conditions have changed the eating habits of individuals and therefore their diet patterns. As a result of the developed food processing techniques and nutritional habits, macro and micronutrients of the diet, fatty acid compositions and pulp content have changed significantly (Cordain et al., 2005; Carrera-Bastos, Fontes, & Lindeberg, 2011). Today, this diet pattern, which changes with the consumption of packaged and processed carbohydrates and fast food consumption and with the excessive consumption of sugary and carbonated beverages, is called "western type diet". Compared to other nutritional approaches, the Western-type diet, has a high content of energy, SFA, TFA, sugar and pre-packaged products with added sugar, pulp, MUFA, PUFA, vitamins and minerals are characterized by insufficient nutritional patterns (Odermatt, 2011).

As a result of close to 6500 cohort, case-control and cross-sectional studies conducted on humans, it was found that there was a relationship between the content of the diet and the inflammatory markers found in the blood. The effects of some nutrients in the nutritional pattern of the individual on the inflammatory markers such as Interleukin-1 β (IL-1 β), Interleukin-4 (IL-4), Interleukin-6 (IL-6), Interleukin-10 (IL-10), Tumor Necrous Factor-α (TNF-α) and C-Reactive Protein (CRP) were investigated and "Dietary Inflammation Index (DII)" was developed. While total fat, SFA and simple sugar content found in an individual's nutrition pattern had pro-inflammatory effects; anti-inflammatory properties of MUFA, PUFA and pulp intake have been reported (Shivappa, Steck, Hurley, Hussey, & Hebert, 2014). In addition, high energy density of the diet and the energy received from the need to trigger more inflammatory processes are reported (Bawaked et al., 2017).

Inflammation is a physiological response to infectious agents and tissue damage. Inflammation is not a disease, but a system that must be in balance for a healthy life, and is the response of the immune system to attacks from outside or inside the body (Libby, 2007). Adipose tissue has an important role in inflammation. Adipose tissue is not only an energy storage organ but also an important endocrine organ and secretes the inflammatory markers such as IL-1β, IL-6, TNF-α, CRP, and adipokines such as adiponectin, leptin and resistin (Shivappa, 2014).

Inflammation is divided into acute and chronic inflammation. Acute inflammatory response represents the process of wound healing and tissue regeneration, which will normally improve within a few days. When the inflammatory process does not proceed appropriately, a low-grade chronic inflammatory response develops. Low-grade chronic inflammation are defined as a metabolic process characterized by increase of the acute phase proteins such as CRP and the pro-inflammatory cytokines such as TNF-α, IL-1 β and IL-6, e-selectin, TGF-β, TLR-4 in plasma and by infiltration of macrophage and T cell and of chemotactic pro-inflammatory chemokines such as monocyte chemotactic protein-1 (MCP-1) in insulin-dependent tissues cells. In this process, increased pro-inflammatory cytokines in plasma and tissues can begin to cause metabolic damage and lead to the formation of chronic diseases (Elenkov & Chrousos, 2012; Calder et. al., 2013; Huang, Zourdos, Jo, & Ormsbee, 2013; Heber & Henning, 2014; Leon-Pedroza et al., 2015).

Chronic inflammation is associated with the formation of many diseases such as especially obesity, insulin resistance, metabolic syndrome, Type 2 Diabetes mellitus (DM), cardiovascular diseases, and cancer. Owing to the control of regulatory mechanisms, the inflammatory response is suppressed and the concentrations of pro-inflammatory cytokines are reduced by the release of cytokines with anti-inflammatory characteristics such as IL-4 and IL-10 (Duncan et al., 2003; Bastard et al., 2006; Alemany, 2013; Kaptoge et al., 2014; Silveria et al., 2018).

When the role of chronic inflammation in metabolic diseases is investigated, it is seen that dietary content and feeding habits have an effect on inflammation indicators (Göktaş, 2016). In studies conducted in humans, it has been shown that dietary components taken by meal with high energy content and glycemic index by food consumption frequency and food consumption records affect the indicators of inflammation such as CRP, IL-6 and TNF-α (Nettleton et al., 2006; Esmaillzadeh et al., 2007). Excessive intake of certain nutrients such as dietary triglycerides, SFA and simple sugar (monosaccharides such as glucose and fructose and disaccharides such as sucrose or tea sugar) is known to induce the onset of postprandial inflammatory response and release of CRP. While omega-3 fatty acids suppress inflammation, omega-6 fatty acids have a pro-inflammatory effect (Margioris, 2009; Calder et al., 2011; Calder et. al., 2013).

In the researches, the level of inflammatory markers such as IL-6, TNF-α and CRP, and adiponectin levels are affected by the dietary pattern of individuals, especially Glycemic Index (GI) / Glycemic Burden (GY) of the diet, fatty acid composition and some vitamin content, and minerals (Lopez-Garcia et al., 2004; Esmaillzadeh et al., 2007; Yannakoulia et al., 2008; Galland, 2010; Calder et al., 2011; Barbaresko, Koch, Schulze, & Nöthlings, 2013). Refined starch, sugars, saturated fats and transyacids have been shown to stimulate pro-inflammatory cytokine release by stimulating the immune system (Giugliano, Ceriello, & Esposito, 2006).

It has been reported that adequate dietary fiber intake prevents inflammation achieving glycemic control by reducing body fat and by lowering cholesterol (Chen, Chen, Wang, Qin, & Bai, 2018). Western diet, rich in red and processed meat, high-fat dairy products, low dietary fiber intake and refined cereals, has been found to be pro-inflammatory and associated with increased plasma CRP and IL-6 levels. Mediterranean diet, rich in whole grains, vegetables and fruits, containing omega-3 fatty acids and olive oil, was associated with low levels of inflammation. In a study conducted with Japanese individuals, increased consumption of fruits, vegetables, soy products and fish was reported to be inversely related to serum CRP levels (Nanri et al., 2008). In another study, it was shown that increasing the consumption of whole-grain products and low-fat dairy products and reducing the consumption of refined grains were positively associated with serum adiponectin levels in healthy Greek women (Yannakoulia et al., 2008).

Metabolic syndrome is characterized by increased blood pressure, blood glucose, triglyceride levels, central obesity and low plasma HDL cholesterol (Alberti et al., 2013). Metabolic syndrome is associated with low-level chronic inflammation. Abdominal obesity, along with increased pro-inflammatory cytokines and adipokines, contributes to the development of metabolic syndrome. Energy and carbohydrate-restricted, low-fat, rich in MUFA and omega-3 fatty acids, high-quality protein, antioxidant vitamins and minerals (A, E and C selenium, zinc) containing diet is reported to prevent metabolic syndrome by reducing inflammation (Andersen & Fernandez, 2013).

MACRONUTRIENTS

The building blocks in the composition of nutrients are called nutrients. In general, the nutritional pattern consists of macro and micronutrients found in the diet. Carbohydrates, fats and proteins are the main macro nutrients in the diet that play a role in physiological mechanisms in the body. An adequate and balanced nutrition pattern implies that an individual's adequate energy intake and the need for macro and micronutrients are met (Baysal, 2012).

While the amount and origin of edible nutrients plays an important role in the development of low-grade chronic inflammation (Pang, Xie, Chen, & Hu, 2014), the effects of macronutrients on inflammation are extensively investigated (Bressan & Hermsdorff, 2008; Goletzke et al., 2014; Pang et al., 2014; B´edard, Lamarche, Corneau, Dodin, & Lemieux, 2015; Corley, Kyle, Starr, McNeill, & Deary, 2015; Okreglicka, 2015; Ozawa, Shipley, Kivimaki, Singh-Manoux, & Brunner, 2017).

CARBOHYDRATES

Carbohydrates having the closed formula of $C_n(H_2O)_n$ by the combination of carbon, hydrogen and oxygen atoms are the most important macro nutrients that meet the body's energy needs (Baysal, 2012). Carbohydrates are aldehyde or ketone derivatives of polyhydroxy alcohols or their polymers (Aksoy, 2016).

Glucose, a simple six-carbon sugar, is moderately sweet. It usually occurs as a result of the destruction of starch in the organism. Glucose, the carbohydrate form circulating in the blood, is considered the body's fuel. Glucose plays an important role in amino acid synthesis, production of proteins and lipid metabolism. The normal level of glucose in the blood is 70-100 mg / dl. The decrease in this amount is called hypoglycemia and the increase is called hyperglycemia (Aksoy, 2016).

Fructose is a monosaccharide that structurally has the same chemical formula as glucose, but which contains the ketone group at the second carbon instead of the aldehyde group in the first carbon (Forshee et al., 2007). Honey, fresh vegetables and fruits are the natural sources of fructose in the diet, while high fructose corn syrup (synthetic fructose) and sucrose are the sources of added sugar (Makarem, Bandera, Nicholson, & Parekh, 2018). Particularly in the last 40 years, the use of fructose as a sweetener in beverages containing high fructose corn syrup (CFM) or sucrose has increased (Malik & Hu, 2015). Compared to other sweeteners, high fructose corn syrup, which has a high degree of sweetness and low cost, is frequently used in the food industry (Duffey & Popkin, 2008).

Saccharose, or sucrose or tea sugar, is a disaccharide formed by the combination of a glucose and a fructose molecule. Starch-based sugar (SBS) is a product in which the glucose contained in the starch hydrolyzate obtained from corn is converted into fructose with the help of enzymes. The most commonly used forms are known to be SBS-55 (55% fructose, 41% glucose, 4% glucose polymers) and SBS-42 (42% fructose, 53% glucose, 5% glucose polymers) (Forshee et al., 2007).

Epidemiological and intervention studies show that the type and amount of carbohydrates in the diet may have an effect on low-grade chronic inflammation in individuals. While whole grains and carbohydrated foods with high pulp content such as vegetables and fruits are effective in preventing inflammation, simple sugars (fructose, sucrose), carbonated drinks containing them, and processed carbohydrated foods (high fructose / glucose corn syrup) may have adverse effects, leading to the onset of inflammation or the chronicity of an already inflammatory response (Calder et al., 2011).

In a study, it was found that consumption of glucose (80 g / day), sucrose (80 g / day) and fructose (80 g / day) taken for 3 weeks increased CRP and adiponectin levels in healthy individuals (Aeberli et al., 2011). In parallel, in another study, it was shown that CRP levels increased in healthy individuals for 10 weeks as a result of consumption of sweetened drinks with high fructose corn syrup (18% energy) and sucrose (18% energy) (Angelopoulos, Lowndes, Sinnett, & Rippe, 2016).

It was determined that glucose uptake causes acute oxidative stress and inflammation at cellular and molecular level. Refined carbohydrates lose their content of pulp, vitamins, minerals and essential fatty acids as they are overprocessed. High consumption of refined carbohydrates leads to rapid changes in blood glucose and insulin levels, leading to an increase in the feeling of hunger and free fatty acid levels (Mohanty et al., 2000; Esposito et al., 2002; Foster-Powell, Holt, & Brand-Miller, 2002; Dandona, Chaudhuri, Ghanim, & Mohanty, 2007).

Esposito et al. (2002) have shown that acute hyperglycemia formed by three consecutive intravenous injections of glucose bolus each of per 2 hours, caused a significant increase in pro-inflammatory cytokines such as TNF-α, IL-6 and IL-18 in both control and glucose tolerance impaired subjects.

Vos, Kimmons, Gillespie, Welsh, & Blanck (2008) has reported that fructose consumption is highest among adolescents aged 12-18 years. Dietary nutrition with high fructose has been shown to cause glucose intolerance and insulin resistance, type 2 diabetes, obesity, hypertension and cardiovascular disease (Ross, Bartness, Mielke, & Parent, 2009).

It has been shown that increased triglyceride levels in plasma and liver due to high fructose consumption increase reactive oxygen species production by increasing β-oxidation of fatty acids. The imbalance between the increase of reactive oxygen species and their detoxification from serum, tissue and organs can lead to oxidative stress. Oxidative stress leads to the release of pro-inflammatory molecules such as TNF-α, IL-1β, IL-6, and CRP by producing an inflammatory response in tissues and organs (Baena et al., 2015; Harvey, 2011).

In recent years, the effect of different carbohydrate species on postprandial glucose, insulin response and inflammatory markers have been investigated. Both experimental and observational studies show that whole grain and / or high dietary fiber intake is effective in lowering serum levels of inflammatory markers such as IL-6, TNF-α, CRP (Chuang et al., 2011; Jaacks, 2014). However, different types of carbohydrate and fiber have different effects on postprandial glucose and insulin response. In this context, Jenkins (1981) proposed the concept of GI in order to determine the glycemic response of carbohydrates in different foods.

GI is a physiological carbohydrate classification system based on the glycemic response given after consuming a food containing carbohydrate, compared to a response to a reference food such as white bread containing the same amount of carbohydrate or glucose solution (Jenkins, 1981). GL is determined by multiplying the GI of a food by the amount of carbohydrate present in each serving, divided by 100 (Salmerón et al., 1997). GI is a comparative measure of the effects of nutrients on blood glucose levels. GY is the effect of edible amount of a carbohydrate-containing food on blood sugar (Akbulut, Eşingen, Bingöl, & Bayraktar, 2013).

High GI foods (white bread, white rice, soda, crackers, refined breakfast cereals, instant oats, baked plain potatoes, mashed potatoes, raisins, watermelons, sugar, sugary drinks) are quickly digested and cause significant fluctuations in blood sugar levels. In response to a rapid and sudden increase in blood sugar, large amounts of insulin are secreted from the pancreas. Unprocessed fresh foods such as whole grains, legumes, fruits and vegetables have a low GI. Low GI foods (100% stone bread, steel-cut oats, 100% whole grain, brown rice, quinoa, white and whole wheat pasta, sweet potatoes, apples, bananas, strawberries, oranges, legumes, yogurt, milk) are digested and absorbed by blood sugar insulin gradually increases.

Studies have shown a positive correlation between dietary GI and GL and inflammation biomarkers (Jenkins, 1981; Levitan et al., 2008). In a study, a 10-unit increase in GI of the diet was reported to cause a 29% increase in serum CRP (Du et al., 2008). Characteristically high refined carbohydrates and / or low-fiber carbohydrates, such as foods with a high GI value, are the main dietary factors affecting inflammation (Ricker & Haas, 2017).

Studies have reported the mechanism by which high GI diets cause inflammation. High GI diets exert hyperglycemia-stimulating activity that increases pro-inflammatory cytokines including IL-6 and TNF-α and stimulates oxidative stress in both healthy and impaired glucose tolerance subjects (Dandona et al., 2007; Esposito et al., 2002). Cross-sectional studies in healthy middle-aged women report a strong positive relationship between dietary GI and GL and plasma CRP (Levitan et al., 2008; Liu et al., 2002). In addition, intervention studies have shown that low GI and low GL diets lower plasma CRP in overweight and obese adults (Wolever et al., 2008; Göğebakan et al., 2011; Neuhouser et al., 2012).

A low-GI diet reduces the body's absorption of glucose, reducing hyperglycemia and hyperinsulinemia, leading to a reduction in systemic inflammation. In studies of overweight and obese subjects, a low GI (Bouche et al., 2002; Qi et al., 2006) or low GL diet (Neuhouser et al., 2012; Heggen et al., 2012; Joslowski et al., 2015) had caused weight loss and improved insulin sensitivity, leading to a reduction in pro-inflammatory cytokines. Considering the known benefits of low GI diet, it is recommended by various health care providers, including preventing or managing diabetes and coronary heart disease, and a possible weapon against obesity (Augustin et al., 2015; Wolever et al., 2008).

The pulp content of the diet; It affects the relationship between carbohydrate quality and systemic inflammation. Dietary total pulp was inversely related to IL-6 and TNF-α, which are important inflammatory markers (Ma et al., 2008). Dietary fiber reduces lipid oxidation and thus has an anti-inflammatory effect on the body. Low-fiber diet causes hyperglycemia and increases the level of pro-inflammatory cytokines such as IL-6, IL-18 and TNF-α. IL-6 plays a primary role in CRP production. Therefore, an increase in IL-6 levels leads to an increase in serum CRP levels (Ma et al., 2008; Silva & Pais de Lacerda, 2012).

It is known that dietary fiber increases insulin sensitivity, decreases postprandial hyperglycemia, improves blood lipids and decreases blood pressure as well as decreasing the level of inflammatory markers in the body (Anderson et al., 2009). Epidemiological studies have shown that whole grain cereals are inversely related to diabetes and chronic vascular disease risk markers such as insulin sensitivity, fasting insulin and C-peptide (McKeown, Meigs, Liu, Wilson, & Jacques, 2002; Liese et al., 2003; Jensen et al., 2006).

In an intervention study in which the effect of dietary fiber intake on the inflammatory marker CRP was observed; The serum CRP levels of the group receiving high pulp (48.0 g) were significantly lower than those receiving low pulp (30.2 g) (Johansson-Persson, 2014). Serum CRP levels of the individuals decreased significantly as a result of 8 weeks of intervention with low calorie (1200-1600 kcal/day) rich in complex carbohydrates (whole grain, bulgur, legumes) (Razad et al., 2014).

The type of carbohydrate in the meal may affect the level of circulating anti-inflammatory cytokines. High pulp content of the meal increases adiponectin release (Esposito et al., 2003). In a cross-sectional study of seven hundred and eighty diabetic men, it was shown that a high-fiber, low-GY diet may increase serum adiponectin concentration in diabetic individuals, in accordance with this data (Qi et al., 2005). Yannakoulia et al. (2008) showed that a diet model rich in whole grain products is positively associated with circulating adiponectin concentration, although not significant.

Carbohydrates, which are an important part of the nutritional pattern, can have an effect on inflammation depending on the amount and type of consumption. While carbohydrates with high pulp content such as whole grains, fruits and vegetables in diet is beneficial for health; sucrose, fructose, high fructose / glucose corn syrup, glucose added products may have adverse health effects depending on the amount and duration of consumption.

PROTEINS AND INFLAMMATION

Proteins are macronutrients that play a role in the important biochemical mechanisms of the body obtained from plant and animal sources in the diet. The recommended daily diet intake (RDI) for protein is 0.8 g / kg body weight. In sports medicine, more protein consumption is recommended for athletes, and the recommended protein intake is 1.4-2 g / kg daily (Campbell et al., 2007). Older people also require higher levels of proteins in their daily diet to prevent or alleviate sarcopenia and osteopenia. Because dietary protein increases calcium absorption and has anabolic effects on muscle and bone cells (Hunt, Johnson & Fariba Roughead, 2009).

It has been shown that a high protein diet (20% of energy) can help combat dyslipidemia, thereby reducing the risk of cardiovascular disease, increasing tissue sensitivity to insulin, and a potentially effective strategy in the fight against obesity, metabolic syndrome and hypertension (Cordain, Eaton, Brand Miller, Mann, & Hill, 2002; O'Keefe & Cordain, 2004; Hodgson, Burke, Beilin, & Puddey, 2006; Larsen et al., 2010).

The amount of protein in the daily diet, its source (vegetable protein, animal protein) and the amino acid composition of the diet play a role in the formation of an inflammatory response (Baysal, 2012). Meat, milk and products; The oxidation of proteins and amino acids in their structures during packaging, processing, storage and cooking causes oxidative stress in the intestinal lumen and causes inflammation (Estévez & Luna, 2017). While the consumption of animal-derived protein in western-type diet causes metabolic syndrome and increased plasma inflammatory markers (Van Horn et al., 2012), consumption of plant-derived protein improves the plasma lipid profile with phytoestrogen components in soy protein content and inhibits insulin resistance (Bhathena & Velasquez, 2002).

Several studies have found that high red meat consumption is positively associated with serum CRP concentration (Azadbakht & Esmaillzadeh, 2009; Montonen, 2013). The results of the DIOGenes (Diet, Obesity and Genes) study show that altering the protein content of the diet affects the level of inflammatory markers, particularly CRP concentration (Göğebakan et al., 2011). In western type nutrition, the presence of red meat and processed meat products as a source of protein was found to be associated with increased CRP levels in serum (Montonen et al. 2013). According to a study examining the relationship between macronutrients in the diet and serum CRP levels; The consumption of protein sources containing high cholesterol and saturated fat such as eggs, red meat, whole-fat dairy products has been found to be associated with high CRP levels. In the same study, there was a significant positive correlation between fat, protein, cholesterol intake and serum CRP levels (Khayyatzadeha et al., 2017).

Azadbakht, Atabak, and Esmaillzadeh (2008), in a randomized controlled parallel study in individuals with Type 2 diabetes, reported that a significant decrease in serum CRP levels in the soy protein given group. In another study, it was stated that the addition of eggs to the diet caused a significant decrease in CRP level and this effect was associated with the effect of lutein on the egg content to reduce the inflammatory response. In the same study, serum adiponectin levels were significantly increased in the egg consuming group. The increase in adiponectin level has been explained that the antioxidant components (lutein and zeaxanthin) in the egg content reduce the effect of inflammatory cytokines capable of inhibiting adiponectin expression (Ratliff et al., 2008).

FATS AND INFLAMMATION

Fats constitute 20-35% of the energy in daily diet is another macro nutrient that has the potential to induce inflammation. The majority of dietary fat is in the form of triacylglycerol (95%), with a small amount of free fatty acids and phospholipids (Baysal, 2012).

Fatty acids (FA) are divided into three main categories: 1) saturated fatty acids (SFA), 2) monounsaturated fatty acids (MUFA), 3) polyunsaturated fatty acids (PUFA). In addition, PUFAs are biologically available in two ways: omega-6 PUFA, also known as omega-6 and omega-3 PUFA, also known as omega-3. The trans isomers of most SFA and fatty acids are harmful to health when over-consumed, while MUFA and some PUFA-containing fats are healthy. In addition, balanced consumption of omega-6 and omega-3 PUFA is an important factor in reducing the risk of chronic disease and maintaining health. The main sources of diet omega-3 PUFA are fish and seafoods as well as vegetable oils such as rapeseed and flaxseed (Kris-Etherton, Harris, & Appel, 2002; Sekuła, Figurska, Barysz, & Ołtarzewski, 2008).

The type of fatty acid consumed may have an effect on the markers of inflammation and oxidative stress associated with chronic diseases in the body and vascular endothelial adhesion molecules. (Ruiz-Nunez, Dijck-Brouwer, & Muskiet, 2016; Nishida & Otsu, 2017). SFA, MUFA, PUFA and trans fatty acids may play a role in the formation of immune response through different mechanisms on inflammation. While omega-3 fatty acids induce anti-inflammatory gene expression, omega-6 fatty acids have a pro-inflammatory effect (Calder, 2011; Minihane et al., 2015).

Dietary saturated fatty acids and omega-6 / omega-3 ratio are higher than recommended increases inflammation (Margioris, 2009). While western-type nutrition with high omega-6 / omega-3 (15/1) increased inflammation, reducing this ratio to 2-3/1 has been shown to suppress inflammation in patients with rheumatoid arthritis (Simopoulos, 2002). In a study by Lopez-Garcia (2005), plasma C-reactive protein ($p < 0.001$) and IL-6 ($p < 0.05$) levels were significantly higher in the group with the highest percentage of total energy ($2.1 \pm 0.4\%$) from trans fatty acids.

The American Heart Association (AHA) emphasizes that the total amount of fat from a healthy diet should be limited to 25-35%, saturated fat <7%, trans fatty acids <1%, and cholesterol intake <300 mg (Stone, 2014).

Saturated Fatty Acids (SFA)

SFA, a source of animal nutrients in the diet, is a nutrient whose intake levels increase with consumption of processed products (Weigert et al., 2004; Innis, 2007). Palm oil in processed foods ready for consumption and nutrients of animal origin (milk and dairy products, meat and meat products, etc.) are the main sources of saturated fatty acids taken from diet. (Lee, 2013).

The total amount of fat taken from diet has the potential to induce inflammation in the body (Ruiz-Nunez, 2014; Fritsche, 2015). It is reported that inflammation increases as the increased saturation rate of fatty acids, not only the total amount of fat in the diet (Calder & Grimble, 2002; Nergiz-Unal, 2016). Dietary high saturated fatty acids have been shown to activate the inflammatory response process through the toll-like receptor and in particular by TLR-4 and nuclear kappa B factor (NF-κB) pathways (Lee et al., 2003; Weigert et al., 2004; Bressan, Hermsdorff, Zulet, & Mart´ınez, 2009; Navarro et al., 2016). Similarly, studies in humans and laboratory animals have also shown similar inflammatory responses and increased pro-inflammatory cytokine levels. In a study, it was shown that saturated fatty acid content of diet was positively correlated with serum CRP level and every 1% decrease in energy from saturated fats caused 0.14 mg / L decrease in serum CRP level (Klein-Platat et al., 2005; Arya et al., 2006; Milanski et al., 2009).

High SFA uptake by diet in cell culture and animal studies has been shown to induce metabolic stress in organs and tissues, stimulating the production and release of pro-inflammatory markers (Enos et al., 2013; Enos et al., 2014; Suganami et al., 2007; Sui et al., 2016). In an in vitro cell culture study, SFA (0.5 mmol / L) applied to primary hepatocytes was found to activate NF-κB, stimulating nod-like receptor-3 (NLRP3) inflammasome and increasing IL-1β release (Sui et al., 2016). Similarly, in adipocyte and monocyte / macrophage cell culture studies, it was found that saturated fatty acids increased the release of TNF-α from inflammatory markers by activating the TLR-4 pathway by NF-κB activation (Suganami et al., 2007). In a similar study, it was shown that it stimulates endoplasmic reticulum stress with TLR-2 and TLR-4 in the hippocampus of diet-fed mice containing high saturated fatty acids (5% g / feed) for 8 weeks, and consequently stimulates the release of pro-inflammatory markers (Milanski et al. 2009).

When human studies were evaluated, it has been shown that the increase in SFA consumption in daily diet was associated with increased levels of plasma acute phase proteins (CRP, e-selectin, fibrinogen) and pro-inflammatory cytokines (TNF-α, IL-1β, IL-6) and endothelial damage markers (ICAM-1, VCAM-1) using epidemiological data. It was determined that consuming 8-12% of total energy intake from saturated fatty acids for 5 weeks in male subjects increased plasma CRP and IL-6 levels, but did not affect E-selectin and fibrinogen levels (King, Egan, & Geesey, 2003). In another human study, plasma pro-inflammatory and oxidative stress markers were not affected in overweight / obese individuals as a result of a diet containing high saturated fatty acids (25% energy) for 4 weeks (Marina et al., 2014).

Similarly, in a study of 54 obese individuals, it was reported that the diet rich in isocaloric saturated fatty acids did not increase IL-6 and IL-1β levels from pro-inflammatory cytokines (Teng, Chang, Vethakkan, Nesaretnam, & Sanders, 2017). In addition, it was reported that the diet given after the test meal containing high saturated fatty acids given to slightly obese / obese individuals (n = 11) acutely increased ICAM-1 levels but did not affect the levels of inflammatory markers (Peairs, Rankin, & Lee, 2011).

In conclusion, dietary high saturated fatty acids activate inflammatory processes in cell culture and animal studies, but studies on human organs or studies on their organs are quite limited.

TFA, whose consumption is increased with processed products similar to saturated fatty acids, can also cause an inflammatory response. A significant association between dietary trans fatty acids consumption and increased plasma pro-inflammatory cytokine (TNFR-2, IL-6), acute phase proteins (e-selectin, CRP) and cell adhesion molecules (sICAM-1, sVCAM-1) has been reported (Lopez-Garcia et al., 2005). Similarly, in an intervention study, it was found that inflammatory markers such as CRP, IL-6, fibrinogen were significantly increased in male individuals fed a diet containing high trans fatty acids (8% energy) for 5 weeks (Baer, Judd, Clevidence, & Tracy, 2004).

Mono Unsaturated Fatty Acids (MUFA)

Monounsaturated fatty acids are a nutrient that has positive effects on overall health and has positive effects on the replacement of saturated fatty acids in the diet (Hamley, 2017). The main sources of MUFA in the form of cis-containing single double bonds are olive oil and nuts such as almonds, walnuts and hazelnuts. MUFA, which meets 15-25% of daily energy intake in the Mediterranean diet, is a nutrient recommended to increase consumption in many national and international guidelines (Casas, Sacanella, & Estruch, 2014). Oleic acid (18: 1ω-9) forms the basic monounsaturated fatty acid in the diet (Calder, 2015).

When their role in chronic diseases is examined, the positive effects of dietary MUFA intake on cardiovascular diseases are emphasized. MUFA, which has positive effects on plasma lipid profile, prevents oxidized LDL formation and decreases LDL, total cholesterol and triglyceride levels (Lapointe, Couillard, & Lemieux, 2006; Hunter, Zhang, & Kris-Etherton, 2010).

Monounsaturated fatty acids have been shown to have positive effects on the release of pro-inflammatory cytokines. Studies have shown an inverse relationship between the consumption of MUFA and acute phase proteins such as plasma CRP, pro-inflammatory cytokines such as TNF-α, IL-1β, IL-6, and endothelial dysfunction markers such as VCAM-1 and ICAM-1 (Esposito et al., 2004; Fuentes et al., 2008; Mena et al., 2009). Two meta-analysis studies have shown that MUFA consumption reduces plasma TNF-α, IL-6 and VCAM-1 levels (Schwingshackl & Hoffmann, 2014; Schwingshackl, Christoph, & Hoffmann, 2015).

Poly Unsaturated Fatty Acids (PUFA)

Omega-3 fatty acid is a rich source of PUFA and acts in the body by converting into eicosapentaenoic acid (EPA) and docosahexaenoic acid (DHA). AHA recommends consuming approximately 220 g of fatty fish twice a week for adequate intake of omega-3 fatty acids. The anti-inflammatory effects of EPA and DHA have been shown to be achieved by reducing the levels of pro-inflammatory proteins such as CRP, TNF-α, IL-6 (Itariu et al., 2012; Kiecolt-Glaser et al., 2012). Lesn'a et al. (2013) found that CRP and IL-8 decreased after replacing a SFA-rich diet (42% of total caloric value) with a PUFA-rich diet (40%) in a three-week randomized crossover study.

There is an inverse relationship between dietary w-3 fatty acid content and markers of inflammation (Calder, 2006; Wall et al., 2010). The results of the MESA (Multi Ethnic Study of Atherosclerosis) study show that w-3 uptake is inversely related to serum IL-6 levels (He et al., 2009). In a study of 405 healthy men and 454 women, EPA and DHA intake from w-3 fatty acids were inversely related to serum TNF-α levels; however, high consumption of both w-3 and w-6 fatty acids were associated with lowering inflammation in the body (Pischon et al., 2003). In the ATTICA study, it was reported that those who consumed at least 300 g of fish per week had 33% lower serum CRP levels than those who did not consume any fish (Zampelas et al., 2005).

Fats, which have an important place in daily nutrition pattern, differ in terms of their chemical structure and dietary sources. Numerous studies aimed at investigating the relationship between fats and inflammation highlight the importance of this macronutrient in modulating several inflammatory biomarkers. Silver et al. (2014) investigated the effect of an hyperlipidemic diet (50% of TCV) with MUFA, PUFA and SFA (50% of TCV) on an equal basis, and reported a decrease in interleukin IL-1α, IL-1β, 1L-12 and IL-17, improved tumor necrosis factor-alpha (TNF-α) and tumor necrosis factor-beta (TNF-β) concentrations and vascular function after two weeks, as well as a 6% increase in fat oxidation, an average of 2.5 kg of body fat decrease, mean 2.5 kg lean mass increase and interferon gamma (IFN-c).

Alpha-linoleic acid from vegetable oils is converted to some degree omega-3 fatty acids during digestion and into longer and more unsaturated EPA and DHA

(Cleland, Gibson, Pedler, & James, 2005). The western diet generally contains too much saturated and trans fatty acids and does not contain enough omega-3 PUFA compared to omega-6 PUFA. High consumption of SFA and trans fatty acids increase the risk of cardiovascular disease by increasing total cholesterol and LDL levels (Stamler, Daviglus, Garside, Dyer, Greenland, & Neaton, 2000).

Greater consumption of omega-3 fatty acids appears to be effective in preventing and alleviating many inflammatory and autoimmune diseases (Simopoulos, 2002). With regard to linoleic acid, after an n-3 supplement with type-2 diabetics (EPA 1.548 mg / d; and others n-3 338 mg / d), for eight weeks, despite of maintaining CRP levels, it resulted in a decrease in IL-2 concentrations and TNF-α. (Malekshahi Moghadam, Saedisomeolia, Djalali, Djazayery, Pooya, & Sojoudi, 2012).

Rajkumar et al. (2014) reported an improvement in pro-inflammatory profile with CRP reduction in overweight patients after n-3 supplementation (EPA 180 mg / day and DHA 120 mg / day) for six weeks. Ito et al. (2014) observed the same effect in dyslipidemic individuals. Itariu et al. (2012), have confirmed a decrease in gene expression of subcutaneous adipose tissue, a decrease in gene expression, a decrease in IL-6 concentration, increased anti-inflammatory eicosanoids in visceral adipose tissue, after eight weeks of n-3 supplementation (EP-460 m /day and DHA 380 mg/d). In another study, the authors observed CRP reduction in men with coronary artery disease after eight weeks of n-3 supplementation (EPA 720 mg and DHA 480 mg) (Agh et al., 2017).

The beneficial mechanism of linoleic acid (n-3 series) is associated with EPA (C20: 5 n-3) and DHA (22: 6 n-3), derivatives of linoleic acid, which have more anti-inflammatory effect than derivatives of arachidonic acid (ARA n-6 PUFA) derived from linoleic acid. Such an effect has been reported in an adult study.

After four months of supplementation (1.4 g/d) there was no increase in ARA metabolites, but an increase in EPA and DHA formation was reported compared to the placebo group (soybean oil)(Cipollina, Salvatore, Muldoon, Freeman, & Scarbohydratespfer, 2014). Therefore, the reduction in inflammation was due to the synthesis of anti-inflammatory metabolites rather than suppression of pro-inflammatory metabolites derived from ARA.

Pro-inflammatory eicosanoids and endocannabinoids formed by increased ARA metabolism due to high LA intake in the diet were found to be associated with the risk of inflammation and the development of certain diseases (Chilton et al., 2014).

It has evidence that 12S-HETE, formed by 12S-LOX and 15-LOX-1 enzyme-catalyzed reactions and known pro-inflammatory and proapoptotic effects, have effects on diabetes. 12S-HETE inhibits insulin secretion in response to glucose, such as cytokines, and induce NAPH oxidase-1 (NOX-1) enzyme, causing damage to pancreatic islet cells. The NOX-1 enzyme allows the formation of reactive oxygen molecules and reduces glucose-stimulated insulin secretion. This effect of 12S-HETE can be blocked by 12S-LOX inhibitors. In addition, a study showed that adipose tissue inflammation and insulin resistance decreased in 15-LOX-1 suppressed mice fed high fat diet (Powell & Rokach, 2014).

ARA metabolites play an active role in the inflammation process. Studies have shown that leukotrienes, one of the metabolites of ARA, contribute to the development of symptoms in inflammatory diseases and also have a possible role in the formation of these diseases (Radmark, Werz, Steinhilber, & Samuelsson, 2014). Among the mediators involved in the pathogenesis of many inflammatory diseases (inflammatory bowel disease, rheumatoid arthritis, psoriasis, atopic dermatitis, etc.), the various products of the COX and LOX pathways of ARA metabolism (PGE2, LTB4, LTC4, 12-HETE, 15-HETE, TXA2, TXB2 and platelet-activating factor), and there are significant increases in their levels, and there is a positive correlation between the level of these mediators and the severity of inflammation (Oktar & Alican, 2000; Aksoy, Şentürk, Cantürk, & Turanlı, 2001; Wisastra & Dekker, 2014).

Adjusting the ratio of SFA, MUFA and PUFA in diet seems to be a more effective strategy than the use of hypolipidemic diets that may have adverse effects on the modulation of inflammation. In addition, higher SFA consumption is related to the increase in inflammatory biomarkers, which is proportional to the amount taken. Therefore, selecting MUFA and PUFA-rich foods and avoiding foods with high SFA content may be beneficial in modulating inflammation and reducing the associated risk of disease.

CONCLUSION

The emergence of chronic diseases, prognosis and the course of acute and chronic complications due to chronic disease are affected by the inflammation status of the organism. This pro-inflammatory response is characterized by a low degree of inflammation that has different characterization from a classical inflammation process and cannot be resolved for a long time.

According to many national and international health guidelines, a healthy and balanced diet pattern is one of the leading modifiable risk factors for the protection of individuals from chronic diseases. Macro and micronutrients of the diet in terms of adequate and balanced, short and long term prevention of chronic diseases, has positive effects on the onset and prognosis.

As a result, carbohydrates, fats and proteins, which are the leading macro nutrients, play an important role in the inflammatory response of the individual according to their daily intake levels, sources and types. Although the diet is rich in complex carbohydrate, pulp, MUFA, PUFA, the reduction of SFA, TFA, simple sugar and processed carbohydrates can lead to positive effects on inflammatory pathways and prevent chronic diseases in the long term.

REFERENCES

Aeberli, I., Gerber, P. A., Hochuli, M., Kohler, S., Haile, S. R., Gouni-Berthold, I., ... Berneis, K. (2011). Low to moderate sugar-sweetened beverage consumption impairs glucose and lipid metabolism and promotes inflammation in healthy young men: A randomized controlled trial. *The American Journal of Clinical Nutrition*, *94*(2), 479–485. doi:10.3945/ajcn.111.013540 PMID:21677052

Agh, F., Mohammadzadeh Honarvar, N., Djalali, M., Nematipour, E., Gholamhoseini, S., Zarei, M., ... Javanbakht, M. H. (2017). Omega-3 fatty acid could increase one of myokines in male patients with coronary artery Disease: A randomized, doubleblind, placebo-controlled trial. *Archives of Iranian Medicine*, *20*(1), 28–33. PMID:28112528

Akbulut, G., Eşingen, S. Ü., Bingöl, F. N., & Bayraktar, A. (2013). Diabetes mellitus'un tıbbi beslenme tedavisine farklı bir bakış: Glisemik indeks mi, glisemik yük mü daha etkindir? *Bozok Tıp Dergisi*, *3*(2), 42–43.

Aksoy, L., Şentürk, N., Cantürk, T., & Turanlı, A. Y. (2001). Deri Hastalıklarında Lökotrienlerin Rolü. *Türkderm*, *35*, 337–340.

Aksoy, M. (2016). *Beslenme Biyokimyası. 5* (pp. 59–62). Ankara: Baskı. Hatipoğlu Yayınevi.

Alberti, K.G., Eckel, R.H., Grundy, S.M., Zimmet, P.Z., Cleeman, J.I., Donato, K.A., ... Smith, S.C. Jr. (2003). Harmonizing the metabolic syndrome: a joint interim statement of the international diabetes federation task force on epidemiology and prevention; national heart, lung, and blood Institute; American heart association; World heart federation; international atherosclerosis society; and international association for the study of obesity. *Circulation, 20*(16), 1640-1645.

Alemany, M. (2013). Relationship between energy dense diets and white adipose tissue inflammation in metabolic syndrome. *Nutrition Research*, *33*(1), 1–11. doi:10.1016/j.nutres.2012.11.013 PMID:23351404

Andersen, C. J., & Fernandez, M. L. (2013). Dietary strategies to reduce metabolic syndrome. *Reviews in Endocrine & Metabolic Disorders*, *14*(3), 241–254. doi:10.100711154-013-9251-y PMID:23943309

Anderson, J. W., Baird, P., Davis, R. H. Jr, Ferreri, S., Knudtson, M., Koraym, A., ... Williams, C. L. (2009). Health benefits of dietary fiber. *Nutrition Reviews*, *67*(4), 188–205. doi:10.1111/j.1753-4887.2009.00189.x PMID:19335713

Angelopoulos, T. J., Lowndes, J., Sinnett, S., & Rippe, J. M. (2016). Fructose Containing Sugars at Normal Levels of Consumption Do Not Effect Adversely Components of the Metabolic Syndrome and Risk Factors for Cardiovascular Disease. *Nutrients*, *8*(4), 179. doi:10.3390/nu8040179 PMID:27023594

Arya, S., Isharwal, S., Misra, A., Pandey, R. M., Rastogi, K., Vikram, N. K., ... Sharma, R. (2006). C-reactive protein and dietary nutrients in urban Asian Indian adolescents and young adults. *Nutrition (Burbank, Los Angeles County, Calif.)*, *22*(9), 865–871. doi:10.1016/j.nut.2006.05.002 PMID:16829027

Augustin, L. S., Kendall, C. W., Jenkins, D. J., Willett, W. C., Astrup, A., Barclay, A. W., ... Poli, A. (2015). Glycemic index, glycemic load and glycemic response: An International Scientific Consensus Summit from the International Carbohydrate Quality Consortium (ICQC). *Nutrition, Metabolism, and Cardiovascular Diseases*, *25*(9), 795–815. doi:10.1016/j.numecd.2015.05.005 PMID:26160327

Azadbakht, L., Atabak, S., & Esmaillzadeh, A. (2008). Soy protein intake, cardiorenal indices, and C-reactive protein in type 2 diabetes with nephropathy. *Diabetes Care*, *31*(4), 648–654. doi:10.2337/dc07-2065 PMID:18184902

Azadbakht, L., & Esmaillzadeh, A. (2009). Red meat intake is associated with metabolic syndrome and the plasma C-reactive protein concentration in women. *The Journal of Nutrition*, *139*(2), 335–339. doi:10.3945/jn.108.096297 PMID:19074209

B'edard, A., Lamarche, B., Corneau, L., Dodin, S., & Lemieux, S. (2015). Sex differences in the impact of the Mediterranean diet on systemic inflammation. *Nutrition Journal*, *14*(1), 46. doi:10.118612937-015-0035-y PMID:25962728

Baena, M., Sanguesa, G., Hutter, N., Sanchez, R. M., Roglans, N., Laguna, J. C., & Alegret, R. (2015). Fructose supplementation impairs rat liver autophagy through mTORC activation without inducing endoplasmic reticulum stress. *Biochimica et Biophysica Acta*, *1851*(2), 107–116. doi:10.1016/j.bbalip.2014.11.003 PMID:25463011

Baer, D. J., Judd, J. T., Clevidence, B. A., & Tracy, R. P. (2004). Dietary fatty acids affect plasma markers of inflammation in healthy men fed controlled diets: A randomized crossover study. *The American Journal of Clinical Nutrition*, *79*(6), 969–973. doi:10.1093/ajcn/79.6.969 PMID:15159225

Barbaresko, J., Koch, M., Schulze, M. B., & Nöthlings, U. (2013). Dietary pattern analysis and biomarkers of low-grade inflammation: A systematic literature review. *Nutrition Reviews*, *71*(8), 511–527. doi:10.1111/nure.12035 PMID:23865797

Bastard, J. P., Maachi, M., Lagathu, C., Kim, M. J., Caron, M., Vidal, H., ... Feve, B. (2006). Recent advances in the relationship between obesity, inflammation, and insulin resistance. *European Cytokine Network*, *17*(1), 4–12. PMID:16613757

Bawaked, R. A., Schroder, H., Ribas-Barba, L., Izquierdo-Pulido, M., Perez-Rodrigo, C., Fito, M., & Serra-Majem, L. (2017). Association of diet quality with dietary inflammatory potential in youth. *Food & Nutrition Research*, *61*(1), 1328961. doi:10.1080/16546628.2017.1328961 PMID:28659737

Baysal, A. (2012). *Beslenme*. Ankara: Hatiboğlu Yayıncılık.

Bhathena, S. J., & Velasquez, M. T. (2002). Beneficial role of dietary phytoestrogens in obesity and diabetes. *The American Journal of Clinical Nutrition*, *76*(6), 1191–1201. doi:10.1093/ajcn/76.6.1191 PMID:12450882

Bouche, C., Rizkalla, S. W., Luo, J., Vidal, H., Veronese, A., Pacher, N., ... Slama, G. (2002). Five week, long glycemic index diet decreases total fat mass and improves plasma lipid profile in moderately overweight nondiabetic men. *Diabetes Care*, *25*(5), 822–828. doi:10.2337/diacare.25.5.822 PMID:11978675

Bressan, J., & Hermsdorff, H. H. M. (2008). *Obesity epidemic, the cause, the treatment.* In E. A. M. Moreira & P. G. Chiarello (Eds.), *Atenção Nutricional: Abordagem dietoter'apica em adulto* (pp. 75–97). Guanabara Koogan, Rio de Janeiro, Brazil.

Bressan, J., Hermsdorff, H. H. M., Zulet, M. A., & Mart'ınez, J. A. (2009). Hormonal and inflammatory impact of different dietetic composition: Emphasis on dietary patterns and specific dietary factors. *Arquivos Brasileiros de Endocrinologia & Metabologia*, *53*(5), 572–581. doi:10.1590/S0004-27302009000500010 PMID:19768248

Calder, P. C. (2006). Polyunsaturated fatty acids and inflammation. *Prostaglandins, Leukotrienes, and Essential Fatty Acids*, *75*(3), 197–202. doi:10.1016/j.plefa.2006.05.012 PMID:16828270

Calder, P. C. (2015). Functional roles of fatty acids and their effects on human health. *JPEN. Journal of Parenteral and Enteral Nutrition*, *39*(1), 18–32. doi:10.1177/0148607115595980 PMID:26177664

Calder, P. C., Ahluwalia, N., Albers, R., Bosco, N., Bourdet-Sicard, R., Haller, D., ... Zhao, J. (2013). A consideration of biomarkers to be used for evaluation of inflammation in human nutritional studies. *British Journal of Nutrition*, *109*(S1), S1–S34. doi:10.1017/S0007114512005119 PMID:23343744

Calder, P. C., Ahluwalia, N., Brouns, F., Buetler, T., Clement, K., Cunningham, K., ... Winklhofer-Roob, B. M. (2011). Dietary factors and low-grade inflammation in relation to overweight and obesity. *BJN, 106*(3), 1–78. PMID:22133051

Calder, P. C., & Grimble, R. F. (2002). Polyunsaturated fatty acids, inflammation and immunity. *European Journal of Clinical Nutrition, 56*(3), 14–19. doi:10.1038j.ejcn.1601478 PMID:12142955

Campbell, B., Kreider, R. B., Ziegenfuss, T., La Bounty, P., Roberts, M., Burke, D., ... Antonio, J. (2007). International Society of Sports Nutrition position stand: Protein and exercise. *Journal of the International Society of Sports Nutrition, 26*(1), 8. doi:10.1186/1550-2783-4-8 PMID:17908291

Carrera-Bastos, P., Fontes, O. & Lindeberg, C. (2011). The western diet and lifestyle and diseases of civilization. *Research Reports in Clinical Cardiology, 15.*

Casas, R., Sacanella, E., & Estruch, R. (2014). The immune protective effect of the Mediterranean diet against chronic low-grade inflammatory diseases. *Endocrine, Metabolic & Immune Disorders Drug Targets, 14*(4), 245–254. doi:10.2174/1871530314666140922153350 PMID:25244229

Chen, J. P., Chen, G. C., Wang, X. P., Qin, L., & Bai, Y. (2018). Dietary Fiber and Metabolic Syndrome: A Meta-Analysis and Review of Related Mechanisms. *Nutrients, 10*(1), 24. doi:10.3390/nu10010024 PMID:29278406

Chilton, F. H., Murphy, R. C., Wilson, B. A., Sergeant, S., Ainsworth, H., Seeds, M., & Mathias, R. A. (2014). Diet-Gene Interactions and PUFA Metabolism: A Potential Contributor to Health Disparities and Human Diseases. *Nutrients, 6*(5), 1993–2022. doi:10.3390/nu6051993 PMID:24853887

Chuang, S. C., Vermeulen, R., Sharabiani, M. T., Sacerdote, C., Saberi Hosnijeh, F., Berrino, F., ... Vineis, P. (2011). The intake of grain fibers modulates cytokine levels in blood. *Biomarkers, 16*(6), 504–510. doi:10.3109/1354750X.2011.599042 PMID:21812595

Cipollina, C., Salvatore, S. R., Muldoon, M. F., Freeman, B. A., & Scarbohydratespfer, F. J. (2014). Generation and dietary modulation of anti-inflammatory electrophilic omega-3 fatty acid derivatives. *PLoS One, 9*(4), e94836. doi:10.1371/journal.pone.0094836 PMID:24736647

Cleland, L. G., Gibson, R. A., Pedler, J., & James, M. J. (2005). Paradoxical effect of n-3-containing vegetable oils on long-chain n-3 fatty acids in rat heart. *Lipids, 40*(10), 995–998. doi:10.100711745-005-1461-6 PMID:16382570

Cordain, L., Eaton, S. B., Brand Miller, J., Mann, N., & Hill, K. (2002). The paradoxical nature of hunter-gatherer diets: Meat based, yet non-atherogenic. *European Journal of Clinical Nutrition*, *56*(S1), 42–52. doi:10.1038j.ejcn.1601353 PMID:11965522

Cordain, L., Eaton, S. B., Sebastian, A., Mann, N., Lindeberg, S., Watkins, B. A., ... Brand-Miller, J. (2005). Origins and evolution of the Western diet: Health implications for the 21st century. *The American Journal of Clinical Nutrition*, *81*(2), 341–354. doi:10.1093/ajcn.81.2.341 PMID:15699220

Corley, J., Kyle, J. A. M., Starr, J. M., McNeill, G., & Deary, I. J. (2015). Dietary factors and biomarkers of systemic inflammation in older people: The Lothian Birth Cohort 1936. *British Journal of Nutrition*, *114*(7), 1088–1098. doi:10.1017/S000711451500210X PMID:26343358

Dandona, P., Chaudhuri, A., Ghanim, H., & Mohanty, P. (2007). Pro-inflammatory effects of glucose and anti-inflammatory effect of insulin: Relevance to cardiovascular disease. *The American Journal of Cardiology*, *99*(4), 15–26. doi:10.1016/j.amjcard.2006.11.003

Du, H., van der A, D. L., van Bakel, M. M. E., van der Kallen, C. J. H., Blaak, E. E., van Greevenbroek, M. M. J., ... Feskens, E. J. M. (2008). Glycemic index and glycemic load in relation to food and nutrient intake and metabolic risk factors in a Dutch population. *The American Journal of Clinical Nutrition*, *87*(3), 655–661. doi:10.1093/ajcn/87.3.655 PMID:18326604

Duffey, K. J., & Popkin, B. M. (2008). High-fructose corn syrup: Is this what's for dinner? *The American Journal of Clinical Nutrition*, *88*(6), 1722–1732. doi:10.3945/ajcn.2008.25825C PMID:19064537

Duncan, B. B., Schmidt, M. I., Pankow, J. S., Ballantyne, C. M., Couper, D., Vigo, A., ... Heiss, G. (2003). Low-grade systemic inflammation and the development of type 2 diabetes: The atherosclerosis risk in communities study. *Diabetes*, *52*(7), 1799–1805. doi:10.2337/diabetes.52.7.1799 PMID:12829649

Lesna, I. K., Suchanek, P., Brabcova, E., Kovar, J., Malinska, H., & Poledne, R. (2013). Effect of different types of dietary fatty acids on subclinical inflammation in humans. *Physiological Research*, *62*(2), 145–152. PMID:23234408

Elenkov, I. J., & Chrousos, G. P. (2012). Stress hormones, proinflammatory and anti-inflammatory cytokines, and autoimmunity. *Annals of the New York Academy of Sciences*, *966*(1), 290–303. doi:10.1111/j.1749-6632.2002.tb04229.x PMID:12114286

Enos, R. T., Davis, J. M., Velazquez, K. T., McClellan, J. L., Day, S. D., Carnevale, K. A., & Murphy, E. A. (2013). Influence of dietary saturated fat content on adiposity, macrophage behavior, inflammation, and metabolism: Composition matters. *Journal of Lipid Research*, *54*(1), 152–163. doi:10.1194/jlr.M030700 PMID:23103474

Enos, R. T., Velazquez, K. T., & Murphy, E. A. (2014). Insight into the impact of dietary saturated fat on tissue-specific cellular processes underlying obesity-related diseases. *The Journal of Nutritional Biochemistry*, *25*(6), 600–612. doi:10.1016/j.jnutbio.2014.01.011 PMID:24742471

Esmaillzadeh, A., Kimiagar, M., Mehrabi, Y., Azadbakht, L., Hu, F. B., & Willett, W. C. (2007). Dietary patterns and markers of systemic inflammation among Iranian women. *The Journal of Nutrition*, *137*(4), 992–998. doi:10.1093/jn/137.4.992 PMID:17374666

Esposito, K., Marfella, R., Ciotola, M., Di Palo, C., Giugliano, F., Giugliano, G., ... Giugliano, D. (2004). Effect of a mediterranean-style diet on endothelial dysfunction and markers of vascular inflammation in the metabolic syndrome: A randomized trial. *Journal of the American Medical Association*, *292*(12), 1440–1446. doi:10.1001/jama.292.12.1440 PMID:15383514

Esposito, K., Nappo, F., Giugliano, F., Di Palo, C., Ciotola, M., Barbieri, M., ... Giugliano, D. (2003). Meal modulation of circulating interleukin 18 and adiponectin concentrations in healthy subjects and in patients with type 2 diabetes mellitus. *The AJCN*, *78*(6), 1135–1140. PMID:14668275

Esposito, K., Nappo, F., Marfella, R., Giugliano, G., Giugliano, F., Ciotola, M., ... Giugliano, D. (2002). Inflammation cytokine concentrations are acutely increased by hyperglycemia in humans: Role of oxidative stress. *Circulation*, *106*, 2067–2072. doi:10.1161/01.CIR.0000034509.14906.AE PMID:12379575

Estévez, M., & Luna, C. (2017). Dietary protein oxidation: A silent threat to human health? *Critical Reviews in Food Science and Nutrition*, *57*(17), 3781–3793. doi:10.1080/10408398.2016.1165182 PMID:27128327

Forshee, R. A., Storey, M. L., Allison, D. B., Glinsmann, W. H., Hein, G. L., Lineback, D. R., ... White, J. S. (2007). A critical examination of the evidence relating high fructose corn syrup and weight gain. *Critical Reviews in Food Science and Nutrition*, *47*(6), 561–582. doi:10.1080/10408390600846457 PMID:17653981

Foster-Powell, K., Holt, S. H., & Brand-Miller, J. C. (2002). International table of glycemic index and glycemic load values: 2002. *The AJCN*, *76*(1), 5–56. PMID:12081815

Fuentes, F., Lopez-Miranda, J., Perez-Martinez, P., Jimenez, Y., Marin, C., Gomez, P., ... Pėrez-Jimėnez, F. (2008). Chronic effects of a high-fat diet enriched with virgin olive oil and a low-fat diet enriched with alpha-linolenic acid on postprandial endothelial function in healthy men. *British Journal of Nutrition*, *100*(1), 159–165. doi:10.1017/S0007114508888708 PMID:18275619

Galland, L. (2010). Diet and Inflammation. *Nutrition in Clinical Practice*, *25*(6), 634–640. doi:10.1177/0884533610385703 PMID:21139128

Giugliano, D., Ceriello, A. & Esposito, K. (2006). The effects of diet on inflammation: emphasis on the metabolic syndrome. *J Am Coll Cardiol, 15*(4), 677-685.

Göğebakan, O., Kohl, A., Osterhoff, M. A., Van Baak, M. A., Jebb, S. A., Papadaki, A., ... Pfeiffer, A. F. (2011). Effects of weight loss and long-term weight maintenance with diets varying in protein and glycemic index on cardiovascular risk factors: The diet, obesity, and genes (DiOGenes) study: A randomized, controlled trial. *Circulation*, *124*(25), 2829–2838. doi:10.1161/CIRCULATIONAHA.111.033274 PMID:22104550

Göktaş, Z. (2016). Pro- ve anti-inflamatuar etkili besinler ve immün sistem. *Türkiye Klinikleri J Nutr Diet-Special Topics, 2*(2).

Goletzke, J., Buyken, A. E., Joslowski, G., Joslowski, G., Bolzenius, K., Remer, T., ... Herder, C. (2014). Increased intake of carbohydrates from sources with a higher glycemic index and lower consumption of whole grains during puberty are prospectively associated with higher IL-6 concentrations in younger adulthood among healthy individuals. *The Journal of Nutrition*, *144*(10), 1586–1593. doi:10.3945/jn.114.193391 PMID:25080538

Hamley, S. (2017). The effect of replacing saturated fat with mostly n-6 polyunsaturated fat on coronary heart disease: A meta-analysis of randomised controlled trials. *Nutrition Journal*, *16*(1), 30. doi:10.118612937-017-0254-5 PMID:28526025

Harvey, R. A. P. D. (2011). *Lippincott's illustrated reviews: Biochemistry* (5th ed.). Philadelphia: Wolters Kluwer Health.

He, K., Liu, K., Daviglus, M. L., Jenny, N. S., Mayer-Davis, E., Jiang, R., ... Herrington, D. (2009). Associations of dietary long-chain n-3 polyunsaturated fatty acids and fish with biomarkers of inflammation and endothelial activation (from the Multi-Ethnic Study of Atherosclerosis [MESA]). *The American Journal of Cardiology*, *103*(9), 1238–1243. doi:10.1016/j.amjcard.2009.01.016 PMID:19406265

Heber, D., & Henning, S. (2014). Biomarkers of Inflammation and the Western Diet. In B. B. Aggarwal (Ed.), *Immunonutrition Interactions of Diet, Genetics, and Inflammation: Taylor & Francis Group*. doi:10.1201/b16661-5

Heggen, E., Klemsdal, T. O., Haugen, F., Holme, I., & Tonstad, S. (2012). Effect of a low fat versus a low glycemic load diet on inflammatory biomarker and adipokine concentrations. *Metabolic Syndrome and Related Disorders*, *10*(6), 437–442. doi:10.1089/met.2012.0012 PMID:22889406

Hodgson, J. M., Burke, V., Beilin, L. J., & Puddey, I. B. (2006). Partial substitution of carbohydrate intake with protein intake from lean red meat lowers blood pressure in hypertensive persons. *The American Journal of Clinical Nutrition*, *83*(4), 780–787. doi:10.1093/ajcn/83.4.780 PMID:16600928

Howarth, N. C., Saltzman, E., & Roberts, S. B. (2001). Dietary fiber and weight regulation. *Nutrition Reviews*, *59*(5), 129–139. doi:10.1111/j.1753-4887.2001.tb07001.x PMID:11396693

Huang, C. J., Zourdos, M. C., Jo, E., & Ormsbee, M. J. (2013). Influence of Physical Activity and Nutrition on Obesity - Related Immune Function. *The Scientific World Journal*. PMID:24324381

Hunt, J. R., Johnson, L. K., & Fariba Roughead, Z. K. (2009). Dietary protein and calcium interact to influence calcium retention: A controlled feeding study. *The American Journal of Clinical Nutrition*, *89*(5), 1357–1365. doi:10.3945/ajcn.2008.27238 PMID:19279077

Hunter, J. E., Zhang, J., & Kris-Etherton, P. M. (2010). Cardiovascular disease risk of dietary stearic acid compared with trans, other saturated, and unsaturated fatty acids: A systematic review. *The American Journal of Clinical Nutrition*, *91*(1), 46–63. doi:10.3945/ajcn.2009.27661 PMID:19939984

Innis, S. M. (2007). Dietary lipids in early development: Relevance to obesity, immune and inflammatory disorders. *Current Opinion in Endocrinology, Diabetes, and Obesity*, *14*(5), 359–364. doi:10.1097/MED.0b013e3282be90b9 PMID:17940463

Itariu, B. K., Zeyda, M., Hochbrugger, E. E., Neuhofer, A., Prager, G., Schindler, K., ... Stulnig, T. M. (2012). Long-chain n-3 PUFAs reduce adipose tissue and systemic inflammation in severely obese nondiabetic patients: A randomized controlled trial. *The American Journal of Clinical Nutrition*, *96*(5), 1137–1149. doi:10.3945/ajcn.112.037432 PMID:23034965

Ito, R., Satoh-Asahara, N., Yamakage, H., Sasaki, Y., Odori, S., Kono, S., ... Shimatsu, A. (2014). An increase in the EPA/AA ratio is associated with improved arterial stiffness in obese patients with dyslipidemia. *Journal of Atherosclerosis and Frombosis*, *21*(3), 248–260. doi:10.5551/jat.19976 PMID:24270918

Jaacks, L. M., Crandell, J., Liese, A. D., Lamichhane, A. P., Bell, R. A., Dabelea, D., ... Mayer-Davis, E. J. (2014). No association of dietary fiber intake with inflammation or arterial stiffness in youth with type 1 diabetes. *Journal of Diabetes and Its Complications*, *28*(3), 305–310. doi:10.1016/j.jdiacomp.2014.01.005 PMID:24613131

Jenkins, D. J., Wolever, T. M., Taylor, R. H., Barker, H., Fielden, H., Baldwin, J. M., ... Goff, D. V. (1981). Glycemic index of foods: A physiological basis for carbohydrate exchange. *The American Journal of Clinical Nutrition*, *34*(3), 362–366. doi:10.1093/ajcn/34.3.362 PMID:6259925

Jensen, M. K., Koh-Banerjee, P., Franz, M., Sampson, L., Grønbæk, M., & Rimm, E. B. (2006). Whole grains, bran, and germ in relation to homocysteine and markers of glycemic control, lipids, and inflammation. *The AJCN*, *83*(2), 275–283. PMID:16469984

Johansson-Persson, A., Ulmius, M., Cloetens, L., Karhu, T., Herzig, K. H., & Onning, G. (2014). A high intake of dietary fiber influences C-reactive protein and fibrinogen, but not glucose and lipid metabolism, in mildly hypercholesterolemic subjects. *European Journal of Nutrition*, *53*(1), 39–48. doi:10.100700394-013-0496-8 PMID:23389112

Joslowski, G., Halim, J., Goletzke, J., Gow, M., Ho, M., Louie, J. C. Y., ... Garnett, S. P. (2015). Dietary glycemic load, insulin load, and weight loss in obese, insulin resistant adolescents. *RESIST Study Clin Nutr*, *34*(1), 89–94. doi:10.1016/j.clnu.2014.01.015 PMID:24534012

Kaptoge, S., Seshasai, S. R., Gao, P., Freitag, D. F., Butterworth, A. S., Borglykke, A., ... Danesh, J. (2014). Inflammatory cytokines and risk of coronary heart disease: New prospective study and updated meta-analysis. *European Heart Journal*, *35*(9), 578–589. doi:10.1093/eurheartj/eht367 PMID:24026779

Khayyatzadeha, S. S., Kazemi-Bajestanic, S. M. R., Bagherniyaa, M., Mehramiza, M., Tayefie, M., Ebrahimic, M., ... Ghayour-Mobarhan, M. (2017). Serum high C reactive protein concentrations are related to the intake ofdietary macronutrients and fiber: Findings from a large representative Persian population sample. *Clinical Biochemistry*, *50*(13-14), 750–755. doi:10.1016/j.clinbiochem.2017.03.016 PMID:28336391

Kiecolt-Glaser, J. K., Belury, M. A., Andridge, R., Malarkey, W. B., Hwang, B. S., & Glaser, R. (2012). Omega3 supplementation lowers inflammation in healthy middle-aged and older adults: A randomized controlled trial. *Brain, Behavior, and Immunity*, *26*(6), 988–995. doi:10.1016/j.bbi.2012.05.011 PMID:22640930

King, D. E., Egan, B. M., & Geesey, M. E. (2003). Relation of dietary fat and fiber to elevation of C-reactive protein. *The American Journal of Cardiology*, *92*(11), 1335–1339. doi:10.1016/j.amjcard.2003.08.020 PMID:14636916

Klein-Platat, C., Drai, J., Oujaa, M., Schlienger, J. L. C. S., & Simon, C. (2005). Plasma fatty acid composition is associated with the metabolic syndrome and low-grade inflammation in overweight adolescents. *The American Journal of Clinical Nutrition*, *82*(6), 1178–1184. doi:10.1093/ajcn/82.6.1178 PMID:16332649

Kris-Etherton, P. M., Harris, W. S., & Appel, L. J. (2002). Fish consumption, fish oil, omega-3 fatty acids, and cardiovascular disease. *Circulation*, *106*(21), 2747–2757. doi:10.1161/01.CIR.0000038493.65177.94 PMID:12438303

Lapointe, A., Couillard, C., & Lemieux, S. (2006). Effects of dietary factors on oxidation of low-density lipoprotein particles. *The Journal of Nutritional Biochemistry*, *17*(10), 645–658. doi:10.1016/j.jnutbio.2006.01.001 PMID:16517144

Larsen, T. M., Dalskov, S. M., van Baak, M., Jebb, S. A., Papadaki, A., Pfeiffer, A. F., ... Astrup, A. (2010). Diet, Obesity, and Genes (Diogenes) Project.: Diets with high or low protein content and glycemic index for weight-loss maintenance. *The New England Journal of Medicine*, *363*(22), 2102–2113. doi:10.1056/NEJMoa1007137 PMID:21105792

Lee, J. H. (2013). Polyunsaturated Fatty acids in children. *Pediatric Gastroenterology, Hepatology & Nutrition*, *16*(3), 153–161. doi:10.5223/pghn.2013.16.3.153 PMID:24224148

Lee, J. Y., Plakidas, A., Lee, W. H., Heikkinen, A., Chanmugam, P., Bray, G., & Hwang, D. H. (2003). Differential modulation of Toll-like receptors by fatty acids: Preferential inhibition by n-3 polyunsaturated fatty acids. *Journal of Lipid Research*, *44*(3), 479–486. doi:10.1194/jlr.M200361-JLR200 PMID:12562875

Leon-Pedroza, J. I., Gonzalez-Tapia, L. A., del Olmo-Gil, E., Castellanos-Rodriguez, D., Escobedo, G., & Gonzalez-Chavez, A. (2015). Low-grade systemic inflammation and the development of metabolic diseases: From the molecular evidence to the clinical practice. *Cirugia y Cirujanos*, *83*(6), 543–551. doi:10.1016/j.circen.2015.11.008 PMID:26159364

Levitan, E. B., Cook, N. R., Stampfer, M. J., Ridker, P. M., Rexrode, K. M., Buring, J. E., ... Liu, S. (2008). Dietary glycemic index, dietary glycemic load, blood lipids, and C-reactive protein. *Metabolism: Clinical and Experimental, 57*(3), 437–443. doi:10.1016/j.metabol.2007.11.002 PMID:18249220

Libby, P. (2007). Inflammatory Mechanisms: The molecular basis of inflammation and disease. *Nutrition Reviews, 65*(12), 140–146. doi:10.1301/nr.2007.dec.S140-S146 PMID:18240538

Liese, A. D., Roach, A. K., Sparks, K. C., Marquart, L., D'Agostino, R. B. Jr, & Mayer-Davis, E. J. (2003). Whole-grain intake and insulin sensitivity: The Insulin Resistance Atherosclerosis Study. *The AJCN, 78*(5), 965–971. PMID:14594783

Liu, S., Manson, J. E., Buring, J. E., Stampfer, M. J., Willett, W. C., & Ridker, P. M. (2002). Relation between a diet with a high glycemic load and plasma concentrations of high-sensitivity C-reactive protein in middle-aged women. *The American Journal of Clinical Nutrition, 75*(3), 492–498. doi:10.1093/ajcn/75.3.492 PMID:11864854

Lopez-Garcia, E., Schulze, M. B., Fung, T. T., Meigs, J. B., Rifai, N., Manson, J. E., & Hu, F. B. (2004). Major dietary patterns are related to plasma concentrations of markers of inflammation and endothelial dysfunction. *AJCN, 80*(4), 1029–1035. PMID:15447916

Lopez-Garcia, E., Schulze, M. B., Meigs, J. B., Manson, J. E., Rifai, N., Stampfer, M. J., ... Hu, F. B. (2005). Consumption of trans fatty acids is related to plasma biomarkers of inflammation and endothelial dysfunction. *The Journal of Nutrition, 135*(3), 562–566. doi:10.1093/jn/135.3.562 PMID:15735094

Ma, Y., Griffith, J. A., Chasan-Taber, L., Olendzki, B. C., Jackson, E., Stanek, E. J., ... Ockene, I. S. (2006). Association between dietary fiber and serum C-reactive protein. *The AJCN, 83*(4), 760–766. PMID:16600925

Ma, Y., Hébert, J. R., Li, W., Bertone-Johnson, E. R., Olendzki, B., Pagoto, S. L., ... Liu, S. (2008). Association between dietary fiber and markers of systemic inflammation in the Women's Health Initiative Observational Study. *Nutrition (Burbank, Los Angeles County, Calif.), 24*(10), 941–949. doi:10.1016/j.nut.2008.04.005 PMID:18562168

Makarem, N., Bandera, E. V., Nicholson, J. M., & Parekh, N. (2018). Consumption of sugars, sugary foods, and sugary beverages in relation to cancer risk: A systematic review of longitudinal studies. *Annual Review of Nutrition, 38*(1), 17–39. doi:10.1146/annurev-nutr-082117-051805 PMID:29801420

Malekshahi Moghadam, A., Saedisomeolia, A., Djalali, M., Djazayery, A., Pooya, S., & Sojoudi, F. (2012). Efficacy of omega-3 fatty acid supplementation on serum levels of tumour necrosis factor-alpha, C-reactive protein and interleukin-2 in type 2 diabetes mellitus patients. *Singapore Medical Journal, 53*(9), 615–619. PMID:23023905

Malik, V. S., & Hu, F. B. (2015). Fructose and Cardiometabolic Health: What the Evidence From Sugar-Sweetened Beverages Tells Us. *Journal of the American College of Cardiology, 66*(14), 1615–1624. doi:10.1016/j.jacc.2015.08.025 PMID:26429086

Margioris, A. N. (2009). Fatty acids and postprandial inflammation. *Current Opinion in Clinical Nutrition and Metabolic Care, 12*(2), 129–137. doi:10.1097/MCO.0b013e3283232a11 PMID:19202384

Marina, A., von Frankenberg, A. D., Suvag, S., Callahan, H. S., Kratz, M., Richards, T. L., & Utzschneider, K. M. (2014). Effects of dietary fat and saturated fat content on liver fat and markers of oxidative stress in overweight/obese men and women under weight-stable conditions. *Nutrients, 6*(11), 4678–4690. doi:10.3390/nu6114678 PMID:25353663

McKeown, N. M., Meigs, J. B., Liu, S., Wilson, P. W., & Jacques, P. F. (2002). Whole-grain intake is favorably associated with metabolic risk factors for type 2 diabetes and cardiovascular disease in the Framingham Offspring Study. *The AJCN, 76*(2), 390–398. PMID:12145012

Mena, M. P., Sacanella, E., Vazquez-Agell, M., Morales, M., Fito, M., Escoda, R., ... Estruch, R. (2009). Inhibition of circulating immune cell activation: A molecular antiinflammatory effect of the Mediterranean diet. *The American Journal of Clinical Nutrition, 89*(1), 248–256. doi:10.3945/ajcn.2008.26094 PMID:19056596

Milanski, M., Degasperi, G., Coope, A., Morari, J., Denis, R., Cintra, D. E., ... Velloso, L. A. (2009). Saturated fatty acids produce an inflammatory response predominantly through the activation of TLR4 signaling in hypothalamus: Implications for the pathogenesis of obesity. *The Journal of Neuroscience, 29*(2), 359–370. doi:10.1523/JNEUROSCI.2760-08.2009 PMID:19144836

Minihane, A. M., Vinoy, S., Russell, W. R., Baka, A., Roche, H. M., Tuohy, K. M., ... Calder, P. C. (2015). Low-grade inflammation, diet composition and health: Current research evidence and its translation. *British Journal of Nutrition, 114*(7), 999–1012. doi:10.1017/S0007114515002093 PMID:26228057

Mohanty, P., Hamouda, W., Garg, R., Aljada, A., Ghanim, H., & Dandona, P. (2000). Glucose challenge stimulates reactive oxygen species (ROS) generation by leucocytes. *Int J Clin Endocrinol Metab*, *85*(8), 2970–2973. doi:10.1210/jcem.85.8.6854 PMID:10946914

Montonen, J., Boeing, H., Fritsche, A., Schleicher, E., Joost, H. G., Schulze, M. B., ... Pischon, T. (2013). Consumption of red meat and whole-grain bread in relation to biomarkers of obesity, inflammation, glucose metabolism and oxidative stress. *European Journal of Nutrition*, *52*(1), 337–345. doi:10.100700394-012-0340-6 PMID:22426755

Nanri, A., Yoshida, D., Yamaji, T., Mizoue, T., Takayanagi, R., & Kono, S. (2008). Dietary patterns and C-reactive protein in Japanese men and women. *The AJCN*, *87*(5), 1488–1496. PMID:18469275

Navarro, S., Kantor, E. D., Song, X., Milne, G. L., Lampe, J. W., Kratz, M., & White, E. (2016). Factors associated with multiple biomarkers of systemic inflammation. *Cancer Epidemiology, Biomarkers & Prevention*, *25*(3), 521–531. doi:10.1158/1055-9965.EPI-15-0956 PMID:26908433

Nergiz-Unal, R. (2016). Diyet Yağı ve Yağ Asitleriyle İmmün Sistem Etkileşimi. *Türkiye Klinikleri J Nutr Diet*, *2*(2), 32–35.

Nettleton, J. A., Steffen, L. M., Mayer-Davis, E. J., Jenny, N. S., Jiang, R., Herrington, D. M., & Jacobs, D. R. Jr. (2006). Dietary patterns are associated with biochemical markers of inflammation and endothelial activation in the Multi-Ethnic Study of Atherosclerosis (MESA). *The American Journal of Clinical Nutrition*, *83*(6), 1369–1379. doi:10.1093/ajcn/83.6.1369 PMID:16762949

Neuhouser, M. L., Schwarz, Y., Wang, C., Breymeyer, K., Coronado, G., Wang, C. Y., ... Lampe, J. W. (2012). A low-glycemic load diet reduces serum C-reactive protein and modestly increases adiponectin in overweight and obese adults. *The Journal of Nutrition*, *142*(2), 369–374. doi:10.3945/jn.111.149807 PMID:22190020

Nishida, K., & Otsu, K. (2017). Inflammation and metabolic cardiomyopathy. *Cardiovascular Research*, *113*(4), 389–398. doi:10.1093/cvr/cvx012 PMID:28395010

O'Keefe, J. H. Jr, & Cordain, L. (2004). Cardiovascular disease resulting from a diet and lifestyle at odds with our Paleolithic genome: How to become a 21st-century hunter-gatherer. *Mayo Clinic Proceedings*, *79*(1), 101–108. doi:10.4065/79.1.101 PMID:14708953

Odermatt, A. (2011). The western-style diet: A major risk factor for impaired kidney function and chronic kidney disease. *American Journal of Physiology. Renal Physiology, 301*(5), F919–F931. doi:10.1152/ajprenal.00068.2011 PMID:21880837

Okreglicka, K. (2015). Health effects of changes in the structure of dietary macronutrients intake in Western societies. *Roczniki Panstwowego Zakladu Higieny, 66*(2), 97–105. PMID:26024397

Oktar, B. K., & Alican, İ. (2000). İnflamatuvar Bağırsak Hastalıklarının Etyopatogenezindeki Olası Mekanizmalar ve Mediyatörler. *Türkiye Tıp Dergisi, 7*(3), 155–161.

Ozawa, M., Shipley, M., Kivimaki, M., Singh-Manoux, A., & Brunner, E. J. (2017). Dietary pattern, inflammation and cognitive decline: Whitehall II prospective cohort study. *Clinical Nutrition (Edinburgh, Lothian), 36*(2), 506–512. doi:10.1016/j.clnu.2016.01.013 PMID:26874911

Pang, G., Xie, J., Chen, Q., & Hu, Z. (2014). Energy intake, metabolic homeostasis, and human health. *Food Science and Human Wellness, 3*(3-4), 89–103. doi:10.1016/j.fshw.2015.01.001

Peairs, A. D., Rankin, J. W., & Lee, Y. W. (2011). Effects of acute ingestion of different fats on oxidative stress and inflammation in overweight and obese adults. *Nutrition Journal, 10*(1), 122. doi:10.1186/1475-2891-10-122 PMID:22059644

Pischon, T., Hankinson, S.E., Hotamisligil, G.S., Rifai, N., Willett, W.C. & Rimm, EB. (2003). Habitual dietary intake of n-3 and n-6 fatty acids in relation to inflammatory markers among US men and women. *Circulation, 108*(2), 155-160.

Powell, W.S. & Rokach, J. (2014). Biosynthesis, biological effects, and receptors of hydroxyeicosatetraenoic acids (HETEs) and oxoeicosatetraenoic acids (oxo-ETEs) derived from arachidonic acid. *Biochimica et Biophysica Acta, 16.*

Qi, L., Rimm, E., Liu, S., Rifai, N., & Hu, F. B. (2005). Dietary glycemic index, glycemic load, cereal fiber, and plasma adiponectin concentration in diabetic men. *Diabetes Care, 28*(5), 1022–1028. doi:10.2337/diacare.28.5.1022 PMID:15855561

Qi, L., Van Dam, R. M., Liu, S., Franz, M., Mantzoros, C., & Hu, F. B. (2006). Whole grain, bran, and cereal fiber intakes and markers of systematic inflammation in diabetic women. *Diabetes Care, 29*(2), 207–211. doi:10.2337/diacare.29.02.06.dc05-1903 PMID:16443861

Radmark, O., Werz, O., Steinhilber, D., & Samuelsson, B. (2014). 5-Lipoxygenase, a key enzyme for leukotriene biosynthesis in health and disease. *Biochimica et Biophysica Acta*, *9*(4C), 2, 3, 5. PMID:25152163

Rajkumar, H., Mahmood, N., Kumar, M., Varikuti, S. R., Challa, H. R., & Myakala, S. P. (2014). Effect of probiotic (VSL#3) and omega-3 on lipid profile, insulin sensitivity, inflammatory markers, and gut colonization in overweight adults: a randomized, controlled trial. Mediators of Inflammation.

Ratliff, J. C., Mutungi, G., Puglisi, M. J., Volek, J. S., & Fernandez, M. L. (2008). Eggs modulate the inflammatory response to carbohydrate restricted diets in overweight men. *Nutrition & Metabolism*, *5*(1), 6. doi:10.1186/1743-7075-5-6 PMID:18289377

Razad, O., Steinvil, A., Rosenzweig, T., Berlinerce, S., Shapirac, I., & Boaz, M. (2014). An eight-week high complex carbohydrate, energy restricted dietary intervention is associated with weight loss and a reduction of inflammation markers. *Bioactive Carbohydrates and Dietary Fibre*, *4*(1), 93–99. doi:10.1016/j.bcdf.2014.07.001

Ricker, M. A., & Haas, W. C. (2017). Anti-inflammatory diet in clinical practice: A review. *Nutrition in Clinical Practice*, *32*(3), 318–325. doi:10.1177/0884533617700353 PMID:28350517

Ross, A. P., Bartness, T. J., Mielke, J. G., & Parent, M. B. (2009). A high fructose diet impairs spatial memory in male rats. *Neurobiology of Learning and Memory*, *92*(3), 410–416. doi:10.1016/j.nlm.2009.05.007 PMID:19500683

Ruiz-Nunez, B., Dijck-Brouwer, D. A., & Muskiet, F. A. (2016). The relation of saturated fatty acids with low-grade inflammation and cardiovascular disease. *The Journal of Nutritional Biochemistry*, *36*, 1–20. doi:10.1016/j.jnutbio.2015.12.007 PMID:27692243

Ruiz-Nunez, B., Kuipers, R. S., Luxwolda, M. F., De Graaf, D. J., Breeuwsma, B. B., Dijck-Brouwer, D. A., & Muskiet, F. A. (2014). Saturated fatty acid (SFA) status and SFA intake exhibit different relations with serum total cholesterol and lipoprotein cholesterol: A mechanistic explanation centered around lifestyle-induced low-grade inflammation. *The Journal of Nutritional Biochemistry*, *25*(3), 304–312. doi:10.1016/j.jnutbio.2013.11.004 PMID:24524903

Salmerón, J., Manson, J. E., Stampfer, M. J., Colditz, G. A., Wing, A. L., & Willett, W. C. (1997). Dietary fiber, glycemic load, and risk of non-insulin-dependent diabetes mellitus in women. *Journal of the American Medical Association*, *277*(6), 472–477. doi:10.1001/jama.1997.03540300040031 PMID:9020271

Schwingshackl, L., Christoph, M., & Hoffmann, G. (2015). Effects of Olive Oil on Markers of Inflammation and Endothelial Function-A Systematic Review and Meta-Analysis. *Nutrients*, *7*(9), 7651–7675. doi:10.3390/nu7095356 PMID:26378571

Schwingshackl, L., & Hoffmann, G. (2014). Mediterranean dietary pattern, inflammation and endothelial function: A systematic review and meta-analysis of intervention trials. *Nutrition, Metabolism, and Cardiovascular Diseases*, *24*(9), 929–939. doi:10.1016/j.numecd.2014.03.003 PMID:24787907

Sekuła, W., Figurska, K., Barysz, A., & Ołtarzewski, M. (2008). Results of the monitoring nutrition in Poland. [in Polish]. *Zywienie Czlowieka i Metabolizm*, *35*, 371–395.

Shivappa, N. (2014). *Dietary inflammatory index and its relationship with inflammation, metabolic biomarkers and mortality*. The Norman J. Arnold School of Public Health University of South Carolina.

Shivappa, N., Steck, S. E., Hurley, T. G., Hussey, J. R., & Hebert, J. R. (2014). Designing and developing a literature-derived, population-based dietary inflammatory index. *Public Health Nutrition*, *17*(8), 1689–1696. doi:10.1017/S1368980013002115 PMID:23941862

Silva, D., & Pais de Lacerda, A. (2012). High-sensitivity C-reactive protein as a biomarker of risk in coronary artery disease. *Revista Portuguesa de Cardiologia [English Edition]*, *31*(11), 733–745. doi:10.1016/j.repc.2012.02.018 PMID:23046630

Silveira, B. K. S., Oliveira, T. M. S., Andrade, P. A., Hermsdorff, H. H. M., Rosa, C. O. B., & Franceschini, S. (2018). Dietary Pattern and Macronutrients Profile on the Variation of Inflammatory Biomarkers: Scientific Update. *Cardiology Research and Practice*, *2018*, 4762575. PMID:29725543

Silver, H. J., Kang, H., Keil, C. D., Muldowney, J. A. III, Kocalis, H., Fazio, S., ... Niswender, K. D. (2014). Consuming a balanced high fat diet for 16 weeks improves body composition, inflammation and vascular function parameters in obese premenopausal women. *Metabolism: Clinical and Experimental*, *63*(4), 562–573. doi:10.1016/j.metabol.2014.01.004 PMID:24559846

Simopoulos, A. P. (2002). Omega-3 fatty acids in inflammation and autoimmune disease. *Journal of the American College of Nutrition*, *21*(6), 495–505. doi:10.1080/07315724.2002.10719248 PMID:12480795

Simopoulos, A. P. (2002). The importance of the ratio of omega-6/omega-3 essential fatty acids. *Biomedicine and Pharmacotherapy*, *56*(8), 365–379. doi:10.1016/S0753-3322(02)00253-6 PMID:12442909

Slavin, J. L. (2005). Dietary fiber and body weight. *Nutrition*, *21*(3), 411–418. doi:10.1016/j.nut.2004.08.018 PMID:15797686

Stamler, J., Daviglus, M. L., Garside, D. B., Dyer, A. R., Greenland, P., & Neaton, J. D. (2000). Relationship of baseline serum cholesterol levels in 3 large cohorts of younger men to long-term coronary, cardiovascular, and all-cause mortality and to longevity. *Journal of the American Medical Association*, *19*(284), 311–318. doi:10.1001/jama.284.3.311 PMID:10891962

Stone, N. J., Robinson, J. G., Lichtenstein, A. H., Merz, C. N. B., Blum, C. B., Eckel, R. H., ... Wilson, P. W. (2014). ACC/AHA guideline on the treatment of blood cholesterol to reduce atherosclerotic cardiovascular risk in adults: A report of the American College of Cardiology/American Heart Association Task Force on Practice Guidelines. *Journal of the American College of Cardiology*, *63*(25 Part B), 2889–2934. doi:10.1016/j.jacc.2013.11.002 PMID:24239923

Suganami, T., Tanimoto-Koyama, K., Nishida, J., Itoh, M., Yuan, X., Mizuarai, S., ... Ogawa, Y. (2007). Role of the Toll-like receptor 4/NF-kappaB pathway in saturated fatty acid-induced inflammatory changes in the interaction between adipocytes and macrophages. *Arteriosclerosis, Thrombosis, and Vascular Biology*, *27*(1), 84–91. doi:10.1161/01.ATV.0000251608.09329.9a PMID:17082484

Sui, Y. H., Luo, W. J., Xu, Q. Y., & Hua, J. (2016). Dietary saturated fatty acid and polyunsaturated fatty acid oppositely affect hepatic NOD-like receptor protein 3 inflammasome through regulating nuclear factor-kappa B activation. *World Journal of Gastroenterology*, *22*(8), 2533–2544. doi:10.3748/wjg.v22.i8.2533 PMID:26937141

Teeman, C. S., Kurti, S. P., Cull, B. J., Emerson, S. R., Haub, M. D., & Rosenkranz, S. K. (2016). Postprandial lipemic and inflammatory responses to high-fat meals: A review of the roles of acute and chronic exercise. *Nutrition & Metabolism*, *13*(1), 80. doi:10.118612986-016-0142-6 PMID:27891165

Teng, K. T., Chang, L. F., Vethakkan, S. R., Nesaretnam, K., & Sanders, T. A. B. (2017). Effects of exchanging carbohydrate or monounsaturated fat with saturated fat on inflammatory and thrombogenic responses in subjects with abdominal obesity: A randomized controlled trial. *Clinical Nutrition (Edinburgh, Lothian)*, *36*(5), 1250–1258. doi:10.1016/j.clnu.2016.08.026 PMID:27642057

Van Horn, L., Tian, L., Neuhouser, M. L., Howard, B. V., Eaton, C. B., Snetselaar, L., ... Lichtenstein, A. H. (2012). Dietary patterns are associated with disease risk among participants in the women's health initiative observational study. *The Journal of Nutrition*, *142*(2), 284–291. doi:10.3945/jn.111.145375 PMID:22190026

Vos, M. B., Kimmons, J. E., Gillespie, C., Welsh, J., & Blanck, H. M. (2008). Dietary fructose consumption among US children and adults: The Third National Health and Nutrition Examination Survey. *Medscape Journal of Medicine*, *10*(7), 160. PMID:18769702

Wall, R., Ross, R. P., Fitzgerald, G. F., & Stanton, C. (2010). Fatty acids from fish: The anti-inflammatory potential of long-chain omega-3 fatty acids. *Nutrition Reviews*, *68*(5), 280–289. doi:10.1111/j.1753-4887.2010.00287.x PMID:20500789

Weigert, C., Brodbeck, K., Staiger, H., Kausch, C., Machicao, F., Haring, H. U., & Schleicher, E. D. (2004). Palmitate, but not unsaturated fatty acids, induces the expression of interleukin-6 in human myotubes through proteasome-dependent activation of nuclear factor-kappaB. *The Journal of Biological Chemistry*, *279*(23), 23942–23952. doi:10.1074/jbc.M312692200 PMID:15028733

WHO. (2019a). World Health Organization. Diet, Nutrition and the Prevention of Chronic Diseases. Retrieved from https://www.who.int/dietphysicalactivity/publications/trs916/en/

WHO. (2019b). World Health Organisation. Healthy diet. Retrieved from http://www.who.int/news-room/fact-sheets/detail/healthy-diet

Wisastra, R., & Dekker, F. D. (2014). Inflammation, Cancer and Oxidative Lipoxygenase Activity are Intimately Linked. *Cancers (Basel)*, *6*(3), 1500–1521. doi:10.3390/cancers6031500 PMID:25037020

Wolever, T. M., Gibbs, A. L., Mehling, C., Chiasson, J. L., Connelly, P. W., Josse, R. G., ... Ryan, E. A. (2008). The Canadian trial of Carbohydrates in Diabetes (CCD), a 1-y controlled trial of low-glycemic index dietary carbohydrate in type 2 diabetes: No effect on glycated hemoglobin but reduction in C-reactive protein. *The American Journal of Clinical Nutrition*, *87*(1), 114–125. doi:10.1093/ajcn/87.1.114 PMID:18175744

Wysham, C. H., & Kirkman, M. S. (2011). Response to Comment on: American Diabetes Association. Standards of Medical Care in Diabetes—2011. *Diabetes Care*, *34*(5), e54–e54. doi:10.2337/dc11-0262

Yannakoulia, M., Yiannakouris, N., Melistas, L., Kontogianni, M. D., Malagaris, I., & Mantzoros, C. S. (2008). A dietary pattern characterized by high consumption of whole-grain cereals and low-fat dairy products and low consumption of refined cereals is positively associated with plasma adiponectin levels in healthy women. *Metabolism: Clinical and Experimental*, *57*(6), 824–830. doi:10.1016/j.metabol.2008.01.027 PMID:18502266

Zampelas, A., Panagiotakos, D. B., Pitsavos, C., Das, U. N., Chrysohoou, C., Skoumas, Y., & Stefanadis, C. (2005). Fish consumption among healthy adults is associated with decreased levels of inflammatory markers related to cardiovascular disease: The ATTICA study. *Journal of the American College of Cardiology*, *46*(1), 120–124. doi:10.1016/j.jacc.2005.03.048 PMID:15992645

Chapter 4
Inflammatory Effects of Micronutrients

Leyla Tevfikoğlu Pehlivan
University of Trakya, Turkey

ABSTRACT

Lifestyle and dietary habits are important factors in different levels of daily food intake and the occurrence of many chronic diseases. Consumption and composition of foods and nutrients, lifestyle, physical activity level, type of occupation, stress, and smoking and alcohol use can affect health in different ways and can trigger inflammation processes. Daily diet plays a major role in the formation of inflammatory responses. With the occurrence of inflammation diseases, the level of food intake changes and it is not possible to provide adequate and balanced nutrition. Especially in the case of inflammation, energy and nutrient intake levels are negatively affected, especially vitamins A, E, D, iron, and folate levels decreased. In studies, it was shown that vitamins A, E, D, K, C, iron, selenium, and zinc show anti-inflammatory properties. The intake of these nutrients in accordance with the requirements is an important step in the prevention and treatment of many diseases. Further research is needed to examine the relationship between different nutrients and energy intake levels.

BACKGROUND

Inflammation is a complex and cellular response of living tissue to injury. Although defined holistically and histologically, it may have local and/or systemic effects. Factors such as age, gender, obesity, smoking, alcohol use, the level of physical activity, and mainly the diet affect the inflammatory response. Many authorities,

DOI: 10.4018/978-1-7998-3594-3.ch004

particularly the World Health Organization (WHO), emphasize that nutrition has a considerable effect on the prevention of noncommunicable diseases. Unhealthy diets and negative behavior patterns in the lifestyle pave the way for the development of cardiovascular diseases, type 2 diabetes, cancer, and other diseases. Consuming food that is rich in trans fats and poor in natural antioxidants and fibers, and which contains refined carbohydrates, simple sugars, saturated fats, and w-3 fatty acids activate innate immunity, decrease the production of anti-inflammatory cytokines while increasing the production of pro-inflammatory cytokines (Casas & Estruch, 2016).

The complex, total and/or synergistic effect of nutrients and the components of nutrients can positively or negatively affect health and inflammatory process. It is difficult to predict the effects of nutrients on health, especially in the long term. While high consumption of certain nutrients such as whole-grain products, vegetables, fruit, fish, fiber, monounsaturated and polyunsaturated fatty acids, vitamins C and E, and carotenoids are associated with low inflammation parameters, saturated and trans-fatty acids, and consumption of high levels of glucose and fatty meals increases postprandial inflammation and triggers the proinflammatory process (Tomkins, 2003).

The inflammatory process is complicated and takes place through the production of many chemical mediators and many cell types that provide immunity to prevent diseases. The inflammatory process consists of the synthesis and release of anti-inflammatory cytokines, inhibition of pro-inflammatory signaling steps, alteration of inflammatory mediators and receptors, and the activation phases of regulatory cells that provide the direct development of inflammatory diseases. In the acute phase response, metabolic changes occur through differences, taking place in many plasma protein concentrations in the short term. These proteins are divided into two groups: positive acute phase proteins, whose levels show an increase in the blood in case of inflammation, such as C-reactive proteins (CRP), haptoglobin, fibrinogen, and α-1 antitrypsin and negative acute-phase proteins, whose levels decrease in the blood, such as albumin, retinol-binding protein (RBP), transthyretin (TTY), and high-density lipoprotein apolipoprotein A1 (high-density lipoprotein apolipoprotein A1-HDL-apo A) (Tomkins, 2003). In addition, tumor necrosis factor-α (TNF-α), interleukin 6 (IL-6), interleukin 18 (IL-18), water-soluble adhesion molecules (E-selectin, intercellular adhesion molecule-1 (ICAM-1) and vascular adhesion molecule-1 (VCAM-1)), which are among pro-inflammatory cytokines, make up the fibrinogen proinflammatory response, while adiponectin is involved in the formation of anti-inflammatory response. These metabolic alterations lead to physiological differences through changes in pulse, fever, and blood pressure levels. In many diseases or disorders such as infection, trauma, type 2 diabetes, cancer, cardiovascular diseases, and obesity, the inflammatory response begins at an acute level, leading to chronic inflammation when this condition persists for weeks and months. The severity of systemic inflammation is associated with CRP level, and a CRP level that is less than 10 mg/L is considered as mild systemic inflammation, between 11 and 80 mg/L as moderate, and greater than 80 mg/L as high (McMillan, Maguire, & Talwar, 2018).

Minerals and vitamins are cofactors of many enzymes in the metabolic processes of cells. Levels of vitamins A, D, E, K, B_1, B_2, B_6, B_{12}, and C and the minerals such as zinc, copper, iron, selenium are of great significance in many inflammatory diseases such as cancer, metabolic syndrome, infection, trauma, type 2 diabetes, digestive system, cardiovascular diseases, and obesity. Besides, the levels of albumin, RBP, and transferrin, which are among the carrier proteins, decrease in inflammation (McMillan et al., 2018; Thurnhams & McCabe, 2012). Clinically, these nutrients and compounds are associated with nutritional status, are affected by inflammation, and their blood levels change (McMillan et al., 2018). In the systemic inflammatory response, the most examined area has been the relationship between CRP marker and many different micronutrient levels. This section has been compiled to demonstrate the effect of the inflammatory response on micronutrients and the inflammatory effects of some micronutrients.

VITAMIN A, RETINOL BINDING PROTEIN, CAROTENOIDS, AND LYCOPENE

Fat-soluble vitamin A and Retinol Binding Protein (RBP) are negative acute phase reactants. Their levels decrease in the presence of inflammation. Louw et al. (1992) investigated patients undergoing orthopedic surgery, plasma vitamin A levels started to decrease with increasing CRP level within 4 hours and a 40% decrease was observed in the first 48 hours postoperatively. Apart from these changes, a decrease in RBP level was observed. Vitamin A and RBP levels were reported to return to normal levels within 7 days without therapeutic support (Louw et al., 1992). Plasma Vitamin A concentration decreased after acute myocardial infarction and then returned to normal level within 3 days without intervention (Labadasias et al., 1987). As a result of routine measurements, Vitamin A levels were found to be inversely correlated with CRP levels in patients with cystic fibrosis due to the presence of fat malabsorption, however, it was found not to be associated with the dietary intake (Duggan, Colin, Agil, Higgins, & Rifai, 1996).

VITAMIN D

There is still disagreement about the relationship between vitamin D and inflammation. Some claim that inflammation reduces 25(OH)D concentration, others postulate that boosting the status of vitamin D decreases inflammation (Henriksen et al., 2017; Mangge et al., 2013). Researchers who support the former that inflammation reduces 25(OH)D concentration posit that inflammation reduces serum 25(OH) D through oxidative stress which leads to the oxidative catabolism of 25 (OH) D. They assume that 25(OH)D is lowered by an oxidative environment by interfering with key vitamin D metabolizing enzymes, disrupting the liver's biosynthesis of 25(OH)D, thus reducing 25(OH)D concentration (Autier, Boniol, Pizot, & Mullie, 2014; Guillot, Semerano, Saidenberg-Kermanac'h, Falgarone, & Boissier, 2010; Adorini, & Penna, 2008).

Inflammation is lowered by vitamin D. In vitro studies show that $1.25(OH)_2D_3$ has powerful anti-inflammatory features (Guo et al., 2013; Korf et al., 2012; Feng et al., 2013). Also, studies on animals show that $1.25(OH)_2D_3$ and its analogs are efficient anti-inflammatories (Erbas et al., 2014; Adzemovic, Zeitelhofer, Hochmeister, Gustafsson, & Jagodic, 2013; Yilmaz et al., 2013). $1.25(OH)_2D_3$ reduces inflammation through multiple mechanisms. $1.25(OH)_2D_3$ influences the innate and adaptive immune systems. This overall effect can be explained as a switch from the more inflammatory T-helper 1 (Th1)/Th17 response to the less inflammatory Th2/Treg profile. In an artificial environment, these impacts lead to decreased production of pro-inflammatory markers such as TNF-α, interferon-gamma (IFN-g), interleukin (IL)-2, IL-12, IL-17, and IL-21, yet this occurs with enhanced production of anti-inflammatory cytokines such as IL (Anarow, 2011).

The inflammatory status of cellular models was reduced by the active form of vitamin D. Vitamin D indirectly alleviated ROS, which are considered a significant factor in the start and development of chronic diseases such as type 2 diabetes (Newsholme et al., 2007). Vitamin D reduced increased Toll-like Receptor (TLR) expression in both immune cells and adipose tissue from overweight and obese individuals. Moreover, TLR activation has been demonstrated in obesity-related insulin resistance and metabolic dysfunction mechanisms. Studies have indicated that TLRs are induced by both endogenous and exogenous factors such as dietary saturated fatty acids and resistin, both of which produce inflammatory changes in circulating immune cells. After that, the TLR transmembrane proteins launch classical signaling cascades which cause the activation of transcription factors, including NFκB and cytokine production. Besides, TLR pathways induce various cellular responses that involve host defense in response to microbial products and then affect energy metabolism. NFκB, that is stimulated, exercise its effect by binding to DNA and producing the transcription of many genes that are involved in many features of innate and adaptive immune responses which include those coding for cytokines, growth factors, adhesion molecules, and various genes controlling cellular differentiation, survival, and propagation. Apparently, evidence claims that 1.25 $(OH)_2$ D_3 has a function to suppress NFκB activity. Vitamin D may act by suppressing NFκB transcriptional activity or by regulating cellular reactive oxygen species (ROS) levels which consequently change NFκB transcriptional activity. Yet, the specific pathway(s) needs confirmation. In the modulation of the transcriptional factor effect, it is also possible to achieve the inhibition of inflammatory signal by means of vitamin D. Besides, vitamin D may cause anti-inflammatory impacts by nongenomic pathways started in plasma membrane vitamin D reseptor (VDR) (Zhang et al., 2012). 1,25$(OH)_2D_3$ bound at the plasma membrane VDR can lead to the activation of one or more second Messenger systems, including phospholipase C (and consequently protein kinase C, by the generation of both diacylglycerol and an increase in intracellular Ca^{2+}), and G protein-coupled receptors. Moreover, non-genomic pathways may collaborate with the classical genomic pathway through cross-talk to have an impact on gene expression (Calton, Keane, Newsholme, & Soares, 2015). Possibly, applying a system biology approach may unveil further action mechanisms. This form of vitamin D, we cannot comment on whether 25(OH) D modulates inflammation. Nevertheless, it is believed that current 25(OH)D levels may be critical as the local tissue concentrations of the active vitamin D metabolite are affected by them (Newison, 2011).

An optimal immune function may require serum 25(OH)D levels as high as 120 nmol/L (Ojaimi et al., 2013). Admittedly, studies reported (Ojaimi et al., 2013; Calton et al., 2015) that the anti-inflammatory benefit of vitamin D was only observed in individuals with 25(OH)D rising to >100 nmol/L. When vitamin D status fell below 100 nmol/L, profitable effects ceased to exist. Recommendations for adequate serum levels of 25 (OH) D can only assess the effect of 25 (OH) D at different doses showing the concentrations of hormone circulating throughout the body through cellular studies. The impact of vitamin D on subsequent cell function was not addressed in this systematic review. Inherent remedial factors such as vitamin D, which aim at immune pathways including NFκB, ROS quenching, and JAK, must be able to incite the adverse effects of inflammation without affecting the defense functions of the host. (Calton et al., 2015).

Anti-inflammatory effects of Vitamin D have been observed in vivo and vitro studies. Vitamin D may reduce inflammation, and oxidative stress caused by inflammation may disturb the metabolism of vitamin D and consequently reduce 5(OH)D. These two are not mutually exclusive. Health professionals should check the benefits and harms of vitamin D on the disease and treat the individuals accordingly by assessing their vitamin D levels in the blood.

VITAMIN E

Chronic inflammation is the significant contributor of the development of chronic diseases such as obesity, cancer and cardiovascular diseases. Overreacting immune response leads to inflammation (McMillan et al., 2018). It is characterized by the production of abundant reactive oxygen/nitrogen species and proinflammatory mediators, such as lipid mediators, particularly leukotrienes and prostaglandins, and cytokines including TNF-α and interleukin-6. Correspondingly, they worsen inflammation and give excessive harm to host tissues. Prostaglandins and leukotrienes are synthesized from arachidonic acid (AA). They have a critical role in mediating the inflammatory response. For example, prostaglandin E2 (PGE2) is produced from COX-1-and COX-2-catalyzed oxidation of AA and is considered to cause pain and fever, besides activating cytokine formation. Leukotriene B4 (LTB4) is also a lipid mediator, which is obtained from AA through the 5-lipoxygenase (5-LOX)-catalyzed reaction in neutrophils. It is one of the most powerful chemotactic agents. Leukotrienes C4 and D4 are also generated by 5-LOX in eosinophils and mast cells. They are known to play major roles in asthma and allergic inflammatory disorders. COX-and 5-LOX-catalyzed eicosanoids are known to develop various cancer types. LTB4 and PGE2 play a major role in inflammation, therefore COXs and 5-LOX have been identified as major targets for drug treatment against chronic diseases. Especially, COX inhibitors, nonsteroidal anti-inflammatory drugs (NSAIDs), have been shown to be efficient in the treatment of inflammatory diseases, reducing the inflammatory response, and preventing cancer. The 5-LOX inhibitor zileuton has clinically been employed in the treatment of asthma. Cytokines have a significant part to play in the control of inflammation and pathogenesis of inflammation-related disorders. For example, IL-6 that is secreted from stimulated macrophages is a proinflammatory cytokine. It makes a contribution to the promotion of carcinogenesis that is associated with cancer, arthritis, and obesity. The anti-IL-6 antibody is employed in the treatment of anti-TNF-α non-responsive arthritis clinically. Nuclear factor (NF)-κB and JAK-STAT 6/3, which are signal transducer and activator of transcription 6/3, are fundamental transcriptional agents. They mediate the response and expression of cytokines and chemokines. NF-κB and STATs are activated by receptor-mediated signaling in immune and other cells types and they bind to consensus target sequences in several promoters and cause expression of numerous genes that involve proinflammatory cytokines as well (Jiang, 2014).

Distinct forms of vitamin E such as γT, δT, and tocotrienols (particularly γTE) have been reported by mechanistic studies to have anti-inflammatory effects by inhibiting COX-2-and 5-LOX-mediated eicosanoids and suppressing NF-κB and JAK–STAT6 or JAK-STAT 3 that signal pathways in many kinds of cells. Studies have reported that long-chain carboxy chromanols, especially 13O-COOHs, inhibit

COXs and 5-LOX more powerfully than unmetabolized vitamin E forms (Galloway, McMillan, & Sattar, 2000).

Superior capacity to get rid of free radicals and prevent lipid oxidation: Inhibition of the release of proinflammatory cytokines and a decrease in the levels of CRP. Gamma-tocopherol reduces proinflammatory NF-kβ and TNF-α activity and prevents prostaglandin synthesis (Helmersson, Arnlöv, Larsson, & Basu et al., 2009).

Intakes of alpha-tocopherol in diet were reversely associated with plasma levels of proinflammatory CRP and IL-6. Also, alpha and gamma-tocopherol was observed to have a synergistic impact on inflammation in a randomized double-blind trial that consisted of subjects with Metabolic Syndrome. In the study, supplementation with 800 mg/day of a combination of alpha- and gamma-tocopherol was found to be more efficient in lowering the levels of plasma CRP and TNF-α than either supplement alone. A considerable decrease in joint stiffness and pain under twice-daily supplementation with 600 mg of alpha-tocopherol was shown in a clinical study; however, plasma inflammatory biomarkers weren't modified (Devaraj, Leonard, Traber, & Jialal, 2008).

VITAMIN K

The pharmaceutical advancement of the anti-inflammatory function of activated protein C, which is a vitamin K–bound protein, is being founded at the limits of inflammation and coagulation (Esmon, 2000). Vitamin K is necessary for the generation of the mature functional protein, whereas it is the role of protein C as a serine protease to limit microthrombus formation in organ tissue beds in sepsis. Vitamin K deficiency has links to several critical chronic diseases that have an inflammatory background. Inflammatory bowel disease, pancreatitis, cystic fibrosis, osteoporosis and chronic kidney disease are among these diseases (Kleinman and Fracchia, 2010; Nakajima et al., 2011; Sikkens et al., 2013).

Nuclear factor kappa-B (NF-κB) can be found in almost all cells. It participates in a range of various biological functions such as inflammation, cell growth, immunity, tumorigenesis and apoptosis, and differentiation. This entails an involvement from birth to death of a cell. This pathway is important for normal cell function, yet it can become over-activated on a wider level or to the extent that may lead to tumorigenesis. Vitamin K has the capacity to regulate the activation of the NF-κB pathway (McCabe, Adams, & Holden, 2013). There are also other signaling pathways which control cell functions. Moreover, there is also significant communication between these pathways.

Studies conducting cell and animal experiments have looked at the way how vitamin K inhibition of IL-6 release following endotoxin challenge can regulate inflammation. These studies used germ-free rats, THP-1 human monocyte-like cells, and murine RAW264.7 macrophage-like cells. They also reported the LPS-stimulated cellular IL-6 mRNA levels reduced significantly. Studies doing vitamin K supplemented animal experiments found that there was a suppression of the hepatic mRNA levels of the inflammation response protein macrophage migration inhibitory factor (MIF), in comparison to animals fed on a vitamin K deficient diet. In this study, supplementation with vitamin K1 was also found to cause a rise in hepatic tissue menaquinone-4 levels. When these in vivo findings are extended in the two cell lines, namely THP-1 and RAW264.7, this indicated that the suppression of LPS-stimulated IL-6 mRNA by vitamin K2 was consistent with the inhibition of NF-κB activity through the restricted phosphorylation of IKK kinases. It was also investigated in these studies whether these events included a classical vitamin K gamma-carboxylation-mediated process. Accordingly, co-culture experiments conducted with warfarin laid out that the inhibitory effects of vitamin K on NF-κB were independent of vitamin K–dependent protein gamma-carboxylation (Hodges, Pitsillides, Ytrebo, & Soper, 2017).

Inflammatory activity of vitamin K is likely to be directed by the inhibition of NF-κB signaling. It is recommended in cell culture experiments that the cells should be primed with vitamin K before they are challenged with agonists. Moreover, there are interesting experimental findings that indicate inhibition of cytokine release in agonist-challenged cell culture and animal models. Given the vitamin K deficiency in chronic diseases, this can reflect on a vitamin K role in organ homeostasis. Thus, efforts to define vitamin K sufficiency based on adequate functional blood clotting factors only can be seen as an over-simplification of the case. Indeed, it needs more consideration (Esmon, 2000).

The value of vitamin K in a therapeutic or a prophylactic role remains as an open question. For example, a seriously ill patient with vitamin K deficiency may not benefit from a vitamin K intervention greatly; however, a patient who has a chronic inflammatory disease may benefit from it. This needs large community studies going on for many years to come up with a conclusion (Hodges et al., 2017).

THIAMIN

Thiamin is usually tested using the indirect enzymatic method of erythrocyte transketolase. Populations who have poor thiamin intakes are known to have low levels of thiamin. Also, there are connections between thiamin deficiency and malaria. Nevertheless, erythrocyte transketolase and acute phase proteins such as CRP have not been compared (Tomkins, 2003).

RIBOFLAVIN

Riboflavin is generally tested by the evaluation of the erythrocyte glutathione reductase activation coefficient. The levels of abnormal riboflavin can be observed in dietary deficiency and malaria. However, we do not know enough about the levels of APPs and change in the status of erythrocyte glutathione reductase activation coefficient (Adelekan & Thumham, 1990).

NIACIN

Niacin levels are estimated indirectly by measuring nicotinamide adenine dinucleotide. The levels of niacin have been observed to be inadequate in patients with HIV. There is an interaction between niacin and certain antiretroviral drugs; nevertheless, no link has been shown with inflammation so far (Tomkins, 2003).

FOLATE

It is well known that serum folate levels decrease during acute inflammation. However, red cell folate levels are much more stable. Besides, they are much less vulnerable to recent changes in dietary intake than the levels of plasma. Chronic inflammation is related to low red cell folate levels similar to subclinical infections. They probably show the real status of micronutrient deficiency (Tomkins, 2003). Inflammatory responses have little impact on general red cell folate levels. Also, these levels are likely to be adequate markers of folate status. According to a study on HIV positive women in Zimbabwe, HIV and alpha1-antichymotrypsin (ACT) were independently related to lower serum folate levels (Friis et al., 2001). Women who had an ACT level of 0.4 g/L had a serum folate level around 1 nmol/L. Low serum folate but normal homocysteine levels can be observed in patients who have atherosclerotic heart diseases (Bunout et al., 2000).

VITAMIN C

Also recognized as vitamin C, ascorbic acid (AA) is a small carbohydrate molecule. It was first classified in the 1920s by Albert von Szent Györgyi, who noticed its role in the prevention and cure of scurvy. This disorder is a pathological life-threatening condition which shows up when people do not have access to fruit or vegetables for a long time (De Tullio, 2010). Natural sources of AA include strawberries, citrus fruits, green leafy vegetables, papaya, etc (Grosso et al., 2013). AA is vitally important to all living things including human beings, animals, and plants. Throughout evolution, some animals such as fish, birds, and a few mammals, including guinea pigs and humans have lost their ability to produce it, whereas some plants and animals species, such as cats and dogs, can biosynthesize it from glucose in the liver (De Tullio, 2010). AA is one of the critical dietary nutrients for the biosynthesis of collagen. Besides, it is a co-factor in the biosynthesis of catecholamines, L-carnitine, cholesterol, some peptide hormones, and amino acids. These functions are implicated in different diseases (Li & Schellhorn, 2007).

On the other hand, the effect of ascorbic acid on the immune system can be listed as follows:

1. Physiological concentrations augment lymphocytes proliferation, while supraphysiological concentrations impede proliferation (Furuya et al., 2008; Bruunsgoard et al., 2003; Calder et al., 2009).
2. It boosts cytokines production and synthesis of immunoglobulins in response to infection (Stephensen et al., 2006).
3. Excess doses may lessen exercise-bound inflammatory reactions.
4. It impacts natural killer and antimicrobial cell activities, lymphocytes proliferation, chemotaxis, and delayed-type hypersensitivity (Zhang, & Farthing, 2000).
5. It inhibits the multiplication of viruses (Zhang, Patchett, Perrett, Domizio, & Farthing, 2000).
6. It realizes the up-regulation of NK cells activity (Ichim et al., 2011).

AA is an antioxidant. Its general activity suggests that conditions related to chronic inflammation and oxidative stress lead to its depletion. Many inflammatory conditions such as type 2 diabetes, gastritis, bowel diseases, and gastrointestinal disorders, lung inflammations, neurodegenerative diseases, obesity, and cardiovascular disease are all linked to a marked reduction in plasma of AA levels in comparison to healthy controls (Ichim et al., 2011).

In summary:

1. Inflammatory bowel diseases;
    - In Crohn's disease and ulcerative colitis, it protects the mucosa from inflammation, while making it less susceptible to oxidative tissue damage (Schmidt et al., 2004; Bernardo et al., 2012).
    - In Coeliac disease, it lowers mucosal inflammatory response to gluten and secretion of proinflammatory cytokines. It inhibits the NF-kB pathway (Romieu, 2005).

2. Lung inflammations
   - It impacts lung function with its protective effects against infection (Biswas, Hwang, Kirkham, & Rahman, 2013; Wu, Huang, Hsu, Wang, & Yeh, 2007; Rossman et al., 2013).
   - It has a positive role in chronic rhinosinusitis (Fisher, Schwarzer, & Illek, 2004; Helms, & Miller, 2006).
   - It has a role in cystic fibrosis transmembrane conductance regulator chloride channel (Bruckdorfer, 2008).
3. Heart diseases
   - It has a protective role against oxidative stress (Wannamethee et al., 2013).
   - It has a part to play in inflammatory and oxidative prevention and modulation related to atrial fibrillation and atherosclerosis (Carnes et al., 2001; Aguirre & May, 2008; Heo & Hyon-Lee, 2013).
4. Neurodegenerative diseases
   - In Alzheimer's disease, it has a protective role against oxidative stress and inflammation. Also, it inhibits apoptosis and cell death in neuroblastoma cells (Huang and May, 2006).
   - In Parkinson's disease, it exhibits neuroprotective effects against oxidative-bound neuronal death (Fitzgerald et al., 2013).
   - No association has been found between AA intake and Amyotrophic Lateral Sclerosis progression (Tawazzi et al., 2011).
   - The role of AA in Multiple Sclerosis remains to be explored (Besler, Comoglu, & Okcu, 2002; Moretti et al., 2013).
5. Obesity and type 2 diabetes
   - It has a role in modulation adipocyte lipolysis and glucocorticoid release from adrenal glands.
   - It also has a part in hyperglycemia improvement and glycosylation in obese diabetic mice.
   - It improves DNA resistance in whole blood WBC against oxidative challenge (Mutlu-Turkoglu et al., 2003; Hasegawa, Niimi, & Odani, 2002; Senen, Adanali, Ayhan, Gorgu, & Erdogan, 2002).
6. Chronic obstructive pulmonary disease (COPD)
   - It has a beneficial effect on skeletal muscle fatigue (Wu et al., 2007; Rossman et all, 2013).

Because of its effects and diversity of regulated pathways, AA is made use of in several fields of medicine such as immunology, toxicology, and radiobiology. AA supplementation enhances the functions of the immune system including lymphocyte proliferation, antimicrobial and natural killer cell activities, chemotaxis, and delayed-type hypersensitivity. AA is not a wonder medicine. Besides, it can cause some unfavorable effects. Moreover, it has a high potential in medicinal chemistry. Particularly, the consumption of AA supplement is reported to cause no considerable side effects to general human health. AA supplement should be used carefully by individuals with a history of kidney stone development and iron overload. The daily recommended doses should not be exceeded as it may result in oxalate crystallization and formation of advanced glycation. It may sometimes result in diarrhea or mild nausea (Wroblewski, 2005).

There is enough information on AA; however, the optimal treatment level for humans is still unknown. AA has some advantages such as simple application, low cost, and minimal or no toxicity. AA is not favored as a single mode of treatment, but it can be used as an auxiliary to regulate immunity, gene expression and other important physiological processes (Sorice et al., 2014).

IRON

The progress in molecular information on iron transport and homeostasis has paved the way for a better understanding of the complex mechanisms involved. It has long been known that iron levels must be strictly managed to provide a fundamental nutrient that is involved in oxygen delivery, metabolism and redox regulation in addition to protecting against excessive levels of a primary toxicant which can create reactive oxygen species (ROS) to produce cellular damage and death. On the contrary to other essential minerals, the balance between iron nutrition and toxicity is sustained by systemic control mechanisms which arrange iron conservation and limit uptake until needs are raised. On the other hand, homeostasis of the majority of other metals is dominated by eliminating excess (Wessling-Resnich, 2010). Eventually, these characteristics of iron and its homeostasis are closely related to the response to inflammation and infection. Therefore, they provide major survival mechanisms which are distinctive in human physiology.

Clinical evidence shows that elevated iron stores worsen susceptibility of the disease and the response to infection and inflammation. Studies have well shown that there is a strong relationship between iron overload and infectious diseases. In tuberculosis, parenteral or oral iron has been found to increase mycobacterial growth (Lounis, Truffot-Pernot, Grosset, Gordeuk, & Boelaert, 2001). Also, morbidity and mortality increase in patients receiving iron supplementation. Indeed, dietary iron is linked to occurrence and death from tuberculosis (Gangaidzo et al., 2001). Host iron status strongly impacts malaria, which is another example of an infectious disease (Koka et al., 2007), and there is an ongoing debate on iron supplementation and how it can be applied in endemic regions. Excess iron related to hereditary hemochromatosis has been reported to cause vulnerability to other infectious pathogens including Vibrio vulnificus and Yersinia enterocolitica (Gerhard et al., 2001; Doherty, 2007). Thalassemic patients with excess iron caused by frequent blood transfusions are reported to develop infections more often (Garcia-Vidal et al., 2008; Ozkalay, Anil, Agus, Helvaci, & Sirti, 2006). Viral infections are also impacted by iron status strongly (Drakesmith & Prentice, 2008). Iron deficiency generally provides relative resistance to infection with high iron status which elevates the disease state. Interestingly, iron deficiency is likely to be a protective adaptive response in some parts of the world where there are soaring infectious diseases (Denic & Agarwal, 2007).

The iron status also impacts inflammatory chronic diseases. Increased iron stores are associated with markers of chronic inflammation and other known risk factors of obesity, metabolic syndrome, and diabetes. Other conditions often related to iron load include atherosclerosis, neurodegeneration, and chronic liver disease. All these findings are important because chronic diseases are widely prevalent in modern society. Besides modified dietary iron or manipulation of iron status can provide simple preventive or therapeutic possibilities. To give an example, reduction of iron stores in diabetics by phlebotomy or iron chelation has presented a kind of enhancement, which puts forward new approaches to the management of the disease. It is noteworthy that iron chelation and deprivation has also been implemented in cancer treatment (Wessling-Resnich, 2010).

The adaptation to iron deficiency provides resistance to infection and enhances the inflammatory condition. This underlies the link between iron and the inflammatory response, which is known as the anemia of inflammation (AI), or called the anemia of chronic disease (ACD). Cartwright et al. documented the properties of the hypoferremic response to inflammation in the 1940s (Cartwright et al., 1946). Currently, we know the iron regulatory hormone hepcidin has a central role in the organized response to lower systemic iron levels. We now know that a considerable amount of stimulatory inputs must be incorporated to strictly control hepcidin gene expression during the inflammatory response to modulate AI and make necessary adjustments to iron homeostasis (Wessling-Resnich, 2010).

Total body iron status generally regulates circulating hepcidin levels and they respond to physiological demands. Iron deficiency and hypoxia are conditions that raise iron demand. They are reflected in low hepcidin, whereas iron loading increases the synthesis of hepcidin. Moreover, infection and inflammation are also linked to increased hepdicin production. Through the acquired anemia of inflammation or chronic disease, these events eventually connect iron homeostasis to the inflammatory response (McMillan et al., 2019).

The upregulation of hepcidin by inflammatory stress response pathways is a key event that triggers systemic iron withdrawal and sequestration due to downregulation of ferroportin. The levels of reduced ferroportin constrain the absorption of dietary iron and promote the retention of iron by the RES. Properties of AI or ACD comprise hypoferremia, normal-to-elevated ferritin levels, and low serum iron-binding capacity. Reduced iron levels lead to iron-restricted erythropoiesis. Mice over-expressing hepcidin repeat this response by developing iron-deficiency anemia. Patients who have glycogen storage disease type 1a (GSD1a) and hepatic adenomas are considered to suffer from anemia resulting from over-expressed hepcidin. When tumors are removed, anemia resolves. This supports the physiological significance of hepcidin. Hepcidin provides a wide contribution; yet, it should be acknowledged that other stress response pathways are also involved in the inflammatory response, such as cytokine-mediated effects which are drawn out by TNF-α and interferon-γ (IFN-γ). Revealing the molecular networks that have a part in this process is of significance in understanding the integration of different pathways into the global response of iron status to inflammation (Wessling-Resnich, 2010).

SELENIUM

Selenium (Se) is a distinct trace element which is available in selenoproteins (SePs) in the form of selenocysteine (Secys). The 21st amino acid Secys is translationally incorporated into UGA codons in combination with the 3-utr Secys-insertion sequence (SECIS). SeP biosynthesis and its functions are crucial for sustaining the life of humans and animals (Köhrle, Jakob, Contempre, & Dumont, 2005). Cellular glutathione peroxidase (GPX) was the first enzyme identified as SeP. Further research identified SeP as a major antioxidant element that acts via enzymes which catalyze redox reactions (Rotruck et al., 1973). Furthermore, the identification of type I iodothyronine deiodinase as Se was a significant discovery for the formation of the connection between Se and thyroid hormones (Berry, Banu, & Larsen, 1991).

As an anti-inflammatory element, the role of Se has connections with its impact on immune cells and on the macrophage signal transduction pathways. Se supplementation has been shown to bring about a significant reduction in the bacterial endotoxin lipopolysaccharide (LPS) induced expression of the main pro-inflammatory genes TNF-α and cyclooxygenase-2 (COX-2) by inhibiting the MAP kinase pathways. Increased TNF-α levels, on the other hand, are likely to induce activation of NF-B at high levels at suppressed levels of Se, while at the same time augmenting CRP secretion by hepatocytes. TNF-α has the capacity of powerfully inducing adhesion molecules, which include endothelial leukocyte adhesion molecule-1 (E-selectin), intercellular adhesion molecule-1 (ICAM-1), and vascular cell adhesion molecule-1 (VCAM-1). These molecules are necessary for progressing endothelial cell proinflammation by involving leukocytes in the endothelium. With this regard, NF- κ B is essential for the transcription of the adhesion molecule genes. In an in vitro study, human umbilical vein endothelial cells (HUVECS) were added Se in the form of sodium selenite, and they were able to notably inhibit TNF-α induced expression of the adhesion molecules. Therefore, increased levels of Se may inhibit NF- κ B through GPx and reduce inflammation. A recent study reported a time-dependent increase in 15-deoxy-Δ 12,14-prostaglandin J 2 (15d-PGJ 2) production. Its formation is known to be mediated by cyclooxygenase-1 (COX-1) by means of selenium added macrophages induced by LPS. This is considered to be an adaptive response to redox regulation and cell protection against proinflammatory gene expression. Another notable anti-inflammatory mechanism of selenium is administered through its function of monocyte adhesion to endothelial cells and movement through tissues. Monocytes are known to stick to the endothelium and turn into macrophages, which are the primary effectors of innate immunity in inflammation. Also, the monocytes adhesion to the endothelial cells is modulated by L-selectin. L-selectin is a member of the selectin family. It facilitates neutrophil movement throughout the inflammatory response which is mediated by several ligands. L -Selectin expression can be notably downregulated by metalloproteinases. By splitting the receptor of L-selectin, they generate a soluble L-selectin which can hinder the sticking of lymphocytes to endothelial cells (Duntas, 2009).

The biological function of sL-selectin has not been established yet; however, decreased levels have been linked to high mortality rates in patients with SIRS (Smalley & Zey, 2005). According to recently published data, Se was found to cause the shedding of L-selectin from monocytes, which leads to degraded differentiation into macrophages; meanwhile, sL-selectin was found to notably increase. These findings have not been pathophysiologically validated yet. However, they may lay out a valid underlying mechanism. Selenium is determined to exert its anti-inflammatory action in patients with sepsis through this mechanism. Apart from this, high doses of Se have the capacity to impair other types of immunity including antiparasitic or allergic asthma responses. This indicates that Se levels can differently impact various kinds of immune response. Functional analysis of SePS polymorphism, – 105G A, considerably spoils SePS expression. This is then followed by higher plasma levels of the cytokines IL-6, IL-1 β, and TNF-α. These results prove that there is a link between SePS and cytokine production. Conversely, recent data could not put forward any role of SePS polymorphisms in the sensitivity to develop immune-mediated diseases. The inflammatory response is modulated by Se through variable and complex mechanisms (Duntas, 2009).

ZINC

Zinc is necessary for the activation of over 300 enzymes or stability of their structures, and there are over 2000 transcription factors which are included in gene expression of zinc-dependent proteins (Prasad, 1993). Zinc is known to be a molecular signal for immune cells, while homeostasis of intracellular zinc levels is sustained by 14 ZIP (SLC 39A) and 10 ZNT (SLC 30A) transporters.

Inflammation causes oxidative stress by augmenting ROS. This leads to the oxidation of LDL. Oxidized LDL stimulates the NF-kB inducible kinase/IK-b kinase/NF-kB by indicating the pathway and upregulates its downstream destination genes such as CRP, adhesion molecules, inflammatory cytokines, inducible nitric oxide synthase, fibrinogen, tissue factor, and cyclooxygenase 2. These cytokines and molecules draw neutrophils, monocytes, macrophages, and platelets, cause coagulation, and start the development of atherosclerosis. Zinc supplementation boosted plasma antioxidant power and lowered plasma inflammatory cytokines and oxidative stress biomarkers in the elderly subjects. Zinc reduced NF-kB activation and its target genes including TNF-α, IL-1b, and VCAM, and augmented the gene expression of A20 and PPAR-a. They are the two zinc finger proteins with anti-inflammatory characteristics in HL-60 and THP-1 cells and HAECs after ox-LDL stimulation. Therefore, zinc was found to reduce the expression of these cytokines and molecules by repression of NF-kB activation through A20 and PPAR-α pathways (Prasad, 2014).

COPPER

Copper can be found and measured in the copper-binding protein complex of ceruloplasmin. It is a positive APP and it is augmented during the acute and chronic inflammatory response. No studies have been found on the interaction between different levels of the acute phase responses and the copper-binding protein levels (Tomkins, 2003).

CONCLUSION

In conclusion, nutrition is an essential part of our lives. The nutritional status and physiological parameters of individuals are correlated and they affect the inflammation process. Future research is recommended to center on the role of specific dietary factors on biomarkers of inflammation as they may modulate inflammation via various mechanisms. Therapeutic lifestyle modifications continue to be the cornerstone in administering inflammation and diseases. Besides, further research should define the anti-inflammatory or pro-inflammatory effects of specific dietary factors. Nutritional deficiencies should be eliminated by providing adequate and balanced nutrition and individuals should be offered health-preserving nutrition recommendations.

REFERENCES

Adelekan, D. A., & Thurnham, D. I. (1990). Plasma ferritin concentrations in anemic children: Relative importance of malaria, riboflavin deficiency, and other infections. *The American Journal of Clinical Nutrition*, *51*(3), 453–456. doi:10.1093/ajcn/51.3.453 PMID:2309651

Adorini, L., & Penna, G. (2008). Control of autoimmune diseases by the vitamin D endocrine system. *Nature Clinical Practice. Rheumatology*, *4*(8), 404–412. doi:10.1038/ncprheum0855 PMID:18594491

Adzemovic, M. Z., Zeitelhofer, M., Hochmeister, S., Gustafsson, S. A., & Jagodic, M. (2013). Efficacy of vitamin D in treating multiple sclerosis-like neuroinflammation depends on developmental stage. *Experimental Neurology*, *249*, 39–48. doi:10.1016/j.expneurol.2013.08.002 PMID:23954214

Aguirre, R., & May, J. M. (2008). Inflammation in the vascular bed: Importance of vitamin C. *Pharmacology & Therapeutics*, *119*(1), 96–103. doi:10.1016/j.pharmthera.2008.05.002 PMID:18582947

Aranow, C. (2011). Vitamin D and the immune system. *Journal of Investigative Medicine*, *59*(6), 881–886. doi:10.2310/JIM.0b013e31821b8755 PMID:21527855

Autier, P., Boniol, M., Pizot, C., & Mullie, P. (2014). Vitamin D status and ill health: A systematic review. *The Lancet. Diabetes & Endocrinology*, *2*(1), 76–89. doi:10.1016/S2213-8587(13)70165-7 PMID:24622671

Bernardo, D., Martínez-Abad, B., Vallejo-Diez, S., Montalvillo, E., Benito, V., Anta, B., ... Garrote, J. A. (2012). Ascorbate-dependent decrease of the mucosal immune inflammatory response to gliadin in coeliac disease patients. *Arranz. Allergologia et Immunopathologia*, *40*(1), 3–8. doi:10.1016/j.aller.2010.11.003 PMID:21420224

Berry, M. J., Banu, L., & Larsen, P. R. (1991). Type I iodothyronine deiodinase is a selenocysteine-containing enzyme. *Nature*, *349*(6308), 438–440. doi:10.1038/349438a0 PMID:1825132

Besler, H. T., Comoğlu, S., & Okcu, Z. (2002). Serum levels of antioxidant vitamins and lipid peroxidation in multiple sclerosis. *Nutritional Neuroscience*, *5*(3), 215–220. doi:10.1080/10284150290029205 PMID:12041878

Biswas, S., Hwang, J. W., Kirkham, P. A., & Rahman, I. (2013). Pharmacological and dietary antioxidant therapies for chronic obstructive pulmonary disease. *Current Medicinal Chemistry*, *20*(12), 1496–1530. doi:10.2174/0929867311320120004 PMID:22963552

Bruckdorfer, K. R. (2008). Antioxidants and CVD. *Proceeding Natural Society*, *67*(2), 214–222. doi:10.1017/S0029665108007052 PMID:18412995

Bruunsgaard, H., Poulsen, H. E., Pedersen, B. K., Nyyssonen, K., Kaikkonen, J., & Salonen, J. T. (2003). Long-term combined supplementation with alpha-tocopherol and vitamin C have no detectable antiinflammatory effects in healthy men. *The Journal of Nutrition*, *133*(4), 1170–1173. doi:10.1093/jn/133.4.1170 PMID:12672938

Bunout, D., Petermann, M., Hirsch, S., de la Mazo, P., Suazo, M., Barrera, G., & Kauffman, R. (2000). Low serum folate but normal homocysteine levels in patients with atherosclerotic vascular disease and matched healthy controls. *Nutrition (Burbank, Los Angeles County, Calif.)*, *16*(6), 434–438. doi:10.1016/S0899-9007(00)00289-6 PMID:10869899

Calton, E. K., Keane, K. N., Newsholme, P., & Soares, M. J. (2015). The impact of vitamin D levels on inflammatory status: A systematic review of immune cell studies. *PLoS One*, *10*(11), e141770. doi:10.1371/journal.pone.0141770 PMID:26528817

Cannell, J. J., Grant, W. B., & Holick, M. F. (2014). Vitamin D and inflammation. *Dermato-Endocrinology*, *6*(1), 1–10. doi:10.4161/19381980.2014.983401 PMID:26413186

Carnes, C. A., Chung, M. K., Nakayama, T., Nakayama, H., Baliga, R. S., Piao, S., ... Van Wagoner, D. R. (2001). Ascorbate attenuates atrial pacing-induced peroxynitrite formation and electrical remodeling and decreases the incidence of postoperative atrial fibrillation. *Circulation Research*, *89*(6), E32–E38. doi:10.1161/hh1801.097644 PMID:11557745

Cartwright, G. E., Lauritsen, M. A., Humphreys, S., Jones, P. J., Merril, I. M., & Wintrobe, M. M. (1946). The Anemia of Infection in The Experimental Production of Hypoferremia and Anemia in Dogs. *The Journal of Clinical Investigation*, *25*(1), 81–86. doi:10.1172/JCI101691

Casas, R., & Estruch, R. (2016). Dietary Patterns, Foods, Nutrients and Chronic Inflammatory Disorders. *Immunologic Research*, *12*(2), 1–10.

De Tullio, M. C. (2010). The Mystery of Vitamin C. *Nature Education*, *3*(9), 48.

Denic, S., & Agarwal, M. M. (2007). Nutritional iron deficiency: An evolutionary perspective. *Nutrition (Burbank, Los Angeles County, Calif.)*, *23*(7-8), 603–614. doi:10.1016/j.nut.2007.05.002 PMID:17583479

Devaraj, S., Leonard, S., Traber, M. G., & Jialal, I. (2008). Gamma-tocopherol supplementation alone and in combination with alpha-tocopherol alters biomarkers of oxidative stress and inflammation in subjects with metabolic syndrome. *Free Radical Biology & Medicine*, *44*(6), 1203–1208. doi:10.1016/j.freeradbiomed.2007.12.018 PMID:18191645

Dhingra, D., Parle, M., & Kulkarni, S. K. (2006). Comparative brain cholinesterase-inhibitng activity of Glycyrrhiza glabra, Myristica fragrans, ascorbic acid, and metrifonate in mice. *Journal of Medicinal Food*, *9*(2), 281–283. doi:10.1089/jmf.2006.9.281 PMID:16822217

Doherty, C. P. (2007). Host-pathogen interactions: The role of iron. *The Journal of Nutrition*, *137*(5), 1341–1344. doi:10.1093/jn/137.5.1341 PMID:17449603

Drakesmith, H., & Prentice, A. (2008). Viral infection and iron metabolism. *Nature Reviews. Microbiology*, *6*(7), 541–552. doi:10.1038/nrmicro1930 PMID:18552864

Duggan, C., Colin, A. A., Agil, A., Higgins, L., & Rifai, N. (1996). Vitamin A status in acute exacerbations of cystic fibrosis. *The American Journal of Clinical Nutrition*, *64*(4), 635–639. doi:10.1093/ajcn/64.4.635 PMID:8839511

Duntas, L. H. (2009). Selenium and inflammation: Underlying anti-inflammatory mechanisms. *Hormonal Metabolic Researches*, *41*(06), 443–447. doi:10.1055-0029-1220724 PMID:19418416

Erbas, O., Solmaz, V., Aksoy, D., Yavasoglu, A., Sagcan, M., & Taskiran, D. (2014). Cholecalciferol (vitamin D_3) improves cognitive dysfunction and reduces inflammation in a rat fatty liver model of metabolic syndrome. *Life Sciences*, *103*(2), 68–72. doi:10.1016/j.lfs.2014.03.035 PMID:24727236

Esmon, C. T. (2000). The anticoagulant and anti-inflammatory roles of the protein C anticoagulant pathway. *Journal of Autoimmunity*, *5*(2), 113–116. doi:10.1006/jaut.2000.0400 PMID:10968895

Feng, X., Lv, C., Wang, F., Gan, K., Zhang, M., & Tan, W. (2013). Modulatory effect of 1,25-dihydroxyvitamin D 3 on IL-1 β-induced RANKL, OPG, TNF-α, and IL-6 expression in human rheumatoid synoviocyte MH7A. *Clinical & Developmental Immunology*, *2013*, 160123. doi:10.1155/2013/160123 PMID:24348674

Fischer, H., Schwarzer, C., & Illek, B. (2004). Vitamin C controls the cystic fibrosis transmembrane conductance regulator chloride channel. *Proceedings of the National Academy of Sciences of the United States of America*, *101*(10), 3691–3696. doi:10.1073/pnas.0308393100 PMID:14993613

Fitzgerald, K. C., O'Reilly, É. J., Fondell, E., Falcone, G. J., McCullough, M. L., Park, Y., ... Ascherio, A. (2013). Intakes of vitamin C and carotenoids and risk of amyotrophic lateral sclerosis: Pooled results from 5 cohort studies. *Annals of Neurology*, *73*(2), 236–245. doi:10.1002/ana.23820 PMID:23362045

Friis, H., Gomo, E., Koestel, P., Ndhlovu, P., Nyazema, N., Krarup, H., & Michaelsen, K. F. (2001). HIV and other predictors of serum folate, serum ferritin, and hemoglobin in pregnancy: A cross-sectional study in Zimbabwe. *The American Journal of Clinical Nutrition*, *73*(6), 1066–1073. doi:10.1093/ajcn/73.6.1066 PMID:11382661

Furuya, A., Uozaki, M., Yamasaki, H., Arakawa, T., Arita, M., & Koyama, A. H. (2008). Antiviral effects of ascorbic and dehydroascorbic acids in vitro. *International Journal of Molecular Medicine*, *22*(4), 541–545. PMID:18813862

Galloway, P., McMillan, D. C., & Sattar, N. (2000). Effect of the inflammatory response on trace element and vitamin status. *Annals of Clinical Biochemistry*, *37*(3), 289–297. doi:10.1258/0004563001899429 PMID:10817241

Gangaidzo, I. T., Moyo, V. M., Mvundura, E., Aggrey, G., Murphree, N. L., Khumalo, H., ... Gourdeuk, V. R. (2001). Association of pulmonary tuberculosis with increased dietary iron. *The Journal of Infectious Diseases*, *184*(7), 936–939. doi:10.1086/323203 PMID:11528590

Garcia-Vidal, C., Upton, A., Kirby, K. A., & Marr, K. A. (2008). Epidemiology of invasive mold infections in allogeneic stem cell transplant recipients: Biological risk factors for infection according to time after transplantation. *Clinical Infectious Diseases*, *47*(8), 1041–1050. doi:10.1086/591969 PMID:18781877

Gerhard, G. S., Levin, K. A., Price Goldstein, J., Wojnar, M. M., Chorney, M. J., & Belchis, D. A. (2001). Vibrio vulnificus septicemia in a patient with the hemochromatosis HFE C282Y mutation. *Archives of Pathology & Laboratory Medicine*, *125*, 1107–1109. PMID:11473471

Grosso, G., Bei, R., Mistretta, A., Marventano, S., Calabrese, G., & Masuelli, L. … Gazzolo, D. (2013). Effects of vitamin C on health: a review of evidence. Frontier in Bioscience (Landmark Ed), 18, 1017-1029.

Guillot, X., Semerano, L., Saidenberg-Kermanac'h, N., Falgarone, G., & Boissier, M. C. (2010). Vitamin D and inflammation. *Joint, Bone, Spine*, *77*(6), 552–557. doi:10.1016/j.jbspin.2010.09.018 PMID:21067953

Guo, J., Ma, Z., Ma, Q., Wu, Z., Fan, P., Zhou, X., ... Wu, E. (2013). 1,25$(OH)_2D_3$ inhibits hepatocellular carcinoma development through reducing secretion of inflammatory cytokines from immunocytes. *Current Medicinal Chemistry*, *20*(33), 4131–4141. doi:10.2174/09298673113209990248 PMID:23992309

Hasegawa, N., Niimi, N., & Odani, F. (2012). Vitamin C is one of the lipolytic substances in green tea. *Phytotherapies. Researches*, *16*(Suppl 1), S91–S92.

Helmersson, J., Ärnlöv, J., Larsson, A., & Basu, S. (2009). Low dietary intake of beta-carotene, alpha-tocopherol and ascorbic acid is associated with increased inflammatory and oxidative stress in a Swedish cohort. *British Journal of Nutrition*, *101*(12), 1775–1782. doi:10.1017/S0007114508147377 PMID:19079838

Helms, S., & Miller, A. (2006). Natural treatment of chronic rhinosinusitis. *Alternative Medicine Review*, *11*(3), 196–207. PMID:17217321

Henriksen, V. T., Rogers, V. E., Rasmussen, G. L., Trawick, R. H., Momberger, N. G., Aguirre, D., & Barker, T. (2014). Proinflammatory cytokines mediate the decrease in serum 25(OH)D concentrations after total knee arthroplasty? *Medical Hypotheses*, *82*(2), 134–137. doi:10.1016/j.mehy.2013.11.020 PMID:24332533

Heo, J. H., Hyon-Lee, & Lee, K.-M. (2013). The possible role of antioxidant vitamin C in Alzheimer's disease treatment and prevention. *American Journal of Alzheimer's Diseases and Other Dementions*, *28*(2), 120–125. doi:10.1177/1533317512473193 PMID:23307795

Hewison, M. (2011). Antibacterial effects of vitamin D. *Nature Reviews. Endocrinology*, *7*(6), 337–345. doi:10.1038/nrendo.2010.226 PMID:21263449

Hewison, M. (2011). Antibacterial effects of vitamin D. *Nature Reviews. Endocrinology*, *7*(6), 337–345. doi:10.1038/nrendo.2010.226 PMID:21263449

Hodges, S. J., Pitsillides, A. A., Ytrebø, L. M., & Soper, R. (2017). Anti-inflammatory actions of vitamin K. doi:10.5772/63891

Huang, J., & May, J. M. (2006). Ascorbic acid protects SH-SY5Y neuroblastoma cells from apoptosis and death induced by betaamyloid. *Brain Research*, *1097*(1), 52–58. doi:10.1016/j.brainres.2006.04.047 PMID:16725131

Ichim, T. E., Minev, B., Braciak, T., Luna, B., Hunninghake, R., Mikirova, N. A., ... Riordan, N. H. (2011). Intravenous ascorbic acid to prevent and treat cancer-associated sepsis? *Journal of Translational Medicine*, *4*, 9–25. PMID:21375761

Calder, P. C., Albers, R., Antoine, J. M., Blum, S., Bourdet-Sicard, R., Ferns, G. A., ... Løvik, M. (2009). Inflammatory disease processes and interactions with nutrition. *British Journal of Nutrition*, *1*, S1–S45. PMID:19586558

Iwamoto, J. (2014). Vitamin K_2 therapy for postmenopausal osteoporosis. *Nutrients*, *6*(5), 1971–1980. doi:10.3390/nu6051971 PMID:24841104

Jiang, Q. (2014). Natural forms of vitamin E: Metabolism, antioxidant, and anti-inflammatory activities and their role in disease, prevention and therapy. *Free Radical Biology & Medicine*, *72*, 76–90. doi:10.1016/j.freeradbiomed.2014.03.035 PMID:24704972

Kleinman, R. E., & Fracchia, M. S. (2010). Vitamin K and cystic fibrosis: Give me a double, please. *The American Journal of Clinical Nutrition*, *92*(3), 469–470. doi:10.3945/ajcn.2010.30138 PMID:20685948

Kochan, I. (1973). The role of iron in bacterial infections, with special consideration of host-tubercle bacillus interaction. *Current Topics in Microbiology and Immunology*, *60*, 1–30. doi:10.1007/978-3-642-65502-9_1 PMID:4197776

Köhrle, J. (2000). The deiodinase family: Selenoenzymes regulating thyroid hormone availability and action. *Cell Mololecules in Life Sciences*, *57*(13), 1853–1863. doi:10.1007/PL00000667 PMID:11215512

Köhrle, J., Jakob, F., Contempre, B., & Dumont, J. E. (2005). Selenium, the thyroid, and the endocrine system. *Endocrinology Reviews*, *26*(7), 944–984. doi:10.1210/er.2001-0034 PMID:16174820

Koka, S., Foller, M., Lamprecht, G., Boini, K. M., Lang, C., Huber, S. M., & Lang, F. (2007). Iron deficiency influences the course of malaria in Plasmodium berghei infected mice. *Biochemistry and Biophysology Research of Community*, *357*(3), 608–614. doi:10.1016/j.bbrc.2007.03.175 PMID:17445762

Korantzopoulos, P., Kolettis, T. M., Kountouris, E., Dimitroula, V., Karanikis, P., Pappa, E., ... Goudevenos, J. A. (2015). Oral vitamin C administration reduces early recurrence rates after electrical cardioversion of persistent atrial fibrillation and attenuates associated inflammation. *International Journal of Cardiology*, *102*(2), 321–326. doi:10.1016/j.ijcard.2004.12.041 PMID:15982504

Korf, H., Wenes, M., Stijlemans, B., Takiishi, T., Robert, S., Miani, M., ... Mathieu, C. (2012). 1,25-Dihydroxyvitamin D_3 curtails the inflammatory and T cell stimulatory capacity of macrophages through an IL-10-dependent mechanism. *Immunobiology*, *217*(12), 1292–1300. doi:10.1016/j.imbio.2012.07.018 PMID:22944250

Krishna, S., Taylor, A. M., Supanaranond, W., Pukrittayakamee, S., ter Kuile, F., Tawfiq, K. M., ... White, N. J. (1999). Thiamine deficiency and malaria in adults from southeast Asia. *Lancet*, *353*(9152), 546–549. doi:10.1016/S0140-6736(98)06316-8 PMID:10028983

Labadarios, D., Brink, P. A., Weich, H. F., Visser, L., Louw, M. E., Shephard, G. S., & van Stuijberg, M. E. (1987). Plasma vitamin A, E, C and B6 levels in myocardial infarction. *South African Medical Journal*, *71*, 561–563. PMID:3576402

Li, Y., & Schellhorn, H. E. (2007). New developments and novel therapeutic perspectives for vitamin C. *The Journal of Nutrition*, *137*(10), 2171–2184. doi:10.1093/jn/137.10.2171 PMID:17884994

Lounis, N., Truffot-Pernot, C., Grosset, J., Gordeuk, V. R., & Boelaert, J. R. (2001). Iron and mycobacterium tuberculosis infection. *Journal of Clinical Virology*, *20*(3), 123–126. doi:10.1016/S1386-6532(00)00136-0 PMID:11166659

Louw, J. A., Werbeck, A., Louw, M. E., Kotze, T. J., Cooper, R., & Labadarios, D. (1992). Blood vitamin concentrations during the acute-phase response. *Critical Care Medicine*, *20*(7), 934–941. doi:10.1097/00003246-199207000-00007 PMID:1617986

Mangge, H., Weghuber, D., Prassl, R., Haara, A., Schnedl, W., Postolache, T., & Fuchs, D. (2013). The role of vitamin D in atherosclerosis inflammation revisited: More a bystander than a player? *Current Vascular Pharmacology*, *13*(3), 392–398. doi:10.2174/15701611113666131209125454 PMID:24329737

McCabe, K. M., Adams, M. A., & Holden, R. M. (2013). Vitamin K status in chronic kidney disease. *Nutrients*, *5*(11), 4390–4398. doi:10.3390/nu5114390 PMID:24212088

McMillan, D. C., Maguire, D., & Talwar, D. (2019). Relationship between nutritional status and the systemic inflammatory response: Micronutrients. *The Proceedings of the Nutrition Society*, *78*(1), 56–67. doi:10.1017/S0029665118002501 PMID:30220267

Moretti, M. L., Budni, J., Dos Santos, D. B., Antunes, A., Daufenbach, J. F., Manosso, L. M., ... Rodrigues, A. L. (2013). Protective effects of ascorbic acid on behavior and oxidative status of restraint-stressed mice. *Journal of Molecular Neuroscience*, *49*(1), 68–79. doi:10.100712031-012-9892-4 PMID:23054587

Murray, M. F. (1999). Niacin as a potential AIDS preventive factor. *Medical Hypotheses*, *53*(5), 375–379. doi:10.1054/mehy.1999.0908 PMID:10616035

Mutlu-Turkoglu, U., Oztezcan, S., Telci, A., Orhan, Y., Aykac-Toker, G., Sivas, A., & Uysal, M. (2003). An increase in lipoprotein oxidation and endogenous lipid peroxides in serum of obese women. *Clinical and Experimental Medicine*, *2*(4), 171–174. doi:10.1007102380300002 PMID:12624707

Nakajima, S., Iijima, H., Egawa, S., Shinzaki, S., Kondo, J., Inoue, T., ... Hayashi, N. (2011). Association of vitamin K deficiency with bone metabolism and clinical disease activity in inflammatory bowel disease. *Nutrition*, *27*(10), 1023–1028. doi:10.1016/j.nut.2010.10.021 PMID:21482072

Newsholme, P., Haber, E. P., Hirabara, S. M., Rebelato, E. L. O., Procopio, J., Morgan, D., ... Curi, R. (2007). Diabetes associated cell stress and dysfunction: Role of mitochondrial and non-mitochondrial ROS production and activity. *The Journal of Physiology*, *583*(1), 9–24. doi:10.1113/jphysiol.2007.135871 PMID:17584843

Ojaimi, S., Skinner, N. A., Strauss, B. J., Sundararajan, V., Woolley, I., & Visvanathan, K. (2013). Vitamin D deficiency impacts on expression of toll-like receptor-2 and cytokine profile: A pilot study. *Journal of Translational Medicine*, *11*(1), 176. doi:10.1186/1479-5876-11-176 PMID:23875738

Ozkalay, N., Anil, M., Agus, N., Helvaci, M., & Sirti, S. (2006). Community-acquired meningitis and sepsis caused by Chryseobacterium meningosepticum in a patient diagnosed with thalassemia major. *Journal of Clinical Microbiology*, *44*(8), 3037–3039. doi:10.1128/JCM.00588-06 PMID:16891537

Prasad, A. S. (1993). *Biochemistry of Zinc*. New York: Plenum Press. doi:10.1007/978-1-4757-9444-1

Prasad, A. S. (2014). Zinc is an antioxidant and anti-inflammatory agent: Its role in human health. *Frontiers In Nutrition*, *1*, 14. doi:10.3389/fnut.2014.00014 PMID:25988117

Romieu, I. (2005). Nutrition and lung health. *The International Journal of Tuberculosis and Lung Disease*, *9*(4), 362–374. PMID:15830741

Rossman, M. J., Garten, R. S., Groot, H. J., Reese, V., Zhao, J., Amann, M., & Richardson, R. S. (2013). Ascorbate infusion increases skeletal muscle fatigue resistance in patients with chronic obstructive pulmonary disease. *The American Journal of Physiology*, *305*(10), R1163–R1170. PMID:24068051

Rotruck, J. T., Pope, A. L., Ganther, H. E., Swanson, A. B., Hafeman, D. G., & Hoekstra, W. G. (1973). Selenium: Biochemical role as a component of glutathione peroxidase. *Science Magazine*, *179*, 558–590. PMID:4686466

Schmidt, R., Luboeinski, T., Markart, P., Ruppert, C., Daum, C., Grimminger, F., ... Günther, A. (2004). Alveolar antioxidant status in patients with acute respiratory distress syndrome. *The European Respiratory Journal*, *24*(6), 994–999. doi:10.1183/09031936.04.00120703 PMID:15572544

Senen, D., Adanali, G., Ayhan, M., Gorgu, M., & Erdogan, B. (2002). Contribution of vitamin C administration for increasing lipolysis. *Aesthetic Plastic Surgery*, *26*(2), 123–125. doi:10.100700266-002-1468-1 PMID:12016497

Sikkens, E. C., Cahen, D. L., Koch, A. D., Braat, H., Poley, J. W., Kuipers, E. J., & Bruno, M. J. (2013). The prevalence of fat-soluble vitamin deficiencies and a decreased bone mass in patients with chronic pancreatitis. *Pancreatology*, *13*(3), 238–242. doi:10.1016/j.pan.2013.02.008 PMID:23719594

Smalley, D. M., & Ley, K. (2005). L-selectin: Mechanisms and physiological significance of ectodomain cleavage. *Journal of Cell and Moleculer Medicine*, *9*(2), 255–266. doi:10.1111/j.1582-4934.2005.tb00354.x PMID:15963248

Sorice, A., Guerriero, E., Capone, F., Colonna, G., Castello, G., & Costantini, S. (2014). Ascorbic acid: Its role in immune system and chronic inflammation diseases. *Mini-Reviews in Medicinal Chemistry*, *14*(5), 444–452. doi:10.2174/1389557514666140428112602 PMID:24766384

Stephensen, C. B., Marquis, G. S., Jacob, R. A., Kruzich, L. A., Douglas, S. D., & Wilson, C. M. (2006). Vitamins C and E in adolescents and young adults with HIV infection. *The American Journal of Clinical Nutrition*, *83*(4), 870–879. doi:10.1093/ajcn/83.4.870 PMID:16600941

Tavazzi, B., Batocchi, A. P., Amorini, A. M., Nociti, V., D'Urso, S., & Longo, S. (2011). ... Lazzarino, G. (2011). Serum metabolic profile in multiple sclerosis patients. *Multiple Sclerosis International*. PMID:22096628

Thurnham, D. I., & McCabe, G. P. (2012). Influence of infection and inflammation on biomarkers of nutritional status with an emphasis on vitamin A and iron. In World Health Organization. Report: Priorities in the assessment of vitamin A and iron status in populations. Geneva, World Health Organization.

Tomkins, A. (2003). Assessing Micronutrient Status in the Presence of Inflammation. *The Journal of Nutrition*, *133*(5), 1649S–1655S. doi:10.1093/jn/133.5.1649S PMID:12730480

Wannamethee, S. G., Bruckdorfer, K. R., Shaper, A. G., Papacosta, O., Lennon, L., & Whincup, P. H. (2013). Plasma vitamin C, but not vitamin E, is associated with reduced risk of heart failure in older men. *Circulation: Heart Failure*, *6*(4), 647–654. doi:10.1161/CIRCHEARTFAILURE.112.000281 PMID:23729199

Wessling-Resnick, M. (2010). Iron Homeostasis and the Inflammatory Response. *Annual Review of Nutrition*, *21*(30), 105–122. doi:10.1146/annurev.nutr.012809.104804 PMID:20420524

Wróblewski, K. (2005). Can the administration of large doses of vitamin C have a harmful effect? *Polish Merkur Lekarsk*, *19*(112), 600–603. PMID:16379336

Wu, T. C., Huang, Y. C., Hsu, S. Y., Wang, Y. C., & Yeh, S. L. (2007). Vitamin E and vitamin C supplementation in patients with chronic obstructive pulmonary disease. *International Journal of Vitamine and Nutrition Reseaches*, *77*(4), 272–279. doi:10.1024/0300-9831.77.4.272 PMID:18271282

Yilmaz, S. S., Hizli, D., Yilmaz, E., Eryilmaz, O. G., Hizli, F., & Haltas, H. (2013). Effect of vitamin D on postoperative adhesion formation in a rat uterine horn adhesion model. *The Journal of Reproductive Medicine*, *58*, 511–516. PMID:24568046

Zhang, Y., Leung, D. Y., Richers, B. N., Liu, Y., Remigio, L. K., Riches, D. W., & Goleva, E. (2012). Vitamin D inhibits monocyte/macrophage proinflammatory cytokine production by targeting MAPK phosphatase-1. *Journal of Immunology*, *188*(5), 2127–2135. doi:10.4049/jimmunol.1102412 PMID:22301548

Zhang, Z. W., & Farthing, M. J. G. (2000). Helicobacter Pylori and gastric malignancy: Importance of oxidants, antioxidants and other cofactors. In R. H. Hunt & G. N. J. Tytgat (Eds.), *Helicobacter pylor: Basic mechanisms to clinical cure* (pp. 513–524). London: Kluwer Academic Publishers. doi:10.1007/978-94-011-3927-4_55

Zhang, Z. W., Patchett, S. E., Perrett, D., Domizio, P., & Farthing, M. J. (2000). Gastric alpha-tocopherol and beta-carotene concentrations in association with Helicobacter pylori infection. *European Journal of Gastroenterology & Hepatology*, *12*(5), 497–503. doi:10.1097/00042737-200012050-00004 PMID:10833091

Chapter 5
Pro-/Anti-Inflammatory Bioactive Proteins and Peptides

Fatma Esra Güneş
University of Marmara, Turkey

ABSTRACT

Bioactive peptides (BP) are specific protein fragments that can affect biological processes or substrates that have a positive impact on functions and conditions on body health. Plant and animal sources that contain physiologically active food proteins, native or processed, are rich sources of bioactive peptides. Bioactive peptides derived from food proteins have been demostrated to have variety of beneficial effects, such as anti-inflammatory and antioxidant properties. BP are accepted the new generation of biologically active regulators; they can prevent oxidation and microbial degradation in foods and furthermore improve quality of life by treating various diseases and disorders. The present review highlights the recent findings on the roles of various food-derived bioactive peptides in inflammation and oxidative stress and discuss the potential benefits and limitations of using these compounds against the burden of chronic diseases.

BACKGROUND

While proteins were just considered as a source of energy and essential nutrient for the body and the health of human, after the discovery and characterisation of proteolytic enzymes, there was generation of protein hydrolysates by means of such enzymes. Protein hydrolysates are defined as complex mixtures of oligopeptides, peptides, and free amino acids that are produced by partial or extensive hydrolysis. Peptides, and free amino acids, are more readily absorbed in the digestive tract when

DOI: 10.4018/978-1-7998-3594-3.ch005

compared to native proteins (García & Manrique, 2019). Recent scientific evidence of research has revealed that many food proteins and peptides exhibit specific biological activities in addition to their established nutritional value (Mine & Shahidi, 2006; Hartmann & Meisel, 2007; Moller, Scholz-Ahrens, Roos, & Schrezenmeir, 2008; Mine, Li-Chan, & Jiang, 2010).

There are many examples of biologically active food proteins with physiological importance that go beyond pure nutritional requirements that concern the available nitrogen for normal growth and development (Kitts & Weiler, 2003).

Bioactive Peptides (BP) (Sharma, Singh, & Rana, 2011; Walther & Sieber, 2011) have been defined as specific protein fragments that can affect biological processes or substrates that have a positive impact on functions and conditions on body health (Kitts & Weiler, 2003; Sánchez & Vazquez, 2017). It is considered as "bioactive" if a dietary component imparts a measurable biological effect at a physiologically realistic level and if it is measured as "bioactivity", it has to have the potential (at least) to affect health in a beneficial way (Schrezenmeir, Korhonen, Williams, Gill, & Shah, 2000; Moller et al., 2008; Moughan & Rutherfurd-Markwick, 2013). Plant and animal sources that contain physiologically active food proteins, native or processed, are rich sources of bioactive peptides (Yoshikawa et al., 2000; Chakrabarti, Jahandideh & Wu, 2014; Malaguti, Dinelli, Leoncini, Bregola, Bosi, Cicero, & Hrelia, 2014; Massaccesi, 2016; Moronta, 2016). BPs are predominantly encrypted inside bioactive proteins. Peptides obtained from proteins from all imaginable sources (vegetable, fungi, animal, or even bacteria in origin) have been generated and characterised based on their structure, functional properties, and the type of bioactivity (García & Manrique, 2019). In addition, there are many physiologically active peptides derived from protease activity from various food protein sources; however, the relationship between structural features and functional activities are not fully explained (Kitts & Weiler, 2003). By far, bovine milk (Torres-Llanez, Vallejo-Cordoba, & Gonzalez-Cordova, 2005; Korhonen & Pihlanto, 2006; Korhonen, 2009; Léonil, 2014; Mohanty, Mohapatra, Misra, & Sahu, 2016), cheese (Pritchard, Phillips & Kailasapathy, 2010), and dairy products (Choi, Sabikhi, Hassan & Anand, 2012), bovine blood (Przybylski, Firdaous, Châtaigné, Dhulster, & Nedjar, 2016), gelatin (Lassoued, Mora, Barkia, Aristoy, Nasri, & Toldra, 2015), meat, eggs, various fish species such as tuna, sardine, herring and salmon are the animal sources that the bioactive proteins and peptides are obtained. Some plant-based sources of BP and proteins are wheat (Kumagai, 2010), maize, soy (Singh, Vij & Hati, 2014), rice (Selamassakul, Laohakunjit, Kerdchoechuen, & Ratanakhanokchai, 2016), mushrooms, pumpkin, sorghum (corn, rice, barley, sunflowers, etc.) and amaranth (Wang & Gonzalez de Mejia, 2005; Silva-Sanchez, de la Rosa, Leon-Galvan, de Lumen, de Leon-Rodriguez & de Mejia, 2008). Currently, more than 1500 distinctive BP have been notified in a database named 'Biopep' (Singh et al., 2014; Sánchez & Vazquez, 2017).

It is reported that the bioactive peptides in the human body can be acquired from two distinctive sources: endogenous bioactive peptides (TEnBP) and exogenous bioactive peptides (ExBP). TEnBP and ExBP was found out to be major role in metabolism. The peptide body bindes to the recycling and reuse of macromolecules, especially proteins. Proteolytic activity, a omnipresent processing in the body, plays a key role in several physiological mechanism just as digestion of dietary proteins, proteolytic cleavage of N-terminal signalling consecutions, and activation of zymogens. Thereby, the idea has emerged that there is area for the body to benefit from proteins in addition to their primary functions, as cryptomic sources of bioactive peptides concern about the dynamic local and systemic environments (Dave, 2019). The biological functions of the peptides, in some instances, are subjected by a definite amino acid sequence, while in other instances, it bases on the relative rate of a particular amino acid or group of amino acids (Siebert, 2001). Just as the amino acid design, charge, hydrophobic properties, weight and length of the peptides, and type of residues at C- and N-terminals. All of these factors influence the functional properties and biological activities of a peptide (Li, He, & Qian, 2011; Bhat, Kumar, & Bhat, 2015; Rizzello, Tagliazucchi, Babini, Sefora Rutella, Taneyo Saa, & Gianotti, 2016, Daliri, Oh, & Lee, 2017; Chalamaiah, Yu, & Wu, 2018; Guha & Majumder, 2018; Chalamaiah, Ulug, Hong, & Wu, 2019). Many BPs share some structural features that include a peptide residue length between 2–20 amino acids (Moller et al., 2008) and the presence of hydrophobic amino acids in addition to proline, lysine or arginine groups (Sánchez & Vazquez, 2017).

Bioactive peptides commonly does not function actively within the native proteins; to obtain their specific "bioactive" functions, proteolysis such as in vivo digestion, in vitro enzymatic hydrolysis, or bacterial fermentation during (Chakrabarti et al., 2014) food processing or ripening or gastrointestinal digestion after food consumption must be released (Kitts & Weiler, 2003; Hartmann & Meisel, 2007; Guha & Majumder, 2018).

During digestion, the BP can be absorbed from the intestine to the blood stream and provided by either local effects in the gastrointestinal system or systemic effects. It was shown in results of pancreatic digestion, KVLPVP peptide obtained from casein that have a much higher angiotensin converting enzyme (ACE) inhibitory activity than that of generated by only L. helveticus proteolysis (KVLPVPQ) (Korhonen & Pihlanto, 2007; Marcone, Belton, & Fitzgerald, 2017).

Some BPs can perform their activity at gastrointestinal level by directly binding to digestive membrane receptors (e.g. opioid receptors) (Massaccesi, 2016; Bouglé & Bouhallab, 2017). Some food proteins (e.g. lactoferrin, wheat albumin, immunoglobulins) fulfill their functions directly in the intestine in their complete form, but what is of even greater importance is the numerous peptides released from proteins by proteolysis occurring during food processing (Moughan & Rutherfurd-Markwick, 2013).

In vivo, gastrointestinal digestion (GI) is the last step for the generation of encrypted peptides responsible for the generation of multiple peptides, including bioactive sequences or by microbial enzymes that are found in the gut or in the food target different cleavage sites in comparison with isolated (Marcone et al., 2017) and in vitro, during food processing or ripening by microbial enzymes (e.g. Lactobacillus helveticus) (Gobbetti, Stepaniak, De Angelis, Corsetti, & Di Cagno, 2002; Dziuba & Dziuba, 2014; Sánchez & Vazquez, 2017).

In vitro enzymatic hydrolysis of food proteins for originating the bioactive function of the peptides is generally performed by using proteolytic enzymes (Sgarbieri, 2017) in the integral hydrolysates, produced as specific, as alcalase, thermolysin, trypsin, papain, flavourzyme, pancreatin, pepsin, chymotrypsin, neutrase and protamex, in proteolysis of food proteins, the fermentation is generally provided by identified as safe (GRAS) different microbial strains, for instance lactic acid bacteria (LAB). (Bhat et al., 2015; Rizzello et al., 2016; Chalamaiah et al., 2018; Chalamaiah et al., 2019). The fermentation processes are involved in affecting flavour development and providing to the occuring of bioactive peptides (Mora, Gallego, & Toldrá, 2018).

Bioactive phosphopeptides are obtained from phosphoproteins that are the phosphocaseins in milk and the proteins composed of phosvitin (60%) and lipovitelin in egg yolk. A subunit of casein contains 1 to 13 phosphoserine residues to stabilize the amorphous calcium phosphate, while an egg yolk protein molecule (phosvitin) contains approximately 120 phosphoserine residues (Castellani, Guérin-Dubiard, David-Briand & Anton, 2004). Phosvitin that contains 90% of all phosphorus in the egg yolk is conceived one of the most phosphorylated proteins found in internal with phosphorus content ranging from 3% to 10% of the molecule and a potential source of bioactive phosphopeptides. It is highly resistant to proteolytic digestion, composed of long continuous segments of oligophosphoserine. It is shown by Goulas et al., (1996) that phosvitin can be to hydrolysis by pepsin, trypsin, and α-chymotrypsin. Pepsin produced 3 peptides: Gly4 – Glu 41 (38 res); Asn 44 – Leu 193 (150 res); and a C-terminal fragment, Leu 193 – Glu 214 (21 res). Action of trypsin resulted in 2 main peptides, Ala 1 – Arg 35 (35 res) and Gln 49 – Arg 212 (164 res). Digestion by α-chymotrypsin released 2 peptides, Gly4 – Gln 49 (46 res) and Ala 50 – Trp 210 (161 res) (Sgarbieri, 2017).

Caseinophosphopeptides (CPPS) and glycomacropeptide (GMP) that have high phosphoserine content and are a mixture of peptides with different molecular masses that about 50% of the CPPs identified the sequence (SerPSerP-SerP-Glu-Glu) as responsible for the property of binding minerals (Bouhallab, 2002) were skilled of increasing the calcium balance by 39% to 70% and could also bind, in addition to Ca, other minerals like Mg, Fe, Ba, Cr, Ni, Se, Co, according to last studies (Scholz-

Ahrens & Schrezenmeir, 2000) CPPs also act as antioxidant at intestinal level, protecting the intestine against oxidative stress and helping to maintain intestinal health (Kitts, 2005). The glycomacropeptide occurs from Kappa casein which due to being water soluble remains in whey after coagulation and separation of caseins, in the milk-clotting process by action of the enzyme chymosin and represents the C-terminal portion of κ-casein (f: 106-169) (Sgarbieri, 2017).

Natural opioids that present the N-terminal sequence (Tyr-Gly-Gly-Phe) are peptides known as enkephalin, endorphin, and dynorphin and are derived respectively from proopiomelanocortin, proenkephalin, and prodynorphin (Bitri, 2004). Opioids are released by all caseins and by some whey proteins. Opioid peptides were obtained from β-casein (f: 60-70), which are the β-casomorphins, and from α-S1-casein (f: 90-96), called α-casomorphins. Unlike the α- and β-caseins, the Kappa-caseins release antagonist opioids or antiopioids. It has been shown that casomorphins can produce analgesia, increase the intestinal transit time of food bolus, and stimulate the absorption of amino acids and electrolytes (Sgarbieri, 2017).

It has been reported that most of peptides and protein hydrolysates from plant and animal origin possess have antioxidant activity. For instance, peptides proceed from soy protein (Wang & De Mejia, 2005; Singh et al., 2014), whey protein, casein, (Phelan, Aherne, Fitz Gerald, & O'Brien, 2009), corn protein (Li et al., 2008), potato protein (Wang & Xiong, 2005), wheat protein, gelatin (Mendis, Rajapakse, Byun & Kim, 2005), egg protein (Bhat et al., 2015a) and muscle protein indicated antioxidant properties (Liu, Xing, Fu, Zhou & Zhang, 2016; Sánchez & Vazquez, 2017).

The antioxidant potential of protein hydrolysates depends on evidenced on the amino acid design and on the disjunction of the tertiary structure of main proteins by enzymatic hydrolysis that end up amelioration in the dissolving accessibility of oxidatively labile amino acid residues. The availability of antioxidant peptide segments in proteins might help to describe why dietary protein intake can support human health beyond the standard nutritional benefits exerted (Elias, Kellerby, & Decker, 2008; Sánchez & Vazquez, 2017).

As well as with the suppression or stimulation of immune responses, the bioactive peptides action mechanism is related to direct interaction with pathogens (Honcock & Sahl, 2006). Studies show that both immunosuppression and immunostimulation can be important in preventing and combating several pathological conditions of the organism, and the biopeptides may act against inflammation, autoimmune diseases, preventing rejection in transplants and improving general health. There are numerous examples in the literature of such interactions, most with peptides derived from milk such as article of Gauthier et al., (2006) noted about the positive effect of peptides on lymphocyte proliferation, especially the effect of milk peptides on antibody production (Sgarbieri, 2017).

Because Nitric Oxide (NO) production is an inflammatory reply to oxidative stress in cells, the overproduction of NO has been reported to play a part in definite inflammatory diseases, as diabetes mellitus, neurodegenerative disorders, and other inflammatory circumstance. It is pointed that the LPS-stimulated macrophage cells produced NO to a degree many times higher than that of untreated cells. Various mechanisms that include the binding to lipid A moiety of LPS and the interference with LPS–CD14 interaction by competition with LPS-binding protein have been suggested for the inhibition of LPS-induced effects on macrophage cell lines by proteins and peptides (Haversen, 2002), and the amino acid sequence of the peptides impact peptide internalization by cells which may change their inhibitory effect. LPS-stimulated RAW264.7 macrophage cells can release large amounts of pro-inflammatory cytokines, such as TNF-x and IL-1. These cytokines can prompt macrophage cells and stimulate the production of other inflammatory cytokines, contributing to different pathophysiological conditions (Chawla, 2011). Downregulation of these cytokines are a significant advance in anti-inflammatory therapy. The downregulation of NO and the pro-inflammatory cytokines TNF- α and IL-1 demostrate a potential anti-inflammatory property of BLG-derived peptides.

It is known that the bioactivity of peptides can be influenced by various factors, including peptide size, composition, and the positioning of the amino acids in the sequence (Hartmann & Meisel, 2007). The occurrence of terminal Leu (L) or Phe (F)—especially C-terminal Leu—has been reported to positively contribute to the antioxidant activity of peptides (Mendis et al., 2005). About 38% of the total amino acids of the identified peptides are composed of hydrophobic and aromatic residues, which possibly contribute to anti-inflammatory properties (Bamdad, 2017a; Bamdad, 2017). In their study, Feng et al., (2019) isolated the antioxidant peptides and described from hydrolysates of walnut meal proteins. The hydrolysates were sequentially purified by ultrafiltration, gel filtration and RP-HPLC to obtain 6 important peptides (VRN, NPAN, AHSVGP, SSE, TY and SGGY) using UPLC-QTOF-MS. TY and SGGY showed stronger ABTS radical scavenging activity and higher ORAC values compared to the other four peptides (Feng, Peng, Wang, Li, Lei, & Xu, 2019).

Reactive oxygen species are often present during the inflammation process. Macrophages and neutrophils that contain the nicotinamide adenine dinucleotide phosphate (NADPH) oxidase complex generate superoxide radicals and hydrogen peroxide to aid in the destruction of foreign agents during the course of inflammation (Young & Mine, 2010).

Most of the dietary proteins demonstrate biological activity in the gastrointestinal tract. These activities range from enhancement of nutrient absorption, inhibition of enzymes, enzyme activity and growth stimulation to the modulation of the immune system in defending against pathogens. A number of proteins have been suggested to facilitate the uptake of essential nutrients. For example, α and β-caseins are thought to enhance calcium uptake by forming soluble casein phosphopeptides during digestion; lactoferrin appears to facilitate iron uptake, whereas other proteins such as vitamin B 12 -binding protein (haptocorrin) and folate-binding protein improve the availability of vitamins. The bioactivities observed for a number of milk proteins such as immunoglobulins and vitamin- or mineral-binding proteins indicate that bioactive proteins are of importance for the development and protection of newborn mammals (Korhonen & Pihlanto, 2006; Walther & Sieber, 2011).

It is known that the in vivo digestion of milk proteins occurs in the stomach under the pepsin, gastric digestive proteinases that digest around 20% proteins. Then, the digested pepsin moves to the duodenum where peptides are further hydrolyzed by pancreatic enzymes. The digestion process is completed by membrane proteases and various peptidases present in the brush border of the small intestine and released by the intestinal microflora. An amino acid residue or a dipeptide from the N- and C-terminal side of oligopeptides are released from these peptidases. Phosphatase(s) found in the brush border of the apical membrane of enterocytes, act(s) in removing phosphate groups, thus giving rise to partial or full peptide dephosphorylation of peptides in different body districts. The phosphorylated sequence is responsible, at the intestinal pH, for binding Ca++, Zn++, and Mg++ and for the in vivo resistance of the complex to gastrointestinal proteases (Pinto, Caira, Cuollo, Lill, Chianese, & Addeo, 2012). However, Fe complexed to β-CN (f15-25)4P was scarcely hydrolyzed in the digestion, suggesting that the coordination of iron ions to CPP blocks the action of both phosphatase and peptidases (Boutrou, Coirre, Jardin & Léonil, 2010). In addition, it was reported brush border enzyme alkaline phosphatase activity could increase the absorption of Fe complexed CPP by releasing Fe from peptides, and Fe complexed to β-CN CPP was absorbed more than Fe complexed to αs1-CN CPP. The variances in protein composition between cow and breast milk may explain some of the differences in the Fe bioavailability of the latter (Kibangou et al., 2005). Iron deficiency, which is a serious nutritional problem, can be decreased by CPP. Fe complexed CPP acts to prevent the formation of poorly absorbed high molecular weight ferric hydroxides. Zinc absorption can also be improved by the formation of Zn complexed to CCP, especially to β-CN (f1-25)4P. Some amount of the mineral CPP complex that was formed in the small intestine was resistant to the digestive and enteric bacteria enzymes and found in the feces of rats fed a casein-based diet (Pinto et al., 2012).

Despite the fact that there is conflicting data in literature on the intestinal absorption of CPP, it seems that the peptides tend to interact directly with the plasma membrane. Another possibility of CPP action on the transmembrane flux of calcium is that CPP might insert themselves into the plasma membrane and form their own calcium selective channels. For the same reason, they may act as calcium-carrier peptides rapidly internalized via endocytosis or other processes and eventually provide ionized calcium in the cytosol (Ferraretto, Signorile, Gravaghi, Fiorilli, & Tettamanti, 2001). The incoming of foreign material, such as CPP, across the mucosal brush-border into the enterocyte is conditioned by the adequate dephosphorylation of peptides by alkaline phosphatase. A more in-depth investigation is needed for the clarification of this issue (Pinto et al., 2012).

Bovine milk is one of the bioactive compound sources. BPs in milk is produced by lysozyme, lactoferrin, immunoglobulins, growth factors and hormones, and may be produced by hydrolysis of native proteins. Milk-derived bioactive peptides are generally encoded and kept ineffective in the primary structure of the milk protein and produced by proteolysis of casein (α-, β-, γ- and κ-casein) and whey proteins (β-lactoglobulin, α-lactalbumin, serum albumin, immunoglobulins, lactoferrin and protease-peptone fractions) (Marcone et al., 2017). These peptides are small in size and have peptidase-resistant carboxyl-terminal proline-proline sequences. Therefore, it coul be considered they are stable and absorbed (Seppo, Jauhiainen, Poussa, & Korpela, 2003). When a whey protein concentrate was treated with trypsin and the obtained peptides were separated using membrane ultrafiltration / nanofiltration, β-lactoglobulin peptides predominated in the hydrolysate (Boutrou, Henry, & Sanchez-Rivera, 2015; Arrutia, Puente, Riera, Menéndez, & González, 2016b; Sánchez & Vazquez, 2017).

Most of these peptides are obtained from the hydrolysis of the major milk proteins through proteolysis, either by using digestive enzymes or by fermentation, although some are naturally occurring and need little or no modification to become active (Moughan & Rutherfurd-Markwick, 2013).

Egg white contains ovoinhibitor, a serine proteinase inhibitor that can reduce enzymatic digestion by trypsin and chymotrypsin. Moreover, it has been demonstrated that certain egg proteins can be absorbed intact. The egg protein bioavailability can be impacted by methods of cooking and preparation of eggs. In studies, it was found that cooked egg proteins were highly digestible (~ 91%) compared to raw egg protein (~ 51%) (Andersen, 2015).

Egg-derived bioactive peptides are generally encoded and ineffective in the primary structure of the egg protein and are produced by proteolysis of the egg protein such as ovalbumin, ovotransferrin, ovomucoid, ovoinhibitor, cystatin, ovomucin, ovoflavoprotein, ovomacroglobulin ovokinin, avidin, ımmunoglobulin and lysozyme (Kitts & Weiler, 2003).

Fish and meat, a source of dietary protein, also contribute to human health through the production of bioactive peptides (Chakrabarti et al., 2014).

The process before consuming meat such as cooking, could facilitate the later generation of bioactive peptides due to denatured proteins being more susceptible to being hydrolysed by the enzymes of the intestinal tract. Proteases that have been used for the hydrolysis of food proteins are obtained from different sources such as of microbial, plant, or animal origin. An enzyme, Flavourzyme from Aspergillus oryzae, and Neutrase and Alcalase from Bacillus subtilis and Bacillus lincheniformis have been the most used in the generation of bioactive peptides in meat and meat products. Proteases from plant origin such as bromelain and papain are enzymes that do the hydrolysis of meat proteins for contribution to meat tenderisation. These enzymes show a wider specificity in comparison with other enzymes such as trypsin or pepsin, cleaving peptide bonds from a wide variety of regions and frequently acting aseither endopeptidases, or as exopeptidases hydrolysing amino acids from N- and C-terminal sites (Toldrá, Reig, Aristoy, & Mora, 2018). Proteolysis by endogenous proteases is the most important event occurring in the ageing of meat that influences its final characteristics with endogenous peptidases as main figures. Lactic acid bacteria such as Lactobacillus sakei, Lactobacillus curvatus, Lactobacillus plantarum and Lactobacillus casei alone or in combination with staphylococci, Kocuria, yeast, or moulds, exert proteolysis through the action of endo- and exopeptidases.

Endopeptidases such as calpains and cathepsins are first responsible for the hydrolysis of proteins into large fragments and oligopeptides, which affect the texture of meat during ageing and the initial steps of curing processes. Later, the activity of exopeptidases such as aminopeptidases and carboxypeptidases will generate small peptides and free amino acids, responsible for the characteristic flavour of dry-cured products (Mora, 2018).

When the chemistry and biological activities of BP from marine organisms such as fish, marine processing waste, and crustaceans, shellfish mollusks, sponges, marine algae, tunicates, coelenterates, ascidians, and mollusks are examined, proteins from these marine organisms are a unique source of protein that can be used as raw material to generate biofunctional peptides (Sánchez & Vazquez, 2017). As waste, the fish processing industry produces more than 60% as by products. To utilize this waste and to add value to different undernourished fish species, protein hydrolysates from fish proteins are being prepared using enzymes (Elias et al., 2008).

Cereal grains that are in human diets such as wheat, barley, rice, rye, oat, millet, sorghum, and corn, are a rich source of BP (Malaguti et al., 2014). GI digestion of soybean seeds and soymilk with regards to BP production using endogenous proteases in vitro has been investigated. Results indicted a large number of BPs produced from soybean proteins demonstrated established activity while others predicted antimicrobial activity, and these peptides also could be formed during food processing.

A large amount of waste is produced during the process in the food industry. For example, as a result of olive oil extraction, two different types of waste material are produced: the solid waste that is a combination of olive pulp, stone, an aqueous liquor, constituted by vegetation water, soft olive tissues, and water added during refinement. These residues are contaminants that are not readily biodegradable and are difficult to process. In a recent study, as a new strategy for the recovery of waste proteins from olive seeds with the potential to produce antioxidant peptides has been investigated (Sánchez & Vazquez, 2017).

Enzymatic hydrolysates of olive were prepared by processing five different proteases: alcalase, thermolysin, neutrase, flavourzyme, and PTN. Among them, alcalase yielded the hydrolysate with the highest antioxidant activity. Fractionated hydrolysates showed a high concentration of short chain peptides, with significantly higher antioxidant and antihypertensive capacities than fractions with higher MWs. The treating of fruits and vegetables produce a significant amount of waste material. These residues can be used to feed animals; however, the majority is discarded. In addition, stones of fruits such as plum (Prunus domestica L.) are rich in proteins and may be a inexpensive source of BP that may be useful (González-García, Marina & García, 2014; Sánchez & Vazquez, 2017).

RELATIONSHIP OF BIOACTIVE PROTEIN AND PEPTIDES WITH INFLAMMATION

Pathogen invasion, injury, tissue damage or infection results in the activiation ofone of the body's defensive responses in the form of inflammation. However, controlled inflammation is essential for normal body function; persistent, chronic inflammation at a low eosis, inflammatory bowel disease, cancer, central nervous system disease, and cardiovascular disease. Chronic inflammation is related generally by the nuclear factor-kappa B (NF-κB) pathway, the mitogen activated protein kinase-c-jun N-terminal kinase (MAPK-JNK) pathway, and the janus kinase signal transducer and activator of transcription (JAK-STAT) pathway, usually under the stimuli of tumor necrosis factor α (TNFα), interleukin-1 (IL-1), and lipopolysaccharides(LPS) (Laveti et al., 2013).

In the classic NF-κB signaling pathway the stimulus (TNFα, IL-1, or LPS) binds to its respective receptor (tumor necrosis factor receptor, TNFR, interleukin-1 receptor, IL-1R, or Toll-like receptors, TLRs) leading to activation of the IκB kinase (IKK) complex in the cytoplasm, which in turn phosphorylates IκBα followed by its subsequent polyubiquitination, proteasomal degradation of IκBα. After release of the homo/heterodimers p50 and RelA (also known asp65) and translocation to the nucleus, these dimers activate transcription of target genes for the inflammatory response. In the MAPK pathway, phosphorylation and activation of MAPK kinase kinase (MAPKKK) leads to phosphorylation of MAPK kinase (MAPKK), which in turn mediates phosphorylation of MAPKs (including extracellular signal-regulated kinase, ERK, JNK, and p38).

Activated MAPKs then phosphorylate a variety of transcription factors (i.e. c-Myc, ATF-2, and c-Jun) leading to diverse cellular activities such as cell proliferation, migration, differentiation, and survival for the ERK1/2 signaling pathway; inflammation for the JNK and p38 signaling pathways (Kim & Choi, 2015). Similarly, when cytokines bind to their corresponding receptors, JAKs are activated leading to phosphorylation of STAT and formation of STAT-STAT dimer. Subsequently, the dimer is translocated to the nucleus and regulates specific gene expression by directly binding to DNA resulting in the inflammatory response (O'Shea, Schwartz, Villarino, Gadina, McInnes & Laurence, 2015; Li, Liu, He & Wu, 2018).

Peroxidation reactions are involved in several pathological processes such as different inflamatory diseases. Dietary proteins and peptides may prevent peroxidation either by their content in amino acid that could stop the peroxidation chain or by their ability to scavenge inducers of peroxidation, such as iron. Food-derived BP have been demostrated to modulate ex vivo the production of proinflammatory mediators in macrophages, by decreasing the production of free radicals, pro-inflammatory interleukins and prostaglandins (Bouglé & Bouhallab, 2017).

Different food-derived bioactive peptides are demostrated to have anti-inflammatory activity both in in vitro cellular systems and in in vivo animal models. Milk-derived tripeptides Val-Pro-Pro (VPP) and Ile-Pro-Pro (IPP) showed anti-inflammation activity through inhibition of the NF-κB pathway, as well as increased release of adiponectin in adipocytes (Chakrabarti & Wu, 2015; Mohanty, Jena, Choudhury, Pattnaik, Mohapatra & Saini, 2016). In addition to the VPP's anti-inflammatory effect, it was reported that interactions mediated through inhibition of either the MAPK-JNK pathway in leukocyte and endothelium or the renin–angiotensin system (RAS) in adipocyte and macrophage. Egg-derived tripeptide Ile-Arg-Trp (IRW)'s anti-inflammatory activity also acted through the NF-κB pathway (Huang, Chakrabarti, Majumder, Jiang, Davidge, & Wu, 2010). Other anti-inflammatory peptides are Val-Pro-Tyr (VPY) and lunasin from soy, and peptide from P. yezoensis (PPY1, a marine algae). Anti-inflammatory peptides identified from food proteins may have a potential role against a wide range of chronic diseases (Li et al., 2018).

Studies on anti-inflammatory effects of food-derived bioactive peptides focus to investigate the interactions between peptides and different signaling pathways in an attempt to minimize inflammation in different chronic diseases. Peptides with known anti-inflammatory mechanisms are summarized in Table 1 (Young & Mine, 2010; Chakrabarti et al., 2014; Sánchez & Vazquez, 2017). This summary explains the effects of these peptides on the expression of pro- and anti-inflammatory cytokines, leading to the modulation of signaling pathways involved in the anti-inflammatory action.

Evidence from recent research have published claims that bioactive peptides exert their anti-inflammatory effect mostly through modulating cytosolic compounds or transcription factors rather than membrane proteins. But, the carrying of these peptides in the cell membrane is unknown yet. Only the anti-inflammatory peptide γ-EC has been proven to bind with the CaSR receptor and subsequently activate the CaSR signaling pathway (Broadhead et al., 2011; Zhang, Kovacs-Nolan, Kodera, Eto & Mine, 2015; Majumder, Mine & Wu, 2016).

Immunomodulatory peptides can enhance immune cell functions, measured as lymphocyte proliferation, natural killer (NK) cell activity, antibody synthesis and cytokine regulation, reduce allergic reactions and enhance mucosal immunity in the gastrointestinal tract (Belovic, Mastilović, Torbica, Stanić & Džinić, 2011). In a study, the activity of DIKTNKPVIF bioactive peptide and its parent protein PH in matter of alleviating proinflammatory events underlying HFD-induced hepatic steatosis was investigated in SAMP8 aging mice feeding a HFD. High-fat diet-promoted changes such as liver steatosis, inflammatory damage, were attenuated by either peptide or parent protein hydrolysate administration which not only enhances lipid metabolism through AMPK activation, but alleviates hepatic proinflammatory response as well. It was concluded that PH and synthesized biopeptide can be used respectively as hepatoprotective agent for counteracting underlying proinflammatory events responsible for hepatosteatosis development and progression in elderly (Dumeus et al., 2018). Moreover, active peptides in autoimmune diseases such as [K6T] P8, a peptide able to inhibit the receptor of IL-15, and Cyclotide [T20K] kalata B1, an active peptide in multiple sclerosis able to block immune-competent cells proliferation, were described. Among peptides active in neurological diseases, a fragment of NCAM protein, named FGL peptide, induced the secretion of IL-4 from microglial cells leading to the increase of CD200 and to the inversion of the age-related decline of hippocampus in vivo. Further, the MHP1 peptide showed an anti-osteoclast activity in ischemic stroke, by suppressing LPS and TNF-α production. One strategy relies on the introduction of conformational constraints, such as mono- or bi-cyclic structuresin order to decrease the conformational flexibility of linear peptides. These modifications often determine an enhancement of membranes permeability and an increase of stability to proteolysis by endo and exopeptidases. Another approach implies the substitution of natural amino acid residues with unnatural ones and/or with N-methyl-_-amino acid, that also increases plasma stability of the lead compound. Further budding peptide technologies, including multifunctional peptides, cell penetrating peptides, and peptide drug conjugates, will facilitate the applicability of peptides as therapeutics in the treatment of inflammation disorders, and even beyond (Manna, Di Natale, Florio & Marasco, 2018).

In previous studies that are about the peptide sequences exhibiting anti-inflammatory activity, even though it has been demostrated the presence of positively charged and hydrophobic amino acids in the peptide sequence, especially in the N and C terminal is considered to play a significant role in anti-inflammatory responses.

Table 1. Food-derived anti-inflammatory peptides/hydrolysates in cell-based and in vivo systems

Source	Protein	Preparation	Active component	Cell tested in	Observed effect	References
Milk	Casein	Bacterial fermentation	VPP Val-Pro-Pro(VPP)Ile-Pro-Pro (IPP)	Endothelial cells and leukocytes Murine colitis Macrophages	Reduced leukocyte Recruitment, Inhibited either MAPK-JNK pathway or renin – angiotensin system	Aihara et al., 2009; Chatterton et al., 2013
	Casein	Corolase hydrolysis *Aspergillus oryzae* Protease hydrolysis	Hydrolysate Hydrolysate	Macrophages Rat adjuvant arthritis	Downregulation of COX-2, NF-κB inhibition reduced arthritic score, anti-inflammatory	Nielsen et al., 2012; Hatori et al., 2008
	Whey protein Lacto bumin	Enzymatic hydrolysis Tryptic hydrolysis	Hydrolysate GLF	Epithelial cells NC/Nga mouse macrophages	Reduced cytokine expression Reduced dermatitis immune-modulating	Piccolomini et al., 2012; Shimizu et al., 2006; Kamau et al., 2010
	Lactoferrin	Enzymatic hydrolysis	Lactoferricin	Synovial cells LPS - stimulated monocytes	Anti-inflammatory, Antiarthritis ⁻ TNF - α, ⁻ IL - 1 β, ⁻ IL - 6, ⁻ IL - 8 protein and mRNA, ⁻ NF -k B	Yan et al., 2013; Haversen et al., 2002
Egg	Ovotransferrin Lysozyme	Thermolysin and pepsin hydrolysis	Ile-Arg-Trp (IRW), IQW muramidase	Human endothelial cells DSS - induced colitis in pigs	Reduced ICAM-1/ VCAM-1 with cytokine treatment Reduced IL-6 and monocyte chemo attractant protein-1 (MCP-1) TNF - α, ⁻ IL - 6, ⁻ IFN - γ, ⁻ IL - 8, ⁻ IL - 17, IL - 4, TGF - β, Foxp3	Majumder et al., 2013; Lee et al., 2009
Fish	Fish protein	Enzymatic hydrolysis	Hydrolysate	Intestinal pithelial cells (human and rat) Murine colitis (DSS/NSAID induced)	Anti-inflammatory, increased proliferation Reduced cytokines, improved healing	Fitzgerald AJ et al., 2005 Marchbank T et al., 2009
Chicken	collagen	Acid treatment followed by *Aspergillus oryzae*protease hydrolysis	Hydrolysate	ApoE knockout mouse SHR (rat)	Reduced Cytokines, improved plasma lipid profile reduced ICAM-1 and decreased blood pressure	Zhang Y et al., 2010
Plant	Soy protein	Fermentation	Chungkookjang	Breast cancer cells	Anti-inflammatory, increased TGF-beta	Hwang JS et al., 2011
	Soy protein	Enzymatic hydrolysis	Lunasin VPY	Macrophage Murine colitis	Reduced cytokines, NF-κB inhibition Reduced cytokines, reduced oxidative stress, and improved histology, Reduced the expression of TNF-a, IFN-g _ IL-1b. Reduced expression of IL-10	deMejia & Dia, 2009; Kovacs-Nolan et al., 2012
	Wheat gluten	*Aspergillus oryzae* protease hydrolysis and fractionation	Pyro-glutamyl leucine	Rat hepatitis Mouse colitis	Anti-inflammatory, İmproved hepatic enzyme profile Improved mucosal histology and less weight loss	Sato et al., 2013; Wada et al., 2013

In recent studies, it has been reported that as the N- and C terminals refer to the N- and C-amino acids only, because unlike tripeptide sequences, it is challenging to determine how many amino acids constitute the middle portion. In addition, the overall positive charge of the peptide may also act as a chemokine (Vogel, Schibli, Jing, Lohmeier-Vogel, & Epand, 2002; Guha & Majumder, 2018). The anti-inflammatory peptides identified so far contained positively charged amino acids like Arg and Lys. However, their location in the peptides was not be stable, that is some of them were found in N terminals, C terminals, as well as some in the middle of the sequence. Peptides like pEL, g-EC, and g-EV contained negatively charged amino acids and still exhibited best antiinflammatory properties, apart from the positively charged amino acids (Zhang et al., 2015). The release of LPS that is a major inducer of inflammation, as a critical component of the cell wall of Gram-negative bacteria, induces the release of proinflammatory cytokines. Studies have shown that peptides, like the human lactoferricin, with highly basic N-terminals or Arg residues at the N-terminals, can bind the LPS released from the bacteria and thus block the inflammation response. However, it was found that two peptides PRRTRMMNGGR, GPR, identified in cooked tuna juice and amaranth protein, respectively, contained Arg in the C-terminals and exhibited anti-inflammatory activity in LPS induced murine macrophages. Therefore, the anti-inflammatory response of these peptides may act through different pathways or the presence of Arg in both C and N terminals may be helpful to reduce LPS induced inflammatory response. Study by Majumder et al., (Majumder et al., 2013) on the egg ovotransferrin peptides also depicted the importance of Arg in the peptide where a difference of only a single amino acid changed the anti-inflammatory activity (Guha & Majumder, 2018).

The hydrophobicity properties availability in the peptides is one of the important factors responsible for the anti-inflammatory reaction. It was found in studies that most of the peptides with anti-inflammatory activity, whether di-, tri-, or oligo-, were rich in hydrophobic amino acids and those are mainly clustered toward the N-terminal, while the C-terminal contained mainly polar groups (Chakrabarti & Wu, 2015; Kwak et al., 2016; Zhao, Wang, Zhang, & Xie, 2016). These studies reported that the presence of the hydrophobic amino acids enhances the interaction between peptide and cell membrane, which may contribute toward modulating the downstream signaling pathways and exhibiting the anti-inflammatory effect (Guha & Majumder, 2018). The molecular weight and the length properties of the peptide also play an important role. It has been demostrated that peptides having low molecular weight can easily cross the intestinal barrier because they are less prone to proteolytic digestion and are easily absorbed in the intestine. In addition, longer peptides have also been reported to have anti-inflammatory activities like lunasin (43 amino acids) and GMP (64 amino acids). In a study conducted by Jacquot et al., they found that murine splenocyte proliferation was stimulated better by longer hydrophobic peptides having 2–3 positively charged amino acids (Jacquot, Gauthier, Drouin & Boutin, 2010). A tri-peptide, RGD (Arg-Gly-Asp; residues 32–34), within the lunasin peptide which is a cell-adhesion module and promotes intracellular accessibility of lunasin by functioning as an extracellular matrix, whereas a stretch of nine Asp residues are present at the C-terminus involved in anti-mitotic functions (Wan, Liu, Sun, Zhang, Chen & Chen, 2017; Guha & Majumder, 2018).

Furthermore, despite structural similarities, which suggested that the relative amino acid position played an essential role in facilitating the interaction with the enzyme as different peptides would be positioned differently on the enzyme, CQV showed better quenching than its analogues QVC and QCV. Molecular docking experiments showed that the peptides interacted with the active site through a series of hydrogen bonds, zinc coordination, and hydrophobic interactions and primarily occupied the S1 and S10 sites of the enzyme (Udechukwu, Tsopmo, Mawhinney, He, Kienesberger & Udenigwe, 2017; Guha & Majumder, 2018).

Together with the physicochemical properties of amino acids, it was also shown that peptide structure may play an significant role in bioactivity. Calcium-induced activation of the calcium sensing receptor (CaSR) plays a role in intracellular signal transduction because of the regular releasing of intracellular calcium. Agonists of CaSR have anti-inflammatory effects and prohibit the TNF-a induced inflammatory pathway (Fujita, Matsuoka, Honda, Kabashima, Hirata & Narumiya, 2011). G-EC and g-EV were found to fully activate CaSR and set off intracellular signaling. Activation of CaSR caused interaction with TNF-α mediated signaling event, thereby inhibiting the JNK and IκBα pathways, exhibiting anti-inflammatory effects (Zhang et al., 2015; Guha & Majumder, 2018).

Milk contains a large amount of caseins and whey proteins, both of which can lead to a series of peptides with bioactive properties after processing, such as enzymatic hydrolysis, digestion and / or fermentation. The direct anti-inflammatory role of VPP has been demonstrated to by its ability to attenuate leukocyte endothelial interactions in vitro, mostly via inhibition of the proinflammatory c-Jun N-terminal kinase (JNK, a MAP kinase type) pathway (Chakrabarti S et al., 2014). Hydrolysates of whey proteins are also promising for inhibiting inflammatory responses in respiratory and intestinal epithelial cells (Iskandar, Dauletbaev, Kubow, Mawji & Lands, 2013).

In a study, when whey protein concentrates (WPC) hydrolyzed by Corolase or thermolysin were examined for antioxidant activity by ORAC assay, Thermolysin hydrolyzed WPC was the strongest hydrolysate with radical scavenging activity and several peptides were identified in this hydrolysate. Lactoferrin is a milk protein with antimicrobial properties, which also exerts anti-inflammatory effects on activated macrophages. The bioactive peptide lactoferricin after hydrolysis of lactoferrin provides anti-inflammatory effects on human cartilage and synovial cells, suggesting potential benefits in arthritis management. Milk proteins also contribute much in the context of antioxidant peptides. YFYPEL, a hexapeptide isolated from pepsin hydrolysate of bovine casein, showed antioxidant activity by scavenging superoxide, DPPH, and hydroxyl radicals in vitro. Ovine κ-casein antioxidant activity also increased by 3-fold upon hydrolysis with pepsin, trypsin, and chymotrypsin. This casein hydrolysate further inhibited lipid peroxidation and several peptides contributing to antioxidant activity were identified. Goat milk casein showed enhanced free radical scavenging and metal ion chelating activity following hydrolysis by a combination of neutral and alkaline proteases (Chakrabarti et al., 2014). β-casein peptides EAMAPK and AVPYPQ, identified in Stracchino cheese digested under simulated GI conditions, reduced ROS levels and activated Nrf2 response in H2O2-treated epithelial IEC-6 cells (Pepe et al., 2016; Fernández-Tomé, Hernández-Ledesma, Chaparro, Indiano-Romacho, Bernardo & Gisbert, 2019).

Goat milk proteins were hydrolysed to caseins (GCP), whey proteins (GWP) and protein fractions containing multiple soluble peptides by pepsin. Compared to bovine milk, proteins and peptides derived from goat milk secreted by digestive enzymes, especially that showed reduced allergenicity. Hydrolysates of whey (P-GWP) and casein (P-GCP) proteins showed strong superoxide anion (O2 · -) scavenging activity. The results show that soluble peptides obtained by digestion with pepsin possess remarkable ability to scavenge superoxide radicals (Ahmed, El-Bassiony, Elmalt, & Ibrahim, 2015). In addition, it has been reported, that digestion of casein produces phosphorylated peptides that exhibit both hydrophilic and lipophilic antioxidant activity due to both metal ion sequestering and quenching of ROS (Sánchez & Vazquez, 2017; Bouglé & Bouhallab 2017) and casein increases ex vivo the stimulated production of IL-2 by human T helper-1 (Th-1) lymphocytes (Guha & Majumder, 2018).

Peptides derived from milk proteins have shown antioxidant properties that prevent peroxidation of essential fatty acids. For instance, the addition of a Leu or Pro residue to the N-terminus of a His-His, dipeptide will enhance antioxidant activity and facilitate further synergy with non-peptide antioxidants [e.g. butylated hydroxytoluene (BHT)] (Kitts & Weiler, 2003).

Fermentation of milk proteins using lactic acid bacteria (LAB) is an attractive approach to generate functional foods enriched with BP given the low cost and positive nutritional image associated with fermented milk products (Sánchez & Vazquez, 2017).

Peptides released during milk fermentation by lactic bacteria modulate the proliferation of human lymphocytes, by controlling the production of certain cytokines and stimulating the phagocytic activity of macrophages. It was also demostrated that immunomodulatory peptides from milk can alleviate atopic allergic reactions in humans and strengthen the immunity of the gastrointestinal tract mucosa (Korhonen & Pihlanto, 2006; Sgarbieri, 2017).

The milk-derived peptides, IPP and VPP, are rich in Pro, these peptides have great potential to show ACE-inhibitory and anti-inflammation activities and are more resistant to intestinal digestion and when consumed orally, they are easily absorbed. Apart from IPP and VPP, other antiinflammatory tri-peptides were also found to have at least one Pro in their structure such as VPY, PAY, and GPR. The presence of proline and the hydrophobic amino acids in the peptide seemed to increase the activity of these peptides (Ichikawa, Morifuji, Ohara, Matsumoto, Takeuchi, & Sato, 2010). The anti-inflammatory activity of VPY was linked to the intestinal peptide transporter, PepT1. It was reported that the expression of PepT1 increases during inflammation and it was linked to nucleotide binding oligomerization domain-containing protein-2 (NOD2) involved in inflammatory responses. Thus, PepT1 has a role in internalizing peptides involved in anti-inflammation, and it was found that VPY could easily be transported and exhibited antiinflammatory properties (Kovacs-Nolan et al., 2012). This might be due to the unique structural composition of VPY. The anti-inflammatory peptide FLV, which has been reported to reduce obesity-linked inflammatory responses, also showed a similar mode of action. PepT2 transporter has been shown to have a major role in the uptake of FLV. The transporter is primarily expressed in adipose tissue and the expression of PepT2 was highly up-regulated in the presence of inflammatory mediators linked to obesity (Kwak et al., 2016). Both VPY and FLV share the same structural composition, that is, one aromatic amino acid and two hydrophobic amino acids, which indicates a strong relationship between the structure of the peptides and its ability to be taken up by the transporter proteins (Guha & Majumder, 2018).

Colostrinin (CLN), contains about 22% proline, and originally this high proline content may confer significant resistance to digestion as proline-rich polypeptide and consists of at least 32 different, occurs naturally in milk, and acts immunoregulatory properties. In addition, CLN shows to have a wide variety of functions including immunomodulation (B and T cell activation), promoting cell proliferation, improving wound healing and having antioxidant, antihypertension and neuroprotective activities (Moughan & Rutherfurd-Markwick, 2013).

Several immunomodulatory peptides derived from α-lactalbumin have been shown to exhibit a range of functions including stimulation of phagocytosis and respiratory burst, protection of mice against K. pneumoniae infection and enhancement of human peripheral blood lymphocyte proliferation (Kamau, Cheison, Chen, Liu, & Lu, 2010; Moughan & Rutherfurd-Markwick, 2013).

The oligopeptide lactoferricin, derived from lactoferrin, stimulated the production of human neutrophil-activating Interleukin-8 (IL-8) by human polymorphonuclear leukocytes. Bovine lactoferricin also promoted phagocytic activity in human neutrophils (Sgarbieri, 2017).

In vitro studies with Lf have shown that the intact protein can inhibit lymphocyte proliferation, while the peptide lactoferricin (residues 17–41 of LF) can suppress IL-6 production by a human monocyte cell line following stimulation with LPS, stimulate the release of IL-8 from human polymorphonuclear leucocytes and promote the phagocytic activity of human neutrophils (Moughan & Rutherfurd-Markwick, 2013).

Roos et al. (1994) demostrated the effects of dietary supplementation with Lf on immune response by giving 0.9 g Lf prior to and following an influenza vaccination in a double-blind placebo-controlled study which resulted in an increased percentage of granulocytes (of total leukocytes). In this study, the phagocytic activity of the granulocytes from the Lf-supplemented group was higher one day after vaccination (Moughan & Rutherfurd-Markwick, 2013)

In addition to the Caseinophosphopeptides (CPPs) with antioxidant activity has been attributed to the high contents of histidine and some hydrophobic amino acids, several peptides are contained in the primary sequences of the αS1-caseins, β-caseins, κ-caseins, and β-LG. In addition, a hexapeptide, Tyr-Phe-Tyr-Pro-Gln-Leu, with antioxidant activity was released from αS1-casein (f: 144-149) by the proteolytic action of pepsin in vitro (Pihlanto, 2011; Sgarbieri, 2017).

The Glycomacropeptide (GMP) and its derivatives are shown to exercise various immunomodulatory functions, such as immunosuppressive effects on the production of IgG antibodies, and to stimulatory effects on the proliferation of phagocytic activities in human cells similar to macrophages. Whey Protein Concentrate (WPC) enriched with the Glycomacropeptide (GMP) suppressed the secretion of Interleukin-4 (IL-4) and of Interferon-Gamma (INF-γ) in culture of mouse lymphocytes. The GMP also induced the production of the family of Interleukins-1 (IL-1) in Mouse macrophage cells. (Sgarbieri, 2017).

Egg, source for many bioactive compounds, is another nutritious dietary component. It was shown that egg tripeptides (IRW and IQW) are produced from ovotransferrin (an egg white component), which is effective in reducing cytokine-induced inflammatory protein expression in the vascular endothelium, at least in part by modulation of the NF-κB pathway. These beneficial effects require the presence of an intact tripeptide as the corresponding dipeptides and constituent amino acids alone failed to replicate the anti-inflammatory functions, indicating a structure-function relationship between the tripeptide structure and blockade of inflammation (Majumder et al., 2013; Chakrabarti et al., 2014).

In the study that was focused on the effect of cooking methods and GI digestion on the antioxidant activity of peptides obtained from avian egg showed that fresh egg yolk has higher antioxidant activity than fresh egg white and whole eggs. Cooking of eggs decreased the antioxidant activity whereas simulated GI digestion increased it. Boiled egg white hydrolysate showed the highest efficacy and a total of 63 peptides have been identified, indicating the formation of new antioxidant peptides (Andersen, 2015).

Three ovomucin hydrolysates have been prepared and desalted, and only the salt-free alcalase hydrolysate increased the proportion of low-MW peptides exhibiting anti-inflammatory activity. This biological activity was comparable to anti-inflammatory activity in dermal fibroblasts. The anti-inflammatory activity of low-MW peptides was regulated through the inhibition of tumour necrosis-mediated nuclear factor κB pathway (Sun, Chakrabarti, Fang, Yin & Wu 2016; Sánchez & Vazquez, 2017). The antioxidant activity of ovotransferrin was enhanced by the rupture of its structure, allowing the approach of amino acid residues that scavenge free radicals and form chelates with pro-oxidant metals. Fourteen peptides were isolated and characterized from ovotransferrin. Two tetrapeptides – Trp-Asn-Ile-Pro and Gly-Trp-Asn-Ile – showed higher antioxidant activity, suggesting that (Trp-Asn-Ile) should represent the nucleus responsible for the high antioxidant activity of these peptides (Sgarbieri, 2017).

The antioxidant activities of water-soluble fractions of a Spanish dry-cured ham extract of a fractionated peptide extract have been described by size-exclusion chromatography. Some of the fractions exhibited large 1, 1-diphenyl-2-picrylhydrazyl radical-scavenging activity, ranging from 39 to 92% as well as superoxide ion quenching ability with values from 41.7 to 50.3% of the antioxidant activity that suggest the presence of peptides with antioxidant activity. The antioxidant peptides Leu-His-Tyr, Leu-Ala-Arg-Leu, Gly-Gly-Glu, Gly-Ala-His, Gly-Ala-Trp-Ala, Pro-His-Tyr-Leu and Gly-Ala-Leu-Ala-Ala-His were obtained from sardinelle (Sardinella aurita) industrial wastes generated using crude enzyme extract from sardine (Sardina pilchardus). The first tripeptide showed the highest DPPH radical scavenging activity, and possibly the presence of amino acids His-Tyr sequence may significantly contribute to the antioxidant activity of the peptides. Glutathione, a tripeptide (γ-Glu-Cys-Gly), protects cells from free radicals. The dipeptide carnosine (β-alanyl-histidine), and its related dipeptides anserine (β-alanyl-1-methylhistidine) and balenine (β-alanyl-3-methylhistidine), have high antioxidant and pH-buffering properties in muscle cells. It is usually found in large amounts in chickens, during the processes inflammation and infection processes. This protein also has immunomodulating effects on chicken macrophages and heterophil-granulocytes and may prevent proliferation of mouse spleen lymphocytes (Sánchez & Vazquez, 2017).

A significant number of recent publications reports the presence of peptides with antioxidant action in hydrolysates from fish proteins and in by-products of the fishery industry. Je et al., (2007) obtained peptides from dark muscles of a variety of tuna (Thunnus obesus) through the enzymatic action of several proteases and evaluated their antioxidant potential. A peptic hydrolysate with potent antioxidant action was obtained, from which it was possible to isolate the peptide (Leu-Asn-

Leu-Pro-Thr-Ala-Val-Tyr-Met-Val-Tyr), with strong free radical scavenging action and antioxidant effect on inhibition of peroxidation of unsaturated fatty acids. The scavenging power of this peptide was also tested in cellular systems, showing high degree of effectiveness. Ranathunga et al. (2006) isolated from the marine species Conger (Conger myriaster) a peptide that presented high antioxidant action, with the following structure: Leu-Gly-Leu-Asn-Gly-Asp-Asp-Val-Asn (MM 1,060Da) (Sgarbieri, 2017).

A wide range of antioxidant peptides has been identified from marine organisms including oyster, shrimp, squid, blue mussel and a variety of fish species (tuna, sardine, hoki, sole, and pacific hake) after hydrolysis with different enzymes. A fish hydrolysate preparation has been shown to induce proliferation and migration in intestinal epithelial cells, which may contribute to anti-inflammatory and healing properties (Chakrabarti et al., 2014). Puffer fish hydrolysate produced strong antioxidant action as shown by the ORAC assay compared to many other fish sources (Harada, Maeda, Hasegawa, Tokunaga, Tamura, & Koizumi, 2010). Both the salmon protein hydrolysate and peptide fractions inhibited the oxidation of linoleic acid. Flounder fish muscle hydrolyzed with α-chymotrypsin has been also reported to possess strong antioxidant activities by scavenging free radicals in vitro. Blue mussel (Mytilus edulis) is a source of antioxidant peptides after hydrolysis by the enzyme neutrase could scavenge 30% of DPPH radicals (Chakrabarti et al., 2014).

21 peptides were determined from the hydrolysate of bivalve mollusks Mactra veneriformis. Furthermore, the sequences were established using MS/MS fragmentation data In the GI system, shellfish is another potential source for antioxidant peptide production. The GI digests of oyster (Crassostrea gigas) yielded an active 1.6 kDa peptide with the amino acid sequence of Leu-Lys-Gln-Glu-Leu-Glu-Asp-Leu-Leu-Glu-Lys-Gln-Glu. This peptide inhibited peroxidation of lipids and neutralized hydroxyl and superoxide radicals (4-29Ngo and Kim, 2013). Other the peptide Leu-Val-Gly-Asp-Glu-Gln-Ala-Val-Pro-Ala-Val-Cys-Val-Pro (1.59 kDa), with potent antioxidant activity, was isolated from the GI digest of mussel muscle protein in a different study. The molecular diversity of marine peptides, as well as information about their anti-inflammatory properties and mechanisms of action, have been described, along with the anti-inflammatory effects of novel BP from sponges, bacterium, and microalgae (Kim & Wijesekara, 2010).

Soy peptides have shown increased antioxidant activities (Singh et al., 2014) compared to intact proteins (Peña-Ramos & Xiong, 2002). Soy protein hydrolysates prepared from native and heated soy protein isolates using different enzymes had varying degrees of hydrolysis (1.7–20.6%) and antioxidant activities (28–65%) (Sánchez & Vazquez, 2017).

Wheat and barley indicate the greatest diversity and abundance of peptides with potential biological activity among the cereal proteins. Wheat and oat also showed the presence of ACE inhibitory peptides and dipeptidyl peptidase inhibitor, as well as peptides with anti-thrombotic, antioxidant, hypotensive, and opioid activities, and wheat and rice have proteins with peptidic sequences showing anticancer activity (Malaguti et al., 2014). 2,5-Diketopiperazines (DKPs) that also known as cyclic dipeptides have received considerable attention as bioactive compounds can be formed from the N-terminal amino acid residues of a linear peptide or protein and have been identified in various foods, particularly in roasted coffee, cocoa, roasted malt, and fermented foods such as beer. Immunomodulatory peptides obtained from hydrolysates of rice and soybean proteins act to stimulate ROS, which triggers non-specific immune defence systems (Sánchez & Vazquez, 2017).

In studies, within colonic epithelial cells, the soluble peptides from amaranth provided anti-inflammatory effects that might be receptor-mediated. These results indicated that peptides reduced CCL20 production by mucosal and immune cells and hence, raised the use of amaranth peptides as a potential dietary supplement. At the same time, it has been shown that Amaranth hypochondriacus hydrolysates, obtained by the action of pepsin and pancreatin enzymes, inhibited the inflammatory process induced by LPS in human and mouse macrophages. These studies have shown that amaranth peptides inhibited the NF-κB signalling pathway leading to a reduction in the nuclear expression of p50 and p65 NF-kB subunits, and the expression of COX-2 and iNOS (Moronta et al., 2016).

Soybean hydrolysates have yielded several bioactive peptides with anti-inflammatory effects on macrophage cell lines, with preparations from germinated beans eliciting the stronger responses. One of the soybean-derived peptides, lunasin that is believed to contribute to their anti-inflammatory effects, potentially involving antagonism of integrin signaling and downstream proinflammatory cascades, appears to perform widespread anti-inflammatory effects suppression of NF-κB activity, reduction cytokine expression and reduction in cyclooxygenase-2 (COX-2) levels in addition to its antioxidant and anticarcinogenic properties. For example, Chungkookjang, a fermented soybean product from Korea, shows anti-inflammatory effects in breast cancer cells by activation of transforming growth factor (TGF)-beta signaling and downregulation of cytokine/chemokines expression (Hwang, Yoo, Song, Kim, Chun, Matsui & Kim, 2011; Chakrabarti S et al., 2014).

But, it was reported that corn protein hydrolysates were more effective than soy protein hydrolysate and inhibited lipid oxidation by 53% at lower incorporated dosage (200 μg/g) while soy protein hydrolysate reduced oxidation by 20% at much higher dosage (800 μg/g). In a recent study, the antioxidant activity of chickpea albumin hydrolysate through in vitro radical scavenging and reducing power assays has been assayed. Further purification of the hydrolysate fraction with highest antioxidant activity identified RQSHFANAQP as the active component responsible. All of the aforementioned peptides were evaluated for antioxidant activity through in vitro methods (Chakrabarti et al., 2014).

In a study on germinated soybean peptides identified a 5–10 kDa fraction which inhibited LPS induced Prostaglandin D2 (PGD2) and Nitric Oxide (NO) production in RAW 264.7 macrophage cells as in vitro.

The most peptides in that fraction contained at least one glutamine residue and out of those four peptides (that is QEPQESQQ, QQQQQGGSQSQ, PETMQQQQQ, and QQQQQGGSQSQSQKG) that were rich in glutamine might be a crucial amino acid involved in the anti-inflammatory activity (Gonzalez-Montoya, Hernandez-Ledesma, Silvan, Mora-Escobedo & Martínez-Villaluenga, 2017; Guha & Majumder, 2018).

A recent study on rye secalin-derived tripeptides (QCA and CQV) and its analogues (QVC and QCV) showed the dose-dependent inhibition of "A disintegrin and metalloproteinase 17" (ADAM17) or TNF-a converting enzyme (TACE) (Udechukwu et al., 2017). This catalytic inhibition of ADAM17 was zinc-chelation dependent as shown by the cysteine-containing tripeptides which interacted with the zinc cofactor. The sulfhydryl (ASH) group in cysteine is a crucial zinc-binding ligand. Fluorescence quenching experiments showed that the peptides may directly interact with the cysteine rich catalytic domain (Arg215-Asp671) of ADAM17 (Guha & Majumder, 2018).

FUTURE DIRECTIONS

Future studies of bioactive peptides would include exhaustive studies on animals and human volunteers to better comprehend the pharmacokinetics of peptides, testing for potential immunogenicity, characterizing individual components of complex peptide-rich hydrolysates to tease out their specific activities. In addition, basic biomedical research is much essential because it is intended to identify specific receptors and signaling pathways involved in mediating some of these beneficial anti-inflammatory and antioxidant actions.

Few receptors have been identified as involved in bioactive peptide actions, except the renin-angiotensin system. Additional studies on identifying specific peptide sequences and their correspondent receptors may provide occasions for better targeting of inflammation and oxidative stress in a tissue- and organ-specific manner.

It is very important that finding out several mechanisms for enhancing bioavailability of bioactive peptides are also important, and studies into the use of mechanisms to protect bioactive peptides such as microencapsulation, lipid-based carriers, or through mucosal delivery are in progress. The development of these technologies would support that bioactive peptides and proteins are more bioavailable and hence potentially more efficacious.

Because last progresses on characterization of various target pathways reporte that bioactive peptides might function locally through receptors on cell membranes, further studies require exploring their mechanisms of action in vivo. It would also be important studying the effects of bioactive peptides on "master regulators" or "central targets" (i.e. MAPK) and "specific targets" (i.e. IR for T2D, PPAR for obesity) to understand the multifunctional nature of many bioactive peptides. Therefore, integration of advanced omics technologies with bioinformatic analysis is expected to be guide the novel pathways of action of the peptides in vivo.

In humans, some preclinical studies applied for bioactive peptides are promising. However, these efforts are yet in their infancy and clearly need to be further evaluated in healthy humans and patients to decipher their role and optimal administration. Ongoing and future study are expected to provide more evidence-based information about the add of bioactive peptides in human clinical trials before their usage.

CONCLUSION

Encrypted between the chemical structure of proteins present in food matrixes and other natural sources, there is an extensive amount of BP. Enzymatic hydrolysis occurring during digestion or fermentation can release much more BP. Because of these activities, BP has the potential to be used as food ingredients for the treatment or prevention of inflamatory conditions.

Different research is required to identify various food protein derived materials that are available sources of bioactive peptides and to describe the underlying mechanisms of physiological activity attributed to these peptides. Moreover, it is suggested that various technical bioprocesses used to recover different bioactive peptides for specific physiological applications related to health are very important.

REFERENCES

Ahmed, A. S., El-Bassiony, T., Elmalt, L. M., & Ibrahim, H. R. (2015). Identification of potent antioxidant bioactive peptides from goat milk proteins. *Food Research International*, *74*, 80–88. doi:10.1016/j.foodres.2015.04.032 PMID:28412006

Aihara, K., Ishii, H., & Yoshida, M. (2009). Casein-derived tripeptide, Val-Pro-Pro (VPP), modulates monocyte adhesion to vascular endothelium. *Journal of Atherosclerosis and Thrombosis*, *16*(5), 594–603.

Andersen, C. J. (2015). Bioactive Egg Components and Inflammation. *Nutrients*, *7*(9), 7889–7913. doi:10.3390/nu7095372 PMID:26389951

Arrutia, F., Puente, Á., Riera, F. A., Menéndez, C., & González, U. A. (2016a). Influence of heat pre-treatment on BSA tryptic hydrolysis and peptide release. *Food Chemistry, 202*, 40–48. doi:10.1016/j.foodchem.2016.01.107 PMID:26920264

Bamdad, B., Shin, S. H., Suh, J. W., Nimalaratne, C., & Sunwoo, H. (2017). Anti-Inflammatory and antioxidant properties of casein hydrolysate produced using high hydrostatic pressure combined with proteolytic enzymes. *Molecules (Basel, Switzerland), 22*(4), 609–618. doi:10.3390/molecules22040609 PMID:28394279

Belovic, M., Mastilović, J. S., Torbica, A. M., Stanić, D. R., & Džinić, N. R. (2011). Potential of bioactive proteins and peptides for prevention and treatment of mass non-communicable diseases. *Food & Feed Research, 38*(2), 51–61.

Bhat, Z. F., Kumar, S., & Bhat, H. F. (2015). Bioactive peptides of animal origin: A review. *Journal of Food Science and Technology, 52*(9), 5377–5392. doi:10.100713197-015-1731-5 PMID:26344955

Bitri, L. (2004). Optimization study for the production of an opioid-like preparation from bovine casein by mild acidic hydrolysis. *International Dairy Journal, 14*(6), 535–539. doi:10.1016/j.idairyj.2003.10.003

Bouglé, D., & Bouhallab, S. (2017). Dietary bioactive peptides: Human studies. *Critical Reviews in Food Science and Nutrition, 57*(2), 335–343. doi:10.1080/10408398.2013.873766 PMID:26067872

Bouhallab, S., Cinga, V., Aít-Oukhatar, N., Bureau, F., Neuville, D., Arhan, P., ... Bouglé, D. (2002). Influence of various phosphopeptides of caseins on iron absorption. *Journal of Agricultural and Food Chemistry, 50*(24), 7127–7130. doi:10.1021/jf025554v PMID:12428971

Boutrou, R., Coirre, E., Jardin, J., & Léonil, J. (2010). Phosphorylation and Coordination Bond of Mineral Inhibit the Hydrolysis of the β-Casein (1–25) Peptide by Intestinal Brush-Border Membrane Enzymes. *Journal of Agricultural and Food Chemistry, 58*(13), 7955–7961. doi:10.1021/jf100568r PMID:20518500

Boutrou, R., Henry, G., & Sanchez-Rivera, L. (2015). On the trail of milk bioactive peptides in human and animal intestinal tracts during digestion: A review. *Dairy Science & Technology, 95*(6), 815–829. doi:10.100713594-015-0210-0

Broadhead, G. K., Mun, H. C., Avlani, V. A., Jourdon, O., Church, W. B., Christopoulos, A., ... Conigrave, A. D. (2011). Allosteric modulation of the calcium-sensing receptor by γ-glutamyl peptides: Inhibition of PTH secretion, suppression of intracellular cAMP levels, and a common mechanism of action with L-amino acids. T*he Journal of Biological Chemistry, 286,* 8786–8797. doi:10.1074/jbc.M110.149724 PMID:21187282

Castellani, O., Guérin-Dubiard, C., David-Briand, E., & Anton, M. (2004). Influence of physicochemical condition and technological treatments on the ion binding capacity of egg yolk phosvitin. *Food Chemistry*, *85*(4), 569–577. doi:10.1016/j.foodchem.2003.08.002

Chakrabarti, S., Jahandideh, F., & Wu, J. (2014). Food-Derived Bioactive Peptides on Inflammation and Oxidative Stress. Hindawi Publishing Corporation. *BioMed Research International*, 11.

Chakrabarti, S., & Wu, J. P. (2015). Milk-Derived Tripeptides IPP (Ile-Pro-Pro) and VPP (Val-Pro-Pro) Promote Adipocyte Differentiation and Inhibit Inflammation in 3T3-F442A Cells. *PLoS One*, *10*(2), e0117492. doi:10.1371/journal.pone.0117492 PMID:25714093

Chalamaiah, M., Ulug, S. K., Hong, H., & Wu, J. (2019). Regulatory requirements of bioactive peptides (protein hydrolysates) from food proteins. *Journal of Functional Foods*, *58*, 123–129. doi:10.1016/j.jff.2019.04.050

Chalamaiah, M., Yu, W., & Wu, J. (2018). Immunomodulatory and anticancer protein hydrolysates (peptides) from food proteins: A review. *Food Chemistry*, *245*, 205–222. doi:10.1016/j.foodchem.2017.10.087 PMID:29287362

Chatterton, D. E., Nguyen, D. N., Bering, S. B., & Sangild, P. T. (2013). Anti-inflammatory mechanisms of bioactive milk proteins in the intestine of newborns. *The International Journal of Biochemistry & Cell Biology*, *45*(8), 1730–1747. doi:10.1016/j.biocel.2013.04.028 PMID:23660296

Chawla, A., Nguyen, K. D., & Goh, Y. P. S. (2011). Macrophage-mediated inflammation in metabolic disease. *Nature Reviews. Immunology*, *11*(11), 738–749. doi:10.1038/nri3071 PMID:21984069

Choi, J., Sabikhi, L., Hassan, A., & Anand, S. (2012). Bioactive peptides in dairy products. *International Journal of Dairy Technology*, *65*(1), 1–12. doi:10.1111/j.1471-0307.2011.00725.x

Daliri, E. B., Oh, D. H., & Lee, B. H. (2017). Bioactive peptides. *Foods*, *6*(5), 32. doi:10.3390/foods6050032 PMID:28445415

Dave, L. (2019). Human Gastrointestinal Endogenous Proteins: A Recently Discovered Source of Gut Modulatory Peptides. In M. Hayes (Ed.), *Novel Proteins for Food, Pharmaceuticals, and Agriculture Sources, Applications, and Advances*. Hoboken, NJ: Wiley-Blackwell.

deMejia, E. G., & Dia, V. P. (2009). Lunasin and lunasin-like peptides inhibit inflammation through suppression of NF-κB pathway in the macrophage. P*eptides, 30(*12), 2388–2398. doi:10.1016/j.peptides.2009.08.005 PMID:19682518

Dumeus, S., Shibu, M. A., Lin, W. T., Wang, M. F., Lai, C. H., Shen, C. Y., ... Huang, C. Y. (2018). Bioactive Peptide Improves Diet-Induced Hepatic Fat Deposition and Hepatocyte Proinflammatory Response in SAMP8 Ageing Mice. *Cellular Physiology and Biochemistry*, *48*(5), 1942–1952. doi:10.1159/000492518 PMID:30092591

Dziuba, B., & Dziuba, M. (2014). Milk proteins-derived bioactive peptides in dairy products: Molecular, biological and methodological aspects. *Acta Scientiarum Polonorum. Technologia Alimentaria*, *13*(1), 5–25. doi:10.17306/J.AFS.2014.1.1 PMID:24583380

Elias, R. J., Kellerby, S. S., & Decker, E. A. (2008). Antioxidant activity of proteins and peptides. *Critical Reviews in Food Science and Nutrition*, *48*(5), 430–441. doi:10.1080/10408390701425615 PMID:18464032

Feng, L., Peng, F., Wang, X., Li, M., Lei, H., & Xu, H. (2019). Identification and characterization of antioxidative peptides derived from simulated in vitro gastrointestinal digestion of walnut meal proteins. *Food Research International*, *116*, 518–526. doi:10.1016/j.foodres.2018.08.068 PMID:30716976

Fernández-Tomé, S., Hernández-Ledesma, B., Chaparro, M., Indiano-Romacho, P., Bernardo, D., & Gisbert, J. P. (2019). Role of food proteins and bioactive peptides in inflammatory bowel disease. *Trends in Food Science & Technology*, *88*, 194–206. doi:10.1016/j.tifs.2019.03.017

Ferraretto, A., Signorile, A., Gravaghi, C., Fiorilli, A., & Tettamanti, G. (2001). Casein Phosphopeptides Influence Calcium Uptake by Cultured Human Intestinal HT-29 Tumor Cells. *The Journal of Nutrition*, *131*(6), 1655–1661. doi:10.1093/jn/131.6.1655 PMID:11385049

Fitzgerald, A. J., Rai, P. S., Marchbank, T., Taylor, G. W., Ghosh, S., Ritz, B. W., & Playford, R. J. (2005). Reparative properties of a commercial fish protein hydrolysate preparation. *Gut*, *54*(6), 775–781. doi:10.1136/gut.2004.060608 PMID:15888784

Fujita, T., Matsuoka, T., Honda, T., Kabashima, K., Hirata, T., & Narumiya, S. (2011). A GPR40 agonist GW9508 suppresses CCL5, CCL17, and CXCL10 induction in keratinocytes and attenuates cutaneous immune inflammation. *The Journal of Investigative Dermatology*, *131*(8), 1660–1667. doi:10.1038/jid.2011.123 PMID:21593768

García, C. A., & Manrique, I. M. (2019). Meat Proteins as a Potential Source of Bioactive Ingredients for Food and Pharmaceutical Use. In M. Hayes (Ed.), *Novel Proteins for Food, Pharmaceuticals, and Agriculture Sources, Applications, and Advances*. Hoboken, NJ: Wiley-Blackwell.

Gauthier, S. F., Pouliot, Y., & Maubois, J. (2006). Growth factors from bovine milk and colostrum: Composition, extraction and biological activities. *Le Lait*, *86*(2), 99–125. doi:10.1051/lait:2005048

Gobbetti, M., Stepaniak, L., De Angelis, M., Corsetti, A., & Di Cagno, R. (2002). Latent bioactive peptides in milk proteins: Proteolytic activation and significance in dairy processing. *Critical Reviews in Food Science and Nutrition*, *42*(3), 223–239. doi:10.1080/10408690290825538 PMID:12058981

González-García, E., Marina, M. L., & García, M. C. (2014). Plum (Prunus Domestica L.) by-product as a new and cheap source of bioactive peptides: Extraction method and peptides characterization. *Journal of Functional Foods*, *11*, 428–437. doi:10.1016/j.jff.2014.10.020

Gonzalez-Montoya, M., Hernández-Ledesma, B., Silván, J. M., Mora-Escobedo, R., & Martínez-Villaluenga, C. (2017). Peptides derived from in vitro gastrointestinal digestion of germinated soybean proteins inhibit human colon cancer cells proliferation and inflammation. *Food Chemistry*, *242*, 75–82. doi:10.1016/j.foodchem.2017.09.035 PMID:29037738

Goulas, A., Triplett, E. L., & Taborsky, G. (1996). Oligophosphopeptides of varied structural complexity derived from the egg phosphoprotein, phosvitin. *Journal of Protein Chemistry*, *15*(1), 1–9. doi:10.1007/BF01886805 PMID:8838584

Guha, S., & Majumder, K. (2018). Structural-features of food-derived bioactive peptides with anti-inflammatory activity: A brief review. *Journal of Food Biochemistry*, *43*(1), e12531. doi:10.1111/jfbc.12531 PMID:31353488

Harada, K., Maeda, T., Hasegawa, Y., Tokunaga, T., Tamura, Y., & Koizumi, T. (2010). Antioxidant activity of fish sauces including puffer (Lagocephalus wheeleri) fish sauce measured by the oxygen radical absorbance capacity method. *Molecular Medicine Reports*, *3*(4), 663–668. doi:10.3892/mmr_00000313 PMID:21472295

Hartmann, R., & Meisel, H. (2007). Food-derived peptides with biological activity: From research to food applications. *Current Opinion in Biotechnology*, *18*(2), 163–169. doi:10.1016/j.copbio.2007.01.013 PMID:17292602

Hatori, M., Ohki, K., Hirano, S. I., Yang, X. P., Kuboki, H., & Abe, C. (2008). Effects of a casein hydrolysate prepared from Aspergillus oryzae protease on adjuvant arthritis in rats. *Bioscience, Biotechnology, and Biochemistry*, *72*(8), 1983–1991. doi:10.1271/bbb.70792 PMID:18685219

Haversen, L., Ohlsson, B. G., Hahn-Zoric, M., Hanson, L. A., & Mattsby-Baltzer, I. (2002). Lactoferrin down-regulates the LPS-induced cytokine production in monocytic cells via NF-kappa B. *Cellular Immunology*, *220*(2), 83–95. doi:10.1016/S0008-8749(03)00006-6 PMID:12657243

Honcock, R. E., & Sahl, H. G. (2006). Antimicrobial and host-defense peptides as new anti-infective therapeutic strategies. *Nature Biotechnology*, *24*(12), 1551–1557. doi:10.1038/nbt1267 PMID:17160061

Huang, W. Y., Chakrabarti, S., Majumder, K., Jiang, Y. Y., Davidge, S. T., & Wu, J. P. (2010). Egg-Derived Peptide IRW Inhibits TNF-alpha-Induced Inflammatory Response and Oxidative Stress in Endothelial Cells. *Journal of Agricultural and Food Chemistry*, *58*(20), 10840–10846. doi:10.1021/jf102120c PMID:20886881

Hwang, J. S., Yoo, H. J., Song, H. J., Kim, K. K., Chun, Y. J., Matsui, T., & Kim, H. B. (2011). Inflammation related signaling pathways implicating TGFβ are revealed in the expression profiling of MCF7 cell treated with fermented soybean, Chungkookjang. N*utrition and Cancer, 63(*4), 645–652. doi:10.1080/01635581.2011.551987 PMID:21547849

Ichikawa, S., Morifuji, M., Ohara, H., Matsumoto, H., Takeuchi, Y., & Sato, K. (2010). Hydroxyproline-containing dipeptides and tripeptides quantified at high concentration in human blood after oral administration of gelatin hydrolysate. *International Journal of Food Sciences and Nutrition*, *61*(1), 52–60. doi:10.3109/09637480903257711 PMID:19961355

Iskandar, M. M., Dauletbaev, N., Kubow, S., Mawji, N., & Lands, L. C. (2013). Whey protein hydrolysates decrease IL-8 secretion in lipopolysaccharide (LPS)-stimulated respiratory epithelial cells by affecting LPS binding to Toll-like receptor 4. *British Journal of Nutrition*, *110*(1), 58–68. doi:10.1017/S0007114512004655 PMID:23286514

Jacquot, A., Gauthier, S. F., Drouin, R., & Boutin, Y. (2010). Proliferative effects of synthetic peptides from b-lactoglobulin and a-lactalbumin on murine splenocytes. *International Dairy Journal*, *20*(8), 514–521. doi:10.1016/j.idairyj.2010.02.013

Je, J. Y., Qian, Z., Byun, H. G., & Kim, S. K. (2007). Purification and characterization of an antioxidant peptide obtained from tuna backbone protein by enzymatic hydrolysis. *Proc Biochem*, *42*(5), 840–846. doi:10.1016/j.procbio.2007.02.006

Kamau, S. M., Cheison, S. C., Chen, W., Liu, X.-M., & Lu, R.-R. (2010). Alpha lactalbumin:its production technologies and bioactive peptides. *Comprehensive Reviews in Food Science and Food Safety*, *9*(2), 197–212. doi:10.1111/j.1541-4337.2009.00100.x

Kibangou, I. B., Bouhallab, S., Henry, G., Bureau, F., Allouche, S., Blais, A., ... Bouglé, D. L. (2005). Milk Proteins and Iron Absorption: Contrasting Effects of Different Caseinophosphopeptides. *Pediatric Research*, *58*(4), 731–734. doi:10.1203/01.PDR.0000180555.27710.46 PMID:16189201

Kim, E. K., & Choi, E. J. (2015). Compromised MAPK signaling in human diseases: An update. *Archives of Toxicology*, *89*(6), 867–882. doi:10.100700204-015-1472-2 PMID:25690731

Kim, S. K., & Wijesekara, I. (2010). Development and biological activities of marine-derived bioactive peptides: A review. *Journal of Functional Foods*, *2*(1), 1–9. doi:10.1016/j.jff.2010.01.003

Kitts, D. D. (2005). Antioxidant properties of casein-phosphopeptides. *Trends in Food Science & Technology*, *16*(12), 549–554. doi:10.1016/j.tifs.2005.08.009

Kitts, D. D., & Weiler, K. (2003). Bioactive Proteins and Peptides from Food Sources. Applications of Bioprocesses used in Isolation and Recovery. In W. Banks (Ed.), Current Pharmaceutical Design (pp. 1309-13239). Bentham Science Publishers Ltd.

Korhonen, H. (2009). Milk-derived bioactive peptides: From science to applications. *Journal of Functional Foods*, *1*(2), 177–187. doi:10.1016/j.jff.2009.01.007

Korhonen, H., & Pihlanto, A. (2006). Bioactive peptides: Production and functionality. *International Dairy Journal*, *16*(9), 945–960. doi:10.1016/j.idairyj.2005.10.012

Korhonen, H., & Pihlanto, A. (2007). Technological options for the production of health-promoting proteins and peptides derived from milk and colostrum. *Current Pharmaceutical Design*, *13*(8), 829–843. doi:10.2174/138161207780363112 PMID:17430184

Kovacs-Nolan, J., Zhang, H., Ibuki, M., Nakamori, T., Yoshiura, K., Turner, P. V., ... Mine, Y. (2012). The PepT1-transportable soy tripeptide VPY reduces intestinal inflammation. *Biochimica et Biophysica Acta. G, General Subjects*, *1820*(11), 1753–1763.

Kumagai, H. (2010). Wheat proteins and peptides. In Y. Mine, E. Li-Chan, & B. Jiang (Eds.), *Bioactive Proteins and Peptides as Functional Foods and Nutraceuticals* (pp. 289–303). Oxford: Wiley-Blackwell. doi:10.1002/9780813811048.ch20

Kwak, S. J., Kim, C. S., Choi, M. S., Park, T., Sung, M. K., Yun, J. W., ... Yu, R. (2016). The soy peptide phe–leu–val reduces TNFa-induced inflammatory response and insulin resistance in adipocytes. *Journal of Medicinal Food*, *19*(7), 678–685. doi:10.1089/jmf.2016.3685 PMID:27322965

Lassoued, I., Mora, L., Barkia, A., Aristoy, M. C., Nasri, M., & Toldra, F. (2015). Bioactive peptides identified in thornback ray skin's gelatin hydrolysates by proteases from Bacillus subtilis and Bacillus amyloliquefaciens. *Journal of Proteomics*, *128*, 8–17. doi:10.1016/j.jprot.2015.06.016 PMID:26149667

Laveti, D., Kumar, M., Hemalatha, R., Sistla, R., Naidu, V. G., Talla, V., ... Nagpal, R. (2013). Anti-inflammatory treatments for chronic diseases: A review. *Inflammation & Allergy Drug Targets*, *12*(5), 349–361. doi:10.2174/18715281113129990053 PMID:23876224

Lee, M., Kovacs-Nolan, J., Yang, C., Archbold, T., Fan, M. Z., & Mine, Y. (2009). Hen egg lysozyme attenuates infl ammation and modulates local gene expression in a porcine model of dextran sodium sulfate (DSS) - induced colitis. *Journal of Agricultural and Food Chemistry*, *57*(6), 2233–2240. doi:10.1021/jf803133b PMID:19231858

Léonil, J. (2014). Milk bioactive peptides: Their interest for cardiovascular diseases and metabolic syndrome prevention. *Medecine Des Maladies Metaboliques*, *8*, 495–499.

Li, S., Liu, L., He, G., & Wu, J. (2018). Molecular targets and mechanisms of bioactive peptides against metabolic syndromes. *Food & Function*, *9*(1), 42–52. doi:10.1039/C7FO01323J PMID:29188845

Li, X.-X., Han, L. J., & Chen, L. J. (2008). In vitro antioxidant activity of protein hydrolysates prepared from corn gluten meal. *Journal of the Science of Food and Agriculture*, *88*(9), 1660–1666. doi:10.1002/jsfa.3264

Li, Y. W., Li, B., He, J., & Qian, P. (2011). Quantitative structure-activity relationship study of antioxidative peptide by using different sets of amino acids descriptors. *Journal of Molecular Structure*, *998*(1–3), 53–61. doi:10.1016/j.molstruc.2011.05.011

Liu, R., Xing, L., Fu, Q., Zhou, G. H., & Zhang, W. G. (2016). A review of antioxidant peptides derived from meat muscle and by-products. *Antioxidants (Basel, Switzerland)*, *5*, 32. PMID:27657142

Majumder, K., Chakrabarti, S., Davidge, S. T., & Wu, J. (2013). Structure and activity study of egg protein ovotransferrin derived peptides (IRW and IQW) on endothelial inflammatory response and oxidative stress. *Journal of Agricultural and Food Chemistry*, *61*(9), 2120–2129. doi:10.1021/jf3046076 PMID:23317476

Majumder, K., Mine, Y., & Wu, J. (2016). The potential of food protein-derived anti-inflammatory peptides against various chronic inflammatory diseases. *Sci Food Agric*, *96*(7), 2303–2311. doi:10.1002/jsfa.7600 PMID:26711001

Malaguti, M., Dinelli, G., Leoncini, E., Bregola, V., Bosi, S., Cicero, A., & Hrelia, S. (2014). Bioactive peptides in cereals and legumes: Agronomical, biochemical and clinical aspects. *International Journal of Molecular Sciences*, *15*(11), 21120–21135. doi:10.3390/ijms151121120 PMID:25405741

Manna, S. L., Di Natale, C., Florio, D., & Marasco, D. (2018). Peptides as Therapeutic Agents for Inflammatory-Related Diseases. *International Journal of Molecular Sciences*, *19*(9), 2714. doi:10.3390/ijms19092714 PMID:30208640

Marchbank, T., Elia, G., & Playford, R. J. (2009). Intestinal protective effect of a commercial fish protein hydrolysate preparation. *Regulatory Peptides*, *155*(1-3), 105–109. doi:10.1016/j.regpep.2009.02.003 PMID:19323982

Marcone, S., Belton, O., & Fitzgerald, D. J. (2017). Milk-derived bioactive peptides and their health promoting effects: A potential role in atherosclerosis. *British Journal of Clinical Pharmacology*, *83*(1), 152–162. doi:10.1111/bcp.13002 PMID:27151091

Massaccesi, L. (2016) Role of Bioactive components in inflammation and oxidative stress in vascular endothelium [Thesis]. University of Bologna.

Mendis, E., Rajapakse, N., Byun, H. G., & Kim, S. K. (2005). Investigation of jumbo squid (Dosidicus gigas) skin gelatin peptides for their in vitro antioxidant effects. *Life Sciences*, *77*(17), 2166–2178. doi:10.1016/j.lfs.2005.03.016 PMID:15916780

Mine, Y., Li-Chan, E., & Jiang, B. (2010). Biologically Active Food Proteins and Peptides in Health: An Overview. In Y. Mine, E. Li-Chan, & B. Jiang (Eds.), Bioactive Proteins and Peptides as Functional Foods and Nutraceuticals. Academic Press.

Mine, Y., Li-Chan, E., & Jiang, B. (Eds.). (2010). *Bioactive proteins and peptides as functional foods and nutraceuticals* (Vol. 29). John Wiley & Sons.

Mine, Y., & Shahidi, F. (2006). *Nutraceutical Proteins and Peptides in Health and Disease*. New York: CRC - Taylor & Francis.

Mohanty, D., Jena, R., Choudhury, P. K., Pattnaik, R., Mohapatra, S., & Saini, M. R. (2016). Milk derived antimicrobial bioactive peptides: A review. *International Journal of Food Properties*, *19*(4), 837–846. doi:10.1080/10942912.2015.1048356

Mohanty, D. P., Mohapatra, S., Misra, S., & Sahu, P. S. (2016). Milk derived bioactive peptides and their impact on human health - A review. *Saudi Journal of Biological Sciences*, *23*(5), 577–583. doi:10.1016/j.sjbs.2015.06.005 PMID:27579006

Moller, N. P., Scholz-Ahrens, K. E., Roos, N., & Schrezenmeir, J. (2008). Bioactive peptides and proteins from foods: Indication for health effects. *European Journal of Nutrition*, *47*(4), 171–182. doi:10.100700394-008-0710-2 PMID:18506385

Mora, L., Gallego, M., & Toldrá, F. (2018). ACEI-Inhibitory Peptides Naturally Generated in Meat and Meat Products and Their Health Relevance. *Nutrients*, *10*(9), 1259. doi:10.3390/nu10091259 PMID:30205453

Moronta, J., Paola, L., Smaldini, P. L., Docena, G. H., & Añón, M. C. (2016). Peptides of amaranth were targeted as containing sequences with potential anti-inflammatory properties. *Journal of Functional Foods*, *21*, 463–473. doi:10.1016/j.jff.2015.12.022

Moughan, P. J., & Rutherfurd-Markwick, K. (2013). *Food bioactive proteins and peptides: antimicrobial, immunomodulatory and anti-inflammatory effects*. Woodhead Publishing Limited.

Ngo, D. H., & Kim, S. K. (2013). Marine bioactive peptides as potential antioxidants. *Current Protein & Peptide Science*, *14*(3), 189–198. doi:10.2174/1389203711314 9990041 PMID:23721315

Nielsen, D. S., Theil, P. K., Larsen, L. B., & Purup, S. (2012). Effect of milk hydrolysates on inflammation markers and drug-induced transcriptional alterations in cell-based models. *Journal of Animal Science*, *90*(4suppl 4), 403–405. doi:10.2527/jas.53953 PMID:23365393

O'Shea, J. J., Schwartz, D. M., Villarino, A. V., Gadina, M., McInnes, I. B., & Laurence, A. (2015). The JAK-STAT pathway: Impact on human disease and therapeutic intervention. *Annual Review of Medicine*, *66*(1), 311–328. doi:10.1146/annurev-med-051113-024537 PMID:25587654

Pepe, G., Sommella, E., Ventre, G., Scala, M. C., Adesso, S., Ostacolo, C., ... Campiglia, P. (2016). Antioxidant peptides released from gastrointestinal digestion of "Stracchino" soft cheese: Characterization, in vitro intestinal protection and bioavailability. *Journal of Functional Foods*, *26*, 494–505. doi:10.1016/j.jff.2016.08.021

Phelan, M., Aherne, A., FitzGerald, R. J., & O'Brien, N. M. (2009). Casein derived bioactive peptides: Biological effects, industrial uses, safety aspects and regulatory status. *International Dairy Journal*, *19*(11), 643–654. doi:10.1016/j.idairyj.2009.06.001

Piccolomini, A. F., Iskandar, M. M., Lands, L. C., & Kubow, S. (2012). High hydrostatic pressure pre-treatment of whey proteins enhances whey protein hydrolysate inhibition of oxidative stress and IL-8 secretion in intestinal epithelial cells. *Food & Nutrition Research*, 56. PMID:22723766

Pihlanto, A. (2011). Milk protein products-Bioactive peptides. In *Bioactive Peptides* (pp. 879–886). Amsterdam, Netherlands: Elsevier.

Pinto, G., Caira, S., Cuollo, M., Lilla, S., Chianese, L., & Addeo, F. (2012). Bioactive Casein Phosphopeptides in Dairy Products as Nutraceuticals for Functional Foods. In Milk Protein (pp. 3-44). INTECH. doi:10.5772/50725

Pritchard, S. R., Phillips, M., & Kailasapathy, K. (2010). Identification of bioactive peptides in commercial Cheddar cheese. *Food Research International*, *43*(5), 1545–1548. doi:10.1016/j.foodres.2010.03.007

Przybylski, R., Firdaous, L., Châtaigné, G., Dhulster, P., & Nedjar, N. (2016). Production of an antimicrobial peptide derived from slaughterhouse by product and its potential application on meat as preservative. *Food Chemistry*, *211*, 306–313. doi:10.1016/j.foodchem.2016.05.074 PMID:27283637

Ranathunga, S., Rajapakse, N., & Kim, S. K. (2006). Purification and characterization of antioxidative peptide derived from muscle of conger eel (Conger myriaster). *European Food Research and Technology*, *222*(3-4), 310–315. doi:10.100700217-005-0079-x

Rizzello, C. G., Tagliazucchi, D., Babini, E., Sefora Rutella, G., Taneyo Saa, D. L., & Gianotti, A. (2016). Bioactive peptides from vegetable food matrices: Research trends and novel biotechnologies for synthesis and recovery. *Journal of Functional Foods*, *27*, 549–569. doi:10.1016/j.jff.2016.09.023

Roos, N., Mahe, S., Benamouzig, R., Sick, H., Rautureau, J., & Tomé, D. (1995). 15N-labeled immunoglobulins from bovine colostrum are partially resistant to digestion in human intestine. *The Journal of Nutrition*, *125*, 1238–1244. PMID:7738684

Sánchez, A., & Vazquez, A. (2017). Bioactive peptides: A review. *Food Quality and Safety*, *1*(1), 29–46. doi:10.1093/fqs/fyx006

Sato, K., Egashira, Y., Ono, S., Mochizuki, S., Shimmura, Y., Suzuki, Y., ... Sanada, H. (2013). Identification of a hepatoprotective peptide in wheat gluten hydrolysate against Dgalactosamine-induced acute hepatitis in rats. *Journal of Agricultural and Food Chemistry*, *61*(26), 6304–6310. doi:10.1021/jf400914e PMID:23742096

Scholz-Ahrens, K. E., & Schrezenmeir, J. (2000). Effects of bioactive substances in milk on mineral and trace element metabolism with special reference to caseinphosphopeptides. *British Journal of Nutrition*, *84*(S1), 147–153. doi:10.1017/S0007114500002373 PMID:11242459

Schrezenmeir, J., Korhonen, H., Williams, M., Gill, H. S., & Shah, N. P. (2000). Foreword. *British Journal of Nutrition*, *84*(S1), S1. doi:10.1017/S0007114500002178

Selamassakul, O., Laohakunjit, N., Kerdchoechuen, O., & Ratanakhanokchai, K. (2016). A novel multi-biofunctional protein from brown rice hydrolysed by endo/endo-exoproteases. *Food & Function*, *7*(6), 2635–2644. doi:10.1039/C5FO01344E PMID:27186602

Seppo, L., Jauhiainen, T., Poussa, T., & Korpela, R. (2003). A fermented milk high in bioactive peptides has a blood pressure-lowering effect in hypertensive subjects. *The American Journal of Clinical Nutrition*, *77*(2), 326–330. doi:10.1093/ajcn/77.2.326 PMID:12540390

Sgarbieri, V. C. (2017). Food Proteins and Bioactive Peptides. *Functional Diets Food Sci. Nutr.*, (3), 23.

Sharma, S., Singh, R., & Rana, S. (2011). Bioactive peptides: A review. *International Journal Bioautomation*, *15*, 223–250.

Shimizu, N., Dairiki, K., Ogawa, S., & Kaneko, T. (2006). Dietary whey protein hydrolysate suppresses development of atopic dermatitis-like skin lesions induced bymite antigen in NC/Nga mice. *Allergology International*, *55*(2), 185–189. doi:10.2332/allergolint.55.185 PMID:17075256

Siebert, K. J. (2001). Quantitative structure-activity relationship modeling of peptide and protein behavior as a function of amino acid composition. *Journal of Agricultural and Food Chemistry*, *49*(2), 851–858. doi:10.1021/jf000718y PMID:11262040

Silva-Sanchez, C., de la Rosa, A. P. B., Leon-Galvan, M. F., de Lumen, B. O., de Leon-Rodriguez, A., & de Mejia, E. G. (2008). Bioactive peptides in amaranth (Amaranthus hypochondriacus) seed. *Journal of Agricultural and Food Chemistry*, *56*(4), 1233–1240. doi:10.1021/jf072911z PMID:18211015

Singh, B. P., Vij, S., & Hati, S. (2014). Functional significance of bioactive peptides derived from soybean. *Peptides*, *54*, 171–179. doi:10.1016/j.peptides.2014.01.022 PMID:24508378

Sun, X., Chakrabarti, S., Fang, J., Yin, Y., & Wu, J. (2016). Low-molecular weight fractions of Alcalase hydrolyzed egg ovomucin extract exert antiinflammatory activity in human dermal fibroblasts through the inhibition of tumor necrosis factor-mediated nuclear factor κB pathway. *Nutrition Research (New York, N.Y.)*, *36*(7), 648–657. doi:10.1016/j.nutres.2016.03.006 PMID:27333955

Toldrá, F., Reig, M., Aristoy, M. C., & Mora, L. (2018). Generation of bioactive peptides during processing. *Food Chemistry*, *267*, 395–404. doi:10.1016/j.foodchem.2017.06.119 PMID:29934183

Torres-Llanez, M. J., Vallejo-Cordoba, B., & Gonzalez-Cordova, A. F. (2005). Bioactive peptides derived from milk proteins. *Archivos Latinoamericanos de Nutricion*, *55*, 111–117. PMID:16335219

Udechukwu, M. C., Tsopmo, A., Mawhinney, H., He, R., Kienesberger, P. C., & Udenigwe, C. C. (2017). Inhibition of ADAM17/TACE activity by zinc-chelating rye secalin-derived tripeptides and analogues. *RSC Advances*, *42*(7), 26361–26369. doi:10.1039/C6RA26678A

Vogel, H. J., Schibli, D. J., Jing, W., Lohmeier-Vogel, E. M., Epand, R. F., & Epand, R. M. (2002). Towards a structure-function analysis of bovine lactoferricin and related tryptophan- and argininecontaining peptides. *Biochemistry and Cell Biology*, *80*(1), 49–63. doi:10.1139/o01-213 PMID:11908643

Wada, S., Sato, K., Ohta, R., Wada, E., Bou, Y., Fujiwara, M., ... Yoshikawa, T. (2013). Ingestion of low dose pyroglutamyl leucine improves dextran sulfate sodium-induced colitis and intestinal microbiota in mice. *Journal of Agricultural and Food Chemistry*, *61*(37), 8807–8813. doi:10.1021/jf402515a PMID:23964746

Walther, B., & Sieber, R. (2011). Bioactive proteins and peptides in foods. *International Journal for Vitamin and Nutrition Research*, *81*(23), 181–191. doi:10.1024/0300-9831/a000054 PMID:22139569

Wan, X., Liu, H., Sun, Y., Zhang, J., Chen, X., & Chen, N. (2017). Lunasin: A promising polypeptide for the prevention and treatment of cancer. *Oncology Letters*, *13*(6), 3997–4001. doi:10.3892/ol.2017.6017 PMID:28599405

Wang, W. Y., & De Mejia, E. G. (2005). A new frontier in soy bioactive peptides that may prevent age-related chronic diseases. *Comprehensive Reviews in Food Science and Food Safety*, *4*(4), 63–78. doi:10.1111/j.1541-4337.2005.tb00075.x

Yan, D., Chen, D., Shen, J., Xiao, G., vanWijnen, A. J., & Im, H. J. (2013). Bovine lactoferricin is anti-inflammatory and anti-catabolic in human articular cartilage and synovium. *Journal of Cellular Physiology, 228*(2), 447–456. doi:10.1002/jcp.24151 PMID:22740381

Yoshikawa, M., Fujita, H., Matoba, N., Takenaka, Y., Yamamoto, T., Yamauchi, R., ... Takahata, K. (2000). Bioactive peptides derived from food proteins preventing lifestyle-related diseases. *BioFactors (Oxford, England), 12*(1–4), 143–146. doi:10.1002/biof.5520120122 PMID:11216476

Young, D., & Mine, Y. (2010). Anti-inflammatory/oxidative stress proteins and peptides. *Bioactive proteins and peptides as functional foods and nutraceuticals*, 13-27.

Zhang, H., Kovacs-Nolan, J., Kodera, T., Eto, Y., & Mine, Y. (2015). γ-Glutamyl cysteine and γ-glutamyl valine inhibit TNF-α signaling in intestinal epithelial cells and reduce inflammation in amouse model of colitis via allosteric activation of the calcium-sensing receptor. Bio*chim Biophys ActaMol Basis Dis, 1852, 792*–804. doi:10.1016/j.bbadis.2014.12.023 PMID:25558818

Zhang, Y., Kouguchi, T., Shimizu, K., Sato, M., Takahata, Y., & Morimatsu, F. (2010). Chicken collagen hydrolysate reduces proinflammatory cytokine production in C57BL/6.KOR-ApoEsh1 mice. *Journal of Nutritional Science and Vitaminology, 56*(3), 208–210. doi:10.3177/jnsv.56.208 PMID:20651463

Zhao, L., Wang, X., Zhang, X. L., & Xie, Q. F. (2016). Purification and identification of anti-inflammatory peptides derived from simulated gastrointestinal digests of velvet antler protein (Cervus elaphus Linnaeus). *Journal of Food and Drug Analysis, 24*(2), 376–384. doi:10.1016/j.jfda.2015.10.003 PMID:28911592

Chapter 6
Pro-/Anti-Inflammatory Food Supplements:
Probiotics and Prebiotics

Hüseyin Eseceli
https://orcid.org/0000-0002-5912-5479
University of Bandıma Onyedi Eylül, Turkey

ABSTRACT

Probiotics are living microorganisms, meaning "for life" and consist of two parts, "pro" and "biota," and prebiotics are indigestible carbohydrates that increase the number and activities of colon bacteria and the effectiveness of probiotics. Probiotic consumption has been reported to have many positive effects, such as increasing immune response, balancing the colony, and increasing endogenous defense capacity of cells. The aim of prebiotics is to grow probiotic bacteria, thus improving the gastrointestinal and immune systems. Recent studies have shown that probiotics may have an impact on gastrointestinal system diseases. It has been shown to stimulate the proliferation of beneficial microorganisms in prebiotics and assist in the probiotic effect. The most commonly used probiotics and prebiotics are lactic acid bacteria that are types of Lactobacillus and Bifidobacterium. Prebiotics are naturally present in nutrients. Probiotics and prebiotics are used to prevent many diseases.

DOI: 10.4018/978-1-7998-3594-3.ch006

DEFINITION AND HISTORY OF PROBIOTICS

The term probiotic has been used frequently in the last 10-15 years. Elie Metchnikoff, winner of the 1912 Nobel Prize in medicine, reported that the Bulgarian people lived longer than other nations, and that this was due to the intake of dairy products containing living bacteria. Metchnikoff emphasized the positive effects of some bacteria and suggested that it would be possible to replace harmful bacteria with beneficial bacteria by giving beneficial microorganisms. He stated that what prolongs life is beneficial microorganisms found in sour milk (Parkes, 2007; Uriot et al., 2017).

The term probiotic comes from the "pro bios" origin in Greek (pro: for, bios: life) and means "for life". The use of probiotics by humans dates back to ancient times. Fermented dairy products, which are widely known in the Greeks and Romans, have been used especially in the treatment of children and convalescent patients. The term probiotic was first proposed by Vergin in 1954 as an antithetical term (Sekhon, 2010). One year later, Kolb suggested that the undesirable effects of antibiotics could be prevented by probiotics. It was used in 1965 by Lilly and Stillwell, the first to use the term probiotic to describe the development of the product produced by one microorganism. In 1974, Parker described probiotics as organisms that help maintain bowel balance (Fuller, 1992). In 1996, Schaffsma described them as living microorganisms that had positive nutritional effects as well as basic nutritional properties (Schaffsma, 1996).

Today, the definition of probiotics is used and agreed upon by FAO and WHO (2002). According to this definition, probiotics are "living microorganisms that, when taken in sufficient amounts, have beneficial health effects on the host."

PROBIOTIC BACTERIA

So far, many species have been isolated and studied. Probiotic microorganisms may be bacteria or yeast. The most studied and used bacteria are from the family of *Lactobacillus* and *Bifidobacterium* (Roberfroid, 2000). Among these species, *Lactobacillus rhamnosus* GG is the most studied probiotic bacteria on *Saccharomyces boulardii*.

The main probiotic microorganisms are: *Lactobacillus acidophilus*, *L. casei*, *L. lactis*, *L. helveticus*, *L. salivarius*, *L. plantarum*, *L. bulgaricus*, *L. curvatus*, *L. gasseri*, *L. rhamnosus*, *L. johnso-nii*, *L. reuteri*, *L. fermeritum*, *L. delbrueckii*, *L. vaginalis*, *L. cellobiosus*, *L. brevis*, *L. curvatus*, *Bifidobacterium bifidum*, *B. breve*, *B. longum*, *B. thermophilum*, *B. adolescentis*, *B. angulatum*, *B. peseudocatenulatum*, *B. animalis* and *B. infantis*, *Streptococcus thermophilus*, *S. cremoris*, *S. thermophilus*,

S. intermedius, S. lactis, S. diacetilactis, Enterococcus faecium, Saccharomyces boulardii, Aspergillus niger.

Probiotic bacteria can be taken separately as medication or supplementary purposes. They can be mixed with functional foods, they can be added to them or can be found naturally in them (Coşkun, 2014).

CHARACTERISTICS OF PROBIOTIC MICROORGANISMS

Probiotic microorganisms must have certain properties in order to be successful. It should be used safely in humans, should be effective, the product should remain alive during shelf rest and should not have pathogenic properties.

- Reliability for the host
- Regulating immune system
- Obtained from the type of host to be used
- Good identification and typing
- Without pathogen and toxic properties (including enterotoxin and cytokine production, enteroinvasivity, pathogenic adhesion, hemolysis, antibiotic resistance gene transport)
- Resistant to stomach acid and bile pancreatic acids
- Being able to secrete antimicrobial substances
- Resistant to food additives
- Resistant to processing conditions
- Can be attached to the intestinal epithelium
- Temporarily colonize the gastrointestinal tract
- Having beneficial effects on host health
- Inhibit the attachment of pathogenic bacteria
- It should contain high numbers of living microorganisms
- Be able to survive in the intestine, maintain metabolic activity
- Maintain viability during storage and use
- They should be able to adapt to natural flora and not to replace them (Salminen, 2005; Williams 2010; Coşkun, 2014)

Probiotic microorganisms' human origin and living characteristics are relative criteria. Saccharomyces boulardii is used for humans although it is not of human origin. Therefore, the use of the expression "biotherapeutic agent would be more accurate (Sleator, 2008).

THE EFFECTS OF MAIN PROBIOTIC MICROORGANISMS ON OUR HEALTH

Lactobacillus rhamnosus: Reduces mucosal defect-producing effects of cow's milk and rotaviruses. It can also shorten the duration of travel diarrhea caused by rotaviruses and antibiotic-associated diarrhea, strengthen the immune response, and is used in the prevention and treatment of cow's milk-related atopic eczema, vaginosis and vaginitis.

Lactobacillus casei: Reduces severity and duration of diarrhea. Stimulates the immune system in the gastrointestinal tract, alleviates the symptoms of Crohn's disease, has strong antimicrobial properties.

Lactobacillus casei shirota: Prevents diarrhea due to bacteria and viruses. It is the most effective microorganism in lactose intolerance, rotavirus and *Clostridium difficile* diarrhea and antibiotic related diarrhea. Prevents recurrences after superficial bladder cancer surgery.

Lactobacillus acidophilus: Lactic acid secretions, lowers the pH in the intestinal lumen and prevents the growth of pathogens such as salmonella and *E. coli*. Increases antibody response and seroconversion rate. Lowers serum cholesterol levels. It is used to prevent necrotizing enterocolitis, radiation enteritis, vaginosis and vaginitis.

Lactobacillus johnsonii: Reduces helicobacter pylori intensity, inflammation and gastritis activity, strengthens the immune response.

Lactobacillus plantarum: Produces short-chain fatty acids that inhibit the emergence of carcinogenic substances by reducing enzyme activities and are effective in irritable bowel syndrome. Enhances immune response.

Lactobacillus bulgaricus: It is effective in preventing antibiotic related diarrhea.

Lactobacillus reuteri: Used in the treatment of acute childhood diarrhea, vaginosis and vaginitis.

Lactobacillus lactis: Strengthens the immune response and is effective in the prevention and treatment of cow's milk-associated atopic eczema.

Bifidobacteria

Bifidobacterium breve: Activates the humoral immune system by increasing anti-rotavirus IgA and anti-influenza virus antibodies.

Bifidobacterium bifidum: Compete with pathogenic microorganisms in place and nutrients in the lumen, reduce the frequency of diarrhea, and increase seroconversion rate and antibody response. It is effective in preventing the development of necrotizing enterocolitis.

***Bifidobacterium infantis*:** Prevents diarrhea and constipation and is used in irritable bowel syndrome.

***Bifidobacterium animalis*:** Provides normal motility. Reduces the risk of acute diarrhea in children and adults.

Yeast

***Saccharomyces cerevisiae boulardii*:** It prevents travel diarrhea and pathogen-induced colitis and enterocolitis. It reduces the risk and duration of developing antibiotic-associated diarrhea.

Others

***Enterococcus faecalis*:** It is effective in achieving remission and maintenance of ulcerative colitis (Coşkun, 2014).

EFFECT MECHANISM OF PROBIOTICS

The exact mechanism of action of probiotics is not known. The most commonly used microorganisms are *Lactobacilli* and *Bifidobacteria* producing lactic acid, acetic acid and propionic acid and reducing the pH of the intestine, suppressing the growth of pathogenic bacteria and providing balance in the intestinal flora. The mechanism of action varies according to the different probiotics and strains, and varies according to the dose and way of administration. Therefore a mechanism detected in a probiotic bacteria cannot be generalized for all probiotics.

Production of inhibiting substances: Probiotics produce many substances that are effective on gram positive and gram negative microorganisms. Some of these are organic acids, hydrogen peroxide, bacteriocin and bacteriocin-like substances.

Blocking of attachment sites: Probiotics compete with pathogens for attachment sites, preventing them from settling in the intestinal tract.

Competitiveness for nutrients: Probiotics consume nutrients necessary for pathogens, preventing them from staying in the system for a long time. However, in vivo data are needed to prove this mechanism.

Destruction of toxin receptors: This mechanism has been proposed in animals because *S. boulardii* cleaves the toxin receptors of *Clostridium difficile* in the intestinal mucosa and protects the host.

Strengthening the immune system: Recent studies have shown that probiotics protect the host against intestinal diseases by strengthening the specific and nonspecific immune system. Although this mechanism has not been fully elucidated, it is thought that specific cell wall components or cell surfaces have an adjuvant effect and strengthen the humoral immune response (Çakır, 2004).

The probable other beneficial effects of probiotics on our health;

- Reduction of the signs and symptoms of lactose intolerance: intracellular b-galactosidase administration to the intestines
- Preventing rotavirus and antibiotic-associated diarrhea and alleviating symptoms: Competitive exclusion, translocation / barrier effect, strengthening of immune response
- Prevention and treatment of allergies (atopic eczema and food allergies): Translocation / barrier effect, immune exclusion, elimination and regulation
- Reducing the risk associated with mutagenicity and carcinogenicity: Metabolism of mutagens, changes in intestinal micro ecology, changes in intestinal metabolic activity, normalization of intestinal permeability, strengthening of intestinal immunity
- Hypocholesterolemic effect: Deconjugation of bile acids
- Inhibition of Helicobacter pylori and intestinal pathogens: Competitive exclusion, barrier effect, antimicrobial compound production
- Prevention of inflammatory bowel diseases: Competitive exclusion, strengthening of epithelial tight junctions, regulation of intestinal permeability, regulation of immune response, production of antimicrobial compounds, destruction of pathogenic antigens (Coskun, 2014).

DOSAGE OF PROBIOTICS

Probiotics are found in foods or sold as capsules, powder or tablets. Content varies from one product to another as cfu. Therefore, users should read the description of the product to check whether they have taken enough doses.

Dosages of probiotics vary according to products and specific indications. To obtain beneficial effects from probiotics, there is no consensus on the minimum number of microorganisms it should contain (Farnworth, 2008). Typically, a probiotic should contain several billion microorganisms to increase the likelihood of adequate bowel colonization (Cremonini et al., 2002).

A typical daily dose of 1-20 billion cfu was used in the studies for lactobacilli while in most of the studies for *S. boulardii* it was 250-500 mg. The daily doses varying between were examined. The dose for children is half of the adult dose (average

5-10 billion cfu / day) and one fourth of infants. The time of administration may also vary from twice a day to once a week. It should not be concluded that increasing the dose will not be safe. However, it is expensive and unnecessary (Coşkun, 2014).

Products should be stored according to the manufacturer's recommendations, as cooling may be required. In addition; preparations may have a limited shelf life and many preparations may contain several different species, so the dosage may vary depending on the product.

Most probiotics do not consistently colonize the lower parts of the digestive tract, and even after the most established strains are removed, they can be isolated from the stool for 1-2 weeks. Probiotics should be taken regularly to ensure colonization (Williams, 2010).

SIDE EFFECTS AND RELIABILITY OF PROBIOTICS

Probiotics are commonly used orally and are well tolerated. The side effects of probiotics, if developed, are usually mild and are more of a concern to the gastrointestinal tract (such as abdominal discomfort or gas). Other side effects include thirst, constipation, nausea, vomiting, abdominal pain and rash. These symptoms are usually mild and disappear as the probiotic use continues.

As probiotics are living microorganisms, there is a risk of invasive infections in individuals with impaired mucosal epithelial integrity. Invasive infections have been reported in immun ocompromised patients, sick preterm infants and / or children, patients with an intravenous catheter or implanted with any medical device.

Theoretically, one of the potential dangers of probiotics is that they can pass through the gastrointestinal tract, causing systemic infection. Lactobacilli-induced sepsis or endocarditis, *S. boulardii* and fungemia, LGG-induced liver abscess has been reported. Although rare, probiotic-associated bacteremia and fungemia have been reported.

The risk of developing bacteremia after lactobacilli was 1/1 million and the risk of developing fungemia after *S. Boulardii* was 1 / 5.6 million. Another theoretical risk is the possibility that antibiotic resistance will be transmitted to pathogenic bacteria via probiotic microorganisms, which has not yet been observed.

The safety of probiotic use in children is controversial. There are concerns about the development of sepsis through bacterial translocation. The fact that probiotics attach to the intestinal wall may increase the risk of translocation. Bacteremia and fungemia have been reported in children with chronic disease or immunosuppressed children with no sepsis due to probiotic use in healthy children (Coşkun, 2014).

THE EFFECTS OF PROBIOTICS ON DISEASES

The Effects of Probiotics on IBS

Irritable bowel syndrome (IBS) is a condition of recurrent functional abdominal pain with abdominal distention and changes in defecation habits (diarrhea, constipation, or both) and is one of the most common gastrointestinal system problems in both adult and childhood. It is thought that multiple factors may be effective in the etiology of IBS. These include altered bowel motility, visceral hypersensitivity, changes in intestinal permeability, psychosocial stress factors, low-level inflammation in the brain-intestinal axis, changes in intestinal flora, and genetic factors. Small intestinal and colon motility increased in dominant IBS. It has been shown to slow down in IBS patients with constipation at the forefront (Arslan, 2014).

Probiotics can be beneficial for IBS patients by acting on many different mechanisms. These include intestinal mucosal barrier function, colon bacteria, mucosal immune system, visceral sensitivity, production and fermentation of bacteriocins, and regulatory effects on neurotransmitter production.

Randomized controlled trials supported the positive effects of *Bifidobacterium* on IBS. A study of IBS patients showed that patients receiving *B. infantis* for eight weeks had reduced bowel movement difficulties and pain (O'Mahony et al., 2005). In the majority of studies investigating the effects of probiotics in IBS patients, the use of probiotics resulted in a decrease in general IBS complaints and also abdominal pain.

When some probiotics are used for a certain period of time, some IBS patients have symptoms that have a curative effect, especially because there is currently no effective treatment, and because probiotics are safe, it is recommended to use them together with other treatment options. However, the positive effects of probiotics vary depending on the type of probiotic used, dose, duration of use, and the dominant symptom of the patient (Ringel, 2011). Extensive studies including well-defined patient groups, using objective monitoring criteria and studying microbiological and physiopathological effects will shed light on the emergence of clear applications in the use of probiotics in IBS patients.

The Effects of Probiotics on Constipation

The rationale for probiotic use in the treatment of functional constipation is based on the demonstration of differences in intestinal microbiota of healthy individuals and individuals with chronic constipation. Probiotics increase peristalsis by reducing the pH of the colon and shortening the colonic transit time. They are thought to reduce visceral hypersensitivity due to its anti-inflammatory effect on enteric mucosa and also reduce pain and bloating. Probiotics have been tried as an alternative treatment for constipation in recent years. While randomized controlled trials have been reported to be ineffective in some of the studies, some have been shown to be useful in patients with constipation.

Studies on the effect of probiotics and prebiotics are mostly in the IBS group where constipation is predominant and there are few studies on functional constipation. It has been shown that *B.Animalis* is effective on colonic transit in IBS patients with constipation and increases stool frequency. Another strain; *Bifidobacterium infantis* 35624 improves its consistency without affecting the stool frequency. When basal transit time is slow, *bifidobacterium lactis* DN has been shown to reduce transit time in healthy individuals, the elderly and those with irritable bowel syndrome. It is considered to be a direct effect on colonic motility as it is not effective on fecal mass and bile acid content (Yüce, 2014).

Effects of Probiotics on Diarrhea

Most studies on the clinical use of probiotics have been performed in diarrhea cases. Probiotics compete with pathogenic microorganisms in terms of acid formations and nutrients and receptors, preventing their adhesion and feeding to the mucosa. In addition, they show resistance to GIS infections by showing antitoxin effect (Yağcı, 2002).

Diarrhea is seen in 40% of children as one of the important side effects encountered during the use of broad-spectrum antibiotics. It is important to prevent a certain number of the diarrhea cases that may occur due to the large number of children taking antibiotics each year. Studies have shown that *L. rhamnosus* GG and *Saccharomyces boulardii* have beneficial effects in the treatment and prevention of antibiotic-associated diarrhea (Cremonini et al., 2002).

One group of children with a mean age of 4.5 years who received antibiotics for upper respiratory tract infection were given *L. rhamnosus* GG twice daily, and the frequency of diarrhea decreased significantly from 16% to 5% compared to the control group (Arvola et al. (2005).

Acute diarrhea is the most common clinical entity of travel-associated diarrhea. Also; acute gastroenteritis, dysenteric diarrhea and persistent diarrhea.

The effects of probiotics in diarrhea due to viral agents have been shown in many studies and it has been found that they may be beneficial in the treatment of diarrhea and prevention of diarrhea development. In viral diarrhea, especially in the treatment of rotavirus-induced diarrhea, probiotics have been shown to preserve the host's natural flora, increase viral excretion, and shorten viral excretion time, thereby reducing infectiousness and intestinal permeability caused by rotavirus infection.

There are many studies on the effectiveness of probiotics in acute infectious diarrhea with different strains, doses and methodologies. Most of the studies were performed in pediatric age groups. Many studies have concluded that gastroenteritis and acute diarrhea have improved with probiotic use. It is said to cause a reduction in diarrhea durations and defecations.

In a study, lactic acid bacteria were found to reduce the severity and duration of bacterial and viral diarrhea (Hove et al., 1999). Another study found that milk fermented with *Lactobacillus casei subspecie rhamnosus* (LGG) reduced the severity and duration of rotavirus-induced diarrhea, increased IgA secretion and local interferon release in the intestine, and reduced intestinal permeability (Gorbach, 2000).

The Effects of Probiotics on Lactose Intolerance

Lactose is the basic carbohydrate of breastmilk and is absorbed from the mucosa after cleavage of glucose and galactose by lactase (β-galactosidase) located on the small intestine brushy margin. Lactose intolerance develops as a result of the decrease of this enzyme. The majority of the world's population has lactose intolerance. In lactose digestive problems, one or more symptoms such as abdominal pain, nausea, vomiting and bloating are seen after taking lactose-containing foods. Lactose intolerance is affected by factors such as the amount of lactose taken, lactase activity, and fermentation of lactose in the colon. Therefore, probiotics can be used to alter the metabolism or content of the microflora in the colon (He et al., 2008).

Lactase activity, which is high at birth, starts to decrease in childhood and adolescence. Secondary forms are caused by damage to the intestinal mucosa (diarrhea) and reduced surface (resection). Individuals with problems with lactose digestion can tolerate yogurt. This is due to the presence of β-galactosidase activity in bacteria in yogurt. There is beta galactosidase (lactase) enzyme in *S. thermophilus* and *L. Delbrueckii* microorganisms in yoghurt which improves lactose digestion. In addition, fermented milk products are darker than milk, so the transit time from the gastrointestinal tract is longer; this allows for better digestion (Coskun, 2006).

The most commonly used probiotic in lactose intolerance is *L.acidophilus*. In a study, in those applied *L. acidophilus* microorganism compared to control group, there was an increased level of β galactosidase in the stool and decreased lactose amount (Jiang, 1997). It was shown that the number of bacteria and the microbial-derived β galactosidase activity in the feces increased without changing the type of predominant bacteria in feces in patients receiving *B.Animalis* added yoghurt and *B.longum* probiotic bacteria (He et al., 2008).

The Effects of Probiotics on the Immune System

The therapeutic effects of probiotics may be due to differences in strains of lactic acid bacteria and experimental methods used in various studies. The immunostimulatory effects of lactic acid bacteria depend on the degree of contact of lymphoid tissues with bacteria that are temporarily colonized in the intestinal lumen. Thus, the viability of probiotics in the gastrointestinal tract may affect their bacterial immunity.

The survival rates of probiotics in the gastrointestinal tract depend on changes in gastric pH. *L. Acidophilus*, one of the lactobacilli bacteria, is more resistant to gastric acid compared to *L. Bulgaricus*, which is a conventional lactic acid culture. (Gönülateş, 2008).

The proliferation of beneficial bacteria in the intestines prevents the settling of pests. The lymphoid tissue in the mucosal membranes surrounding the digestive organs is an important part of the lymphoid tissue of the human body. T lymphocytes synthesized in the epithelium show a suppressing and cytotoxic effect against antigen. B-cell lymphocytes serve as aids. Large amounts of IgA antibodies are produced on the mucosal surface. This antibody, called secretory IgA, is resistant to the action of proteolytic enzymes and protects the mucosa from harmful agents. IgA in the small intestine and IgA2 in the large intestine are common. In the absence of microflora, the passage of antigen to the mucosa increases. *Bifidobacteria* proliferation in the intestine increased the number of cells expressing IgA and IgM antibodies in circulation. The uptake of probiotic microorganisms was found to increase the barrier of the mucosa to the antigen.

It has been reported that probiotic bacteria increase the humoral immune response, thereby helping the development of immune ability in the intestine. Probiotic bacteria also increase the individual's resistance to pathogen. It has been reported that oral lactobacilli uptake paves the way for the destruction of pathogens in the intestine. In experimental animals, lactic acid bacteria have been shown to increase macrophage production and phagocytic activity (Baysal, 2007).

The Effects of Probiotics on Cholesterol

Although cholesterol is a basic building block for all body tissues, high blood cholesterol levels are one of the most important risk factors for coronary heart disease. The latest treatment modalities for lowering blood cholesterol levels include diet, regular exercise and medication. In recent years, there have been new approaches in dietary practices to lower high cholesterol levels in the blood. Among these applications, the use of probiotic bacteria is also important. The first record of the effects of probiotic bacteria fermented dairy products on blood lipids dates back nearly 30 years ago. Since then, many in vitro and in vivo studies have shown that probiotic products, especially those containing certain species of *Lactobacillus* or *Bifidobacterium*, reduce high cholesterol levels in the blood. Therefore, interest in the use of probiotics in this field continues to increase day by day.

Although the results of the studies are variable, it can be concluded that probiotic use has beneficial effects on total cholesterol and LDL cholesterol levels in individuals with high cholesterol level, high limit or normal.

Cholesterol-lowering effects of probiotics were evaluated by in vitro and in vivo studies. The mechanisms to explain the effect of lowering serum cholesterol levels are as follows:

1. Enzymatic deconjugation of bile salts and excretion of cholesterol with these deconjugated bile acids by feces
2. Binding of probiotics to the cell membrane of the intestines and excretion of fecal excretion in the intestine, decreased cholesterol and blood cholesterol levels absorbed from the digestive tract.
3. Conversion of cholesterol to coprostanol in the intestine, formation of short chain fatty acids
4. Reduction of fatty acid and cholesterol synthesis in the liver by short-chain fatty acids formed by fermentation of non-digestible carbohydrates in the large intestine by probiotic bacteria
5. Excess needs of probiotics in blood are mechanisms such as reducing cholesterol concentration and increasing high density lipoprotein (HDL) concentration by attracting cholesterol to the liver (İşlek, 2014).

It has been found that some lactic acid bacteria reduce the amount of cholesterol in the blood by the production of hydroxy methyl glutaryl coA reductase. After three weeks of use of fermented milk products containing probiotics and prebiotics, it was found that the total cholesterol level decreased by 4.4% and the low density lipoprotein level decreased by 5.3% compared to the control group (Schaafsma, 1998). In another study, similar results were obtained in those fed with fermented yogurt for four to eight weeks (Agerholm, 2000). These studies suggest that prebiotic / probiotic-rich nutrition initiated in childhood may be protective against cardiovascular diseases.

Effects of Probiotics on Inflammatory Bowel Diseases

Chronic inflammatory (inflammatory) bowel diseases, ulcerative colitis and Crohn's disease is divided into two (Oktay, 2001).

Ulcerative colitis: It is an inflammatory disease characterized by ulceration limited to mucosa in the colon (Özden, 2007). In an uncontrolled study of Guslandi et al. (2003), 25 ulcerative colithastas with mesalazine were given 4 weeks of *Sacchoromyces boulardii* yeast and 17 of the 24 patients who completed the study had no disease activity. The probiotic product containing *Bifidobacter breve*, *Bifidobacter bifidum* and *Lactobacillus acidophilus* YIT 0168 was found to be effective in the treatment of ulcerative colitis. According to the results of a year-long study, only three out of 11 patients in the probiotic group and nine out of 10 patients in the placebo group had increased symptoms, but no difference was found in colonoscopic findings (Ishikawa et al. 2003).

Crohn's disease: Crohn's disease is a chronic inflammatory disease of unknown etiology that affects people's gastrointestinal tract from mouth to anus (Güner, 2004). Crohn's disease is characterized by transmural inflammation affecting the gastrointestinal tract. Conventional treatment is carried out by modifying the host immune response. However, regulation of intestinal microflora is also accepted as a new treatment modality. With three *Bifidobacteria* and four types of *lactobacilli Str. salivarius sp.* The effect of a probiotic product containing the Thermophilus combination to prevent recurrence of Crohn's disease lesions postoperatively has been demonstrated in a placebo-controlled study. The one-year study found a significant reduction in the recurrence rate of the lesions in patients treated with the antibiotic-probiotic combination compared to the placebo group (Gionchetti et al. 2003).

They found that 32 patients (20 males, 12 females) with clinical diagnosis of Crohn's disease had low recurrence rates in the group receiving meselamine and *Sacchoromyces boulardii* (Guslandi, Mezzi, Sorghy, & Testoni, 2000).

The Effects of Probiotics on Pouchitis

Pouchitis is defined by inflammation in the ileal region after ileal-anal anastomosis, where irregularities in the intestinal flora play a role as a triggering factor. In a study investigating the effect of Lactobacillus GG on patients with endoscopic and histological inflammation of the sac mucosa, probiotic use was found to induce changes in the sac microflora (Kuisma et al. 2003). In the study using probiotic VSL 3 preparation, 85% of the patients treated with VSL 3 showed a decrease in the effects of the disease after 9 months, and findings of recurrence were observed in all individuals in the placebo group (Mimura, Rizzello & Helwig, 2004).

The Effects of Probiotics on Helicobacter Pylori

Helicobacter pylori (HP) infection causes many diseases in humans. Chronic gastritis, peptic ulcer, gastric adenocarcinoma, gastric MALT lymphoma, sideropenic anemia, idiopathic thrombocytopenic purpura are some of them. The most important reason for failure of HP treatment is antibiotic resistance. The positive effects of probiotics in the treatment of HP are primarily due to the correction of intestinal dysbiosis by antibiotics. An increase in facultative anaerobes occurs during HP eradication therapy. Giving *L. acidophilus* and *B. bifidum* probiotics during treatment may reverse this pathogen bacteria increase. A significant reduction is observed during the standard treatment of triple therapy. Again, giving yogurt containing *L. acidophilus* and *B. bifidum* restores the number of *Bifidobacteria* to their previous levels (Sheu et al., 2002).

It has been shown that probiotics can be used as adjuvants in the treatment of HP infection, gastric mucosal inflammation decreases as a result of the use of LGG for eight weeks, and the effect of antibacterial therapy combined with probiotics increases (Inanç, Şahin, & Çiçek, 2005).

The Effects of Probiotics on Allergic Diseases

Allergic diseases have been increasing rapidly in recent years. This rapid increase cannot be explained by genetic factors alone. It is thought that less exposure of microorganisms in children at an early age increases allergic diseases with effective hygienic practices, reduced family structure, consuming very sterile foods and providing better health services. Probiotics have proven to be effective in allergic inflammation and food allergy. The relationship between microorganisms and antigens in the gastrointestinal tract begins immediately after birth, and thus the gastrointestinal microorganisms become the earliest and greatest stimulant in the development of lymphoid tissue in the intestines. Probiotics improve bowel barrier function in allergic individuals and restore normal intestinal microecology. Some probiotics have been shown to reduce the problems associated with allergic inflammation in vivo and in vitro conditions.

Bifidobacteria and *Lactobacilli* have been found to increase the production of IgA, an antibody that provides protection against antigens causing damage to the intestinal mucosa by reducing immune reactions. In addition, IgE antibodies are produced when the immune system is alarmed due to an alien attack. However, when useful bacteria are present in sufficient amounts, they send biochemical stimuli to the immune system to reduce the production of IgE antibodies. This minimizes the damage to the skin, the minimum risk of inflammation and the minimum histamine transition to the skin provides (Akalin & Unal, 2005).

The presence of beneficial bacteria in the intestinal tract appears to be the best way to eliminate the conditions that cause eczema. As a result of probiotic support to the body, a large number of organisms such as *Lactobacilli* and *Bifidobacteria* can be found in the digestive tract. Lactobacilli are the most commonly used microorganisms in patients with eczema. *L. Salivarius* was administered to patients with eczema for four months and compared with placebo, resulting in decreased eczema severity and improved quality of life (Doege, Grajecki, & Zyriax, 2012). In eczema, the skin contains *Staphylococcus aureus* at a higher rate than healthy skin. Probiotic application directly to the skin against this harmful bacteria is highly effective. The application of L acidophilus in the form of an ointment provides relief to the injured skin, while at the same time improving the health of new skin cells. In such applications, results are obtained in a short time. In addition, the use of a good probiotic ointment containing a large amount of beneficial bacteria instead of using a topical cortisone preparation does not lead to the thinning of the skin. Balancing and supporting the digestive effects in the body, creating new relaxing factors on the skin is considered a new beginning in coping with the irritating and painful skin problems of eczema.

The results of research in the treatment of allergic rhinitis and asthma of probiotic microorganisms are conflicting. Some studies have shown a decrease in symptoms, while others have not shown a positive effect. The best clinical responses of probiotics have been observed in atopic dermatitis cases with food allergy in infancy (Saçkesen, 2014).The results showed that bacteria living in the intestine can also keep the immune system away from allergic reactions. In addition, although intestinal microflora has not been investigated extensively yet, it has been shown to have rare immunomodular properties and these features are indispensable in the fight against atopic and other immunological diseases.

The Effects of Probiotics on Cancer

Since cancer is the second most common cause of death in adults after heart disease, it is an important public health problem. Although the cause of cancer cannot be shown in most patients, it is generally thought to be multifactorial.

Probiotics change the intestinal microflora positively. Probiotic intake increases the number of bifidobacteria and lactobacilli in faeces, decreases the pH of faeces and decreases bacterial enzyme activities related to cancer development. The number of Bifidobacteria in faeces increased in individuals receiving *Bifidobacterium longum*. Again, beta-glucoronidase nitroreductase, azorereductase, glycolic acid hydrolase activities were decreased in fecal areas. The decrease in the activity of these enzymes is indicative of decreased carcinogen production in the large intestine. Large bowel cancer is the result of mutations caused by DNA damage in oncogenes and tumor suppressor genes. Lactobacillus, *Streptococcus* and *Bifidobacterium* fermented dairy products were found to have antimutogenic effects in experimental studies. Lactic acid bacteria and their prebiotics, which proliferate them, neutralize carcinogens that are toxic to genes. Thus, DNA damage in the intestinal tissue is prevented and the protective system is stimulated. These effects of probiotics in colon cancer prevention should be supported by studies on humans (Baysal, 2007).

Clinical studies have shown that probiotics play an active role in preventing cancer. In studies related to treatment, their efficacy is limited. Further studies are needed on this subject.

The Effects of Probiotics on Obesity

Obesity is the accumulation of excess fat in the body due to the imbalance between energy intake and expenditure. Genetic and environmental factors (lifestyle) are the most important risk factors, but they do not account for the rapid increase in obesity prevalence worldwide.

In recent years, it has been understood that intestinal microbiota may play a very important role in the development of obesity. Numerous animal studies have shown that intestinal flora bacteria play an important role in energy balance and lubrication and that they create these effects (dietary energy, lipopolysaccharide mediated chronic inflammation, regulation of the accumulation of fatty acids in tissues and intestinal secretion of peptides, etc.) with different mechanisms. It is consistent with different animal studies that obese people have decreased Bacteroidetes and increased Firmicutes in the intestines. In addition, a decrease in bacterial diversity was observed in the intestines. Interestingly, this change is reversed by diet and weight loss. Furthermore, it has been determined that probiotic use balances intestinal flora and helps weight loss in new studies (Arslan, 2012).

- Helps balance the host's key vital functions including intestinal microorganisms, immunity and diet.
- The change in the composition and activity of intestinal microorganisms affects inflammation, fat storage, and glucose response in obese people.
- Probiotics and prebiotics are associated with specific bacteria in obese.
- Prebiotics reduce obesity and are involved in metabolic stress by modulating appetite and intestinal function (Derman, 2014; Aydın, Açıkgöz, & Şimşek, 2010).

Large and long-term studies are needed to investigate the effects of certain treatments, such as probiotics and pharmacological compounds, on the intestinal microbiota and thus their use in the treatment and prevention of obesity.

PREBIOTIC MICROORGANISMS

Description of Prebiotics and Usage Areas

The definition of prebiotic was first made by Gibson and Roberfroid in 1995. It is emphasized that they are mainly nondigestible compounds and that they produce beneficial effects by affecting beneficial microorganisms (WGO, 2017). Over time, this definition has been updated by different institutions. Most recently, in 2017, prebiotics were defined by ISAPP (prebiotics and prebiotics) as substrates that are selectively used by microorganisms in the host's intestinal microbiota and have beneficial health effects (Ouwehand, Derrien, de Vos, Tiihonen, & Rautonen, 2005). According to the new definition of prebiotics, some nutrient components such as polyphenols, polyunsaturated fatty acids and conjugated fatty acids, as well as nondigestible carbohydrates, may also meet the updated definition as they are selectively used by the host's microbiota and affect health. However, further studies showing health benefits are needed for these new candidates to remain in the prebiotic classification (Gibson et al., 2017).

Prebiotics and dietary fibers share many features, but they are not the same. Both cannot be digested in the gastrointestinal tract, but prebiotics are selectively fermented in the colon, while dietary fibers are fermented by various colon bacteria or may not be fermented at all (Ouwehand et al., 2005). Prebiotics are selectively used by the beneficial microflora (such as *Lactobacillus*, *Bifidobacterium*) in the colon, while inhibiting the proliferation of potential pathogenic microorganisms such as toxin-producing *Clostridium*, proteolytic Bacteriodes and toxigenic *Esherichia coli* (Yılmaz, 2004). The prebiotics identified so far are indigestible carbohydrates and include lactulose, inulin and a number of oligosaccharides. Some starches can also reach the colon in the form of fermentable carbohydrate sources that can be used by intestinal bacteria by avoiding full digestion during passage through the human small intestine (Crittenden, 2001).

The use of prebiotics is more common than probiotics. The minimum criteria for a food content to be evaluated as a prebiotic are:

1. It must be absorbed in the upper part of the gastrointestinal tract and should be resistant to hydrolysis.
2. It should be a selective substrate for beneficial bacteria such as lactobacilli and bifidobacteria present in the colon.
3. Convert colonic microflora to a healthier composition (Gibson & Roberfroid 1995).

Carbohydrate structures that meet these criteria; galactooligosaccharides, polydextrose, lactulose, inulin, oligosaccharides, fructooligosaccharides, soy-oligosaccharides, lacticol, maltitol, sorbitol, mannitol, and starch resistant to sugar alcohols. Some prebiotics and their properties are given in Table 1.

In infant formulas, prebiotic mixtures of specific galactooligosaccharides (GOS) and fructooligosaccharides (FOS), which are similar to oligosaccharides in human breast milk, which stimulate the growth of *Bifidobacteria* and *Lactobacilli* have

*Table 1. Molecular structure of prebiotics, recommended intake amounts and other properties * (Marteau, Seksik, Lepage, & Doré, 2004; Singh, Sharma, Malviya, 2012)*

Prebiotics	Molecular Structure	Some Features	Suggested Amount of Intake (g / day)
Fructo-oligosaccharides (FOS)	(FR) n-GI	• Glu [β Fru (2-1)] n, Fru [β Fru (2-1)] n • The degree of polymerization (n) is 2-8 and the average is 4. • Found in plants such as wheat, onion, banana, chicory and garlic. • Obtained by hydrolysis of inulin by endoinulinase enzyme. • Can be added to various foods such as Biscuits, beverages, yogurt, cereals and sweeteners.	2-12
Galacto-oligosaccharides (GOS)	(GA) n-GI	• α-D-Glu (1-4) [β-D-Gal (1-6)] n • The degree of polymerization (n) is 2-8 and the average is 4. • Found in human milk, cow milk and yogurt. • Produced from lactose by the activity of β-galactosidase, which has hydrolytic enzyme activity. • Increases the sweetness of dairy products and lowers lactose concentration for individuals with lactose intolerance. • Selectively increases the number of *Bifidobacteria* and *Lactobacillus in the* colon.	2-3
Isomalto-oligosaccharides	(Gu)n	• Composed of glucose monomers bound by α (1-4) and α (1-6) glucosidic bonds. • The degree of polymerization is 2-6. • Produced by different methods using carbohydrates such as sucrose, maltose, starch and dextran. • Found in plants such as starch, wheat, barley, corn, rice, potato and so on.	10-20
Inulin	(FR) n-Gu	• Glu- [β-Fru (2-1)] n • Polymerization degree 3-60; and the average is 10-12. • It is naturally found in fruits and vegetables (onions, bananas, garlic, leeks, etc.). • Extract from chicory root and Agave tequilana. • It is stable in medium acidity and is used in the production of fermented dairy products since it does not give a permanent taste to the product and does not cause a change in color. • By applying specific separation technologies, a long chain inulin is produced (inulin HP: polymerization degree of 10-60; and an average of 25). • Inulin is hydrolyzed with inulinase enzyme to produce oligofructose (oligofructose: polymerization degree 2-8 and average 4).	European diet: 2-12 Belgium: 5–8 Spain: 7-12
Xylo-oligosaccharides	(X) n	• β (1-4) are chains of linked xylose molecules and in particular are composed of xylobiosis, xylotriose and xylotetraose. • It is found in bamboo shoots, fruits, vegetables, milk and honey. • Enzymatic hydrolysis of xylan occurs by enzymatic applications of natural lignocellulosic materials, diluted solutions of mineral acids, hydrolytic degradation of xylan with water or steam.	0-7
Polydextrose	(Gun)n	• (α and β) includes all possible combinations of linked (1-2), (1-3), (1-4) and (1-6) glucosidic bonds, but 1-6 (both α and β) are dominant. • The degree of polymerization ranges from 2 to 120 and is a highly branched, randomly bonded glucose polymer having an average of 12.	4-12
Soybean-oligosaccharides	(Ga) n-Gu-Fr	• Oligosaccharides found in soybean consisting of raffinose and staciose.	2-4
Resistant starch	(Gun)n	• It consists of linear parts of α - (1-4) D-Glucan units. • It is a starch resistant to hydrolysis by amylase and pullulanase enzymes. • It occurs naturally in seeds, grains and starchy foods cooked and cooled.	

*: Ga = Galactose; Gu = Glucose; Fr = Fructose; Xy = Xylose

been described. Some reports have shown that complementing infant formulas with these specific GOS and FOS mixtures increases the number of *Bifidobacteria* and total lactobacilli, decreases the number of pathogens, and induces a short chain fatty acid profile similar to that of breastfed infants. The specific GOS and FOS prebiotic mixture also results in a different distribution of bifidobacteria species similar to that of breastfed infants (Harman & Knol, 2006). Prebiotic mixtures can also be used to increase intestinal tolerance to oral feeding. Addition of fructo and galactooligosaccharide to premature infant formula stimulates the proliferation of *Bifidobacteria* and provides soft and frequent defecation (Coskun, 2005). Chicory (Cichorium intybus) and artichoke are rich in prebiotics. The chickpea contains 15-20% inulin and 5-10% oligofructose. Inulin, which is found in most foods, is from chicory or synthesized from sucrose. Oligofruktosis is a partially hydrolyzed form of inulin (Coskun, 2006).

The intestines, particularly the colon, contain a large microbial population. An adult's colon microbiota is estimated to contain more than 40 trillion bacteria of hundreds of species. When these bacteria are considered on the basis of phylum, it is found that those found in the colon are Firmicutes, Bacteroidetes, Proteobacteria, Verrucomicrobia, Actinobacteria and Fusobacteria; among these phyla, the most dominant microbiota is known as Firmicutes and Bacteroidetes, which make up about 90% of the microbiota (WGO, 2017). The composition of the human intestinal ecosystem is influenced by certain physiological factors (e.g. age, genetics and origin, environment, nutritional status, dietary habits), or non-physiological factors such as antibiotic and probiotic use (Lagier, Million, Hugon, Armougom, & Raoult, 2012).

Human Bowel Composition

The prebiotics that reach the colon without digestion are fermented by bacteria present in the colon to produce hydrogen, methane, carbon dioxide, short chain fatty acids (acetate, propionate and butyrate) and lactate; therefore, they may show beneficial effects on the host's health by lowering the pH of the intestine and increasing the number and / or activity of beneficial bacteria such as *Bifidobacterium* and *Lactobacillus* in the intestine (Gibson, Probert, Van Loo, Rastall, & Roberfroid, 2004). Gastrointestinal symptoms such as abdominal distention, cramping, flatulence, and bloating may be seen in prebiotic intakes over 20-30 g per day (Gibson & Roberfroid, 1995). The recommended daily use of prebiotics varies depending on the type of prebiotic and the age and physiological status of the consumer (Lagier et al., 2012). The recommended intake amounts of some prebiotics have been given previously (see Table 1). Gastrointestinal disorders are proportional to the degree of polymerization of fermentable carbohydrates. Longer chain inulin type fructans are generally better tolerated due to less fermentation (Bonnema, Kolberg, Thomas, & Slavin, 2010).

THE POSITIVE EFFECTS OF PREBIOTICS ON OUR HEALTH

The effects of prebiotics on health are realized by different mechanisms. In the fermentation process of prebiotics, short chain fatty acids (acetate, propionate and butyrate) are produced. Acetate is considered to be one of the body's energy sources, is used by skeletal muscle, heart and brain and suppresses fatty acid synthesis in the liver (Coskun, 2014). Probionate stimulates proliferation of normal crypt cells, HT-29 adenocarcinoma has antiproliferative effect in cell culture and reduces cholesterol synthesis (Coskun, 2014). Butyrate is considered to be the energy source of colonocytes, regulates the proliferation and differentiation of colonocytes, by altering gene expression by histone acetylation and DNA methylation, particularly affecting epithelial proliferation and differentiation and apoptotic process. Therefore, it is associated with colitis and colon cancer (Schley & Field, 2002). Butyrate upregulates glutathione-S-transferase and catalase in colon cells, enhances cellular detoxification, suppresses DNA repair mechanisms in cancerous cells. Butyrate also reduces cholesterol synthesis (Marteau et al., 2004). Its beneficial effects on immunological functions have been demonstrated by the ability of short-chain fatty acids to increase lymphocyte and / or leukocyte counts in the intestinal-associated lymphoid tissues (GALT) and peripheral blood, and to stimulate the intra-inflammatory macrophages' phagocytic function by increasing the secretion of IgA from the intestinal-associated lymphoid tissue (Markowiak & Śliżewska, 2017). In addition, short-chain fatty acids can increase the solubility and absorption of minerals such as calcium, magnesium and iron ions. It has been suggested that these short-chain fatty acids may also be effective on appetite by regulating the release of some satiety hormones such as PPY, OXM, CCK and GLP-1 in the gastrointestinal tract (Gibson et al., 2017; Markowiak et al., 2015).

Clinical studies have shown beneficial effects of prebiotics on obesity, type 2 diabetes, metabolic syndrome, dyslipidemia, inflammation, infections, allergy, inflammatory bowel disease (IBD), irritable bowel syndrome (IBS), travel diarrhea, constipation, bone, skin and urogenital health (Marteau et al., 2004; Slavin, 2013; Markowiak & Śliżewska, 2017). The benefits of some prebiotic species on human health are summarized in Table 2 (Gibson et al., 2017).

The results obtained from experimental animals indicate that inulin, oligofructose, gluco-oligosaccharide and galacto-oligosaccharides increase especially calcium and magnesium absorption. Oligofructose intake increases bone density in femur and tibia. Care should be taken in generalizing these results for humans. The beneficial effect of prebiotics on calcium absorption has been demonstrated in humans. However, there are not enough studies on its effects on the absorption of iron, magnesium and zinc. Prebiotic use of different types, different doses and different durations and different amounts of calcium consumption have a role in obtaining conflicting results in studies conducted in humans (Coskun, 2006). It shows bifidogenic effect when 4-10g of fructooligosaccharide is taken daily. One portion of leek meal, one small banana, one small onion and garlic meets the daily prebiotic requirement (Inanç et al., 2005). Inulin and oligofructose have been used for centuries as a nutrient component with no side effects. They are also low in calories. The minimum amount recommended for children is 5 gr (Coşkun, 2006).

Table 2. Effects of Prebiotics on Human Health (Gibson et al., 2017)

Health Benefits	Prebiotics
Metabolic health: obesity; 2 types of diabetes; metabolic syndrome; dyslipidemia; inflammation	Inulin, GOS, FOS
Satiety	FOS
Stimulation of neurochemical producing bacteria in the intestine	GOS
Better absorption of calcium and other minerals, bone health	Inulin, FOS
Allergy	GOS, FOS
IBD	Inulin, Lactulose
Urogenital health;	GOS
Intestinal habit and general intestinal health in infants	GOS, FOS
Infections and vaccine response	FOS, GOS, PDX
IBS	GOS
Travel diarrhea	GOS
Constipation	Inulin
Immune function in elderly	GOS
Skin health	GOS

CONCLUSION AND SUGGESTIONS

Probiotics and prebiotics, which are considered as functional food ingredients, have important effects on human gastrointestinal health. Although many studies have been conducted on the treatment and prevention of gastrointestinal infections with probiotics, comparison of the results of these studies are not possible because of the probiotic microorganism type used, the dose, the human populations used in the studies, or the differences in certain factors such as the in vitro-in vivo status of the studies and the state of the disease. In many studies, it is reported that the beneficial effects of probiotics and prebiotics on intestinal health vary according to microorganism type and strain.

- Further controlled studies may be useful to confirm the health effects of probiotics and prebiotics.
- If probiotics and prebiotics are to be taken as preparations, make sure that the preparations to be used are reliable.

REFERENCES

Agerholm, L., Bell, M., & Grunwald, G. (2000). The effect of a probiotic milk product on plasma cholesterol: A meta analysis of short-term intervention studies. *European Journal of Clinical Nutrition*, *54*(11), 856–860. doi:10.1038j.ejcn.1601104 PMID:11114681

Akalın, A. S., & Ünal, G. (2005). Probiotics and Allergy. *The Journal of Food*, *1*(30), 43–45.

Arslan, N. (2012). Obesity and Probiotics. *Turkiye Klinikleri Pediatric Science*, *8*(3), 102.

Arslan, N. (2014). Use of Prebiotics and Probiotics in Irritable Bowel Syndrome. In A. Kara & T. Coşkun (Eds.), *Theory to Clinic Prebiotics, Probiotics* (pp. 325–341). Istanbul: Academy Publishing.

Arvola, T., Laiho, K., Torkkeli, S., Mykkanen, H., Salminen, S., Maunula, L., & Isolauri, E. (1999). Prophlactic Lactobacillus GG Reduces Antibiotic-Associated Diarrhea in Children with Respiratory Infections: A randomized study. *Pediatrics*, *104*(5), 64. doi:10.1542/peds.104.5.e64 PMID:10545590

Aydın, M., Açıkgöz, İ., & Şimşek, B. (2010). Determination of product consumption and probiotic concept knowledge level in studients of Isparta Suleyman Demirel University. *Electronic Journal of Food Technologies*, *5*(2), 1–6.

Baysal, A. (2007). *Nutrition*. Ankara: Hatiboglu Publishing.

Bonnema, A. L., Kolberg, L. W., Thomas, W., & Slavin, J. L. (2010). Gastrointestinal tolerance of chicory inulin products. *Journal of the American Dietetic Association*, *110*(6), 865–868. doi:10.1016/j.jada.2010.03.025 PMID:20497775

Byrne, C., Chambers, E., Morrison, D., & Frost, G. (2015). The role of short chain fatty acids in appetite regulation and energy homeostasis. *International Journal of Obesity*, *39*(9), 1331–1338. doi:10.1038/ijo.2015.84 PMID:25971927

Çakır, İ., & Çakmakçı, L. (2004). Probiotics: Definition, effect mechanism, selection and safety criteria. *The Journal of Food*, *29*(6), 427–434.

Coşkun, T. (2005). Health benefits of functional foods. *Journal of Child Health and Diseases*, *48*, 69–84.

Coşkun, T. (2006). Pro-, Pre- and Synbiotics. *Journal of Child Health and Diseases*, *49*, 128–148.

Coşkun, T. (2014). Probiotics. In A. Kara & T. Coşkun (Eds.), *Theory to Clinic Prebiotics, Probiotics* (pp. 56–71). Istanbul: Academy Publishing.

Cremonini, F., Di Caro, S., Nista, E. C., Bartolozzi, F., Capelli, G., Gasbarrini, G., & Gasbarrini, A. (2002). Meta-analysis: The effect of probiotic administration on antibiotic-associated diarrhea. *Alimentary Pharmacology & Therapeutics*, *16*(8), 1461–1467. doi:10.1046/j.1365-2036.2002.01318.x PMID:12182746

Crittenden, R., Laitila, A., Forssell, P., Mattö, J., Saarela, M., Sandholm, M. T., & Myllarınen, P. (2001). Adhesion of bifidobacterial to granular starch and its implications in probiotic technologies. *Applied and Environmental Microbiology*, *67*(8), 3469–3475. doi:10.1128/AEM.67.8.3469-3475.2001 PMID:11472921

Derman, O. (2014). Obesity and probiotics. In A. Kara & T. Coşkun (Eds.), *Theory to Clinic Prebiotics, Probiotics* (pp. 257–266). Istanbul: Academy Publishing.

Doege, K., Grajecki, D., Zyriax, B. C., Detinkina, E., zu Eulenburg, C., & Buhling, K. J. (2012). İmpact of maternal supplementation with probiotics during pregnancy on atopic eczema in childhood- a meta- analysis. *British Journal ofNutrition*, *107*(1), 1–6. doi:10.1017/S0007114511003400 PMID:21787448

FAO / WHO. (2002) Guidelines for the evaluation of probiotics in food.

Farnworth, E. R. (2008). The evidence to support health claims for probiotics. *The Journal of Nutrition*, *138*(l), 1250–1254. doi:10.1093/jn/138.6.1250S PMID:18492865

Fuller, R. (1992). *Probiotics: The scientific basis*. London: Chapman and Hall. doi:10.1007/978-94-011-2364-8

Gibson, G. R., Hutkins, R., Sanders, M. E., Prescott, S. L., Reimer, R. A., Salminen, S. J., ... Verbeke, K. (2017). Expert consensus document: The International Scientific Association for Probiotics and Prebiotics (ISAPP) consensus statement on the definition and scope of prebiotics. *Nature Reviews. Gastroenterology & Hepatology*, *14*(8), 491–502. doi:10.1038/nrgastro.2017.75 PMID:28611480

Gibson, G. R., Probert, H. M., Van Loo, J., Rastall, R. A., & Roberfroid, M. B. (2004). Dietary modulation of the human colonic microbiota: Updating the concept of prebiotics. *Nutrition Research Reviews*, *17*(02), 259–275. doi:10.1079/NRR200479 PMID:19079930

Gibson, G. R., & Roberfroid, M. B. (1995). Dietary modulation of the human colonic microflora introducing the concept of probiotics. *The Journal of Nutrition*, *125*(6), 1401–1412. doi:10.1093/jn/125.6.1401 PMID:7782892

Gionchetti, P., Rizzello, F., Helwig, U., Venturi, A., Lammers, K. M., Brigidi, P., ... Campieri, M. (2003). Probiotics for the treatment of postoperative complications following intestinal surgery. *Best Practice & Research. Clinical Gastroenterology*, *17*(5), 821–831. doi:10.1016/S1521-6918(03)00071-4 PMID:14507591

Gönülateş, N. (2008). Investigation of immunomodulatory effects of kefir on humans [Master Thesis]. Suleyman Demirel University.

Gorbach, S. (2000). Probiotics and gastrointestinal health. *The American Journal of Gastroenterology*, *95*(1), 2–4. doi:10.1016/S0002-9270(99)00806-0 PMID:10634218

Güner, A. (2004). Crohn Hastalığının Etiyolojisinde Mycobacterium Paratuberculosis (Mycobacterium Avium SBSP Paratuberculosis). *Erciyes University Journal of Faculty Helth Science*, *13*(1), 48–54.

Guslandi, M., Giollo, P., & Testoni, P. A. (2003). A pilot trial of saccharomyces boulardii in ulcerative colitis. *European Journal of Gastroenterology & Hepatology*, *15*(6), 697–698. doi:10.1097/00042737-200306000-00017 PMID:12840682

Guslandi, M., Mezzi, G., Sorghy, M., & Testoni, P. A. (2000). Sacchoromyces Boulardii in maintenance treatment of Crohn's disease. *Digestive Diseases and Sciences*, *45*(7), 1462–1464. doi:10.1023/A:1005588911207 PMID:10961730

Harman, M., & Knol, J. (2006). Quantitative real-time pcr analysis of fecal lactobacillus species in infants receiving a prebiotic infant formula. *Applied and Environmental Microbiology*, *72*(4), 2359–2365. doi:10.1128/AEM.72.4.2359-2365.2006 PMID:16597930

He, T., Priebe, M. G., Zhong, Y., Harmsen, H. J. M., Raangs, G. C., Antonie, J. M., ... Vonk, R. J. (2008). Effects of yogurt and bifidobacteria supplementation on the colonic microbiota in lactose-intolerant subjects. *Journal of Applied Microbiology*, *104*, 595–604. PMID:17927751

Hove, T., Norgaard, H., & Mortensen, B. (1999). Lactic acid bacteria and the human gastrointestinal tract. *European Journal of Clinical Nutrition*, *53*(5), 339–350. doi:10.1038j.ejcn.1600773 PMID:10369488

Inanç, N., Şahin, H., & Çiçek, B. (2005). The impact of probiotics and prebiotics on health. *Erciyes Medical Journal*, *27*(3), 122–127.

Ishikawa, H., Akedo, I., Umesaki, Y., Tanaka, R., Imaoka, A., & Otani, T. (2003). Randomized controlled trial of the effect of bifido bacteria-fermented milk on ulcerative colitis. *Journal of the American College of Nutrition*, *22*(1), 56–63. doi:10.1080/07315724.2003.10719276 PMID:12569115

Işlek, A., & Artan, R. (2014) Use of Probiotics hypercholesterolemia. In A. Kara & T. Coşkun (Eds.), Theory to Clinic Prebiotics, Probiotics. Istanbul: Academy Publishing.

Jiang, T., & Savaiano, D. A. (1997). In vitro lactose fermentation by human colonic bacteria is modified by Lactobacillus acidophilus supplementation. *The Journal of Nutrition*, *8*(127), 1489–1495. doi:10.1093/jn/127.8.1489 PMID:9237942

Kuisma, J., Mentula, S., Jarvinen, H., Kahri, A., Saxelin, M., & Farkkila, M. (2003). Effect of Lactobacillus rhamnosus GG on ileal pouch inflammation and microbial flora. *Alimentary Pharmacology & Therapeutics*, *17*(4), 509–515. doi:10.1046/j.1365-2036.2003.01465.x PMID:12622759

Lagier, J. C., Million, M., Hugon, P., Armougom, F., & Raoult, D. (2012). Human gut microbiota: Repertoire and variations. *Frontiers in Cellular and Infection Microbiology*, *2*, 136. doi:10.3389/fcimb.2012.00136 PMID:23130351

Markowiak, P., & Śliżewska, K. (2017). Effects of probiotics, prebiotics, and synbiotics on human health. *Nutrients*, *9*(9), 1021. doi:10.3390/nu9091021 PMID:28914794

Marteau, P., Seksik, P., Lepage, P., & Doré, J. (2004). Cellular and physiological effects of probiotics and prebiotics. *Mini-Reviews in Medicinal Chemistry*, *4*(8), 889–896. doi:10.2174/1389557043403369 PMID:15544550

Mimura, T., Rizzello, F., & Helwig, U. (2004). Once daily high dose probiotic therapy (VSL 3) for maintaining remission in recurrent or refractory pouchitis. *Gut*, *53*(1), 108–114. doi:10.1136/gut.53.1.108 PMID:14684584

O'Mahony, L., McCarthy, J., Kelly, P., Hurley, G., Luo, F., Chen, K., ... Quigley, E. M. (2005). Lactobacillus and bifidobacterium in irritable bowel syndrome: Symptom responses and relationship to cytokine profiles. *Gastroenterology*, *128*(3), 541–551. doi:10.1053/j.gastro.2004.11.050 PMID:15765388

Oktay, E. (2001). Inflammatory bowel diseases: Ethiopathogenesis, yopatogenez, symptamatology, diagnosis and complications. In *Gastrointestinal System Diseases Symposium* (pp. 199-206). Istanbul Cerrahpaşa University. Retrieved from http://www.ctf.edu.tr/stek/pdfs/23/2319EO.pdf

Ouwehand, A. C., Derrien, M., de Vos, W., Tiihonen, K., & Rautonen, N. (2005). Prebiotics and other microbial substrates for gut functionality. *Current Opinion in Biotechnology, 16*(2), 212–217. doi:10.1016/j.copbio.2005.01.007 PMID:15831389

Özden, A. (2007). Yogurt and healty life. *Current Gastroenterology, 11*(3), 166–178.

Parkes, G. C. (2007). An overview of probiotics and prebiotics [Review]. *Nursing Standard, 21*(20), 43–47. doi:10.7748/ns2007.01.21.20.43.c4510 PMID:17288356

Ringel, Y., & Ringel, K. T. (2011). The rationale and clinical effectiveness of probiotics in irritable bowel syndrome. *Journal of Clinical Gastroenterology, 45*, 145–148. doi:10.1097/MCG.0b013e31822d32d3 PMID:21992954

Roberfroid, M. B. (2000). Prebiotics and probiotics: Are they functional foods? *The American Journal of Clinical Nutrition, 71*(6), 1682–1687. doi:10.1093/ajcn/71.6.1682S PMID:10837317

Saçkesen, C. (2014). Prebiotics and probiotics in the prevention and treatment of allergic diseases. In A. Kara & T. Coşkun (Eds.), Theory to Clinic Prebiotics, Probiotics (pp. 301-311). Istanbul: Academy Publishing.

Salminen, S. J., Gueimonde, M., & Isolauri, E. (2005). Probiotics that modify disease risk. *The Journal of Nutrition, 135*(5), 1294–1298. doi:10.1093/jn/135.5.1294 PMID:15867327

Schaafsma G. (1996). State-of-the-art concerning probiotic strains in milk products. *IDF Nutrition Newsletter*, (5), 23-24.

Schaafsma, G., Meuling, W. J. A., Van Dokkum, W., & Bouley, C. (1998). Effects of a milk product, fermented by Lactobacillus acidophilus and with fructo-oligosaccharides added, on blood lipids in male volunteers. *European Journal of Clinical Nutrition, 52*(6), 436–440. doi:10.1038j.ejcn.1600583 PMID:9683397

Schley, P., & Field, C. (2002). The immune-enhancing effects of dietary fibres and prebiotics. *British Journal of Nutrition, 87*(6S2), 221–230. doi:10.1079/BJNBJN/2002541 PMID:12088522

Sekhon, B. S. (2010). Prebiotics, probiotics and synbiotics: An overview. *Journal of Pharmaceutical Education and Research, 1*, 13–36.

Sheu, B. S., Wu, J. J., Lo, C. Y., Wu, H. W., Chen, J. H., Lin, Y. S., & Lin, M. D. (2002). Impact of supplement with Lactobacillus-and Bifidobacterium-containing yogurt on triple therapy for Helicobacter pylori eradication. *Alimentary Pharmacology & Therapeutics*, *16*(9), 1669–1675. doi:10.1046/j.1365-2036.2002.01335.x PMID:12197847

Singh, R., Sharma, P. K., & Malviya, R. (2012). Prebiotics: Future trends in health care. *Mediterranean Journal of Nutrition and Metabolism*, *5*(2), 81–90. doi:10.100712349-011-0065-8

Slavin, J. (2013). Fiber and prebiotics: Mechanisms and health benefits. *Nutrients*, *5*(4), 1417–1435. doi:10.3390/nu5041417 PMID:23609775

Sleator, R. D., & Hill, C. (2008). New frontiers in probiotic research. *Letters in Applied Microbiology*, *46*(2), 143–147. doi:10.1111/j.1472-765X.2007.02293.x PMID:18028323

Uriot, O., Denis, S., Junjua, M., Roussel, Y., Dary-Mourot, A., & Blanquet-Diot, S. (2017). Streptococcus thermophilus: From yogurt starter to a new promising probiotic candidate? *Journal of Functional Foods*, *37*, 74–89. doi:10.1016/j.jff.2017.07.038

Williams, N. T. (2010). Probiotics [Review]. *American Journal of Health-System Pharmacy*, *67*(6), 449–458. doi:10.2146/ajhp090168 PMID:20208051

World Gastroenterology Organisation. *Global Guidelines Probiotics and Prebiotics* [Internet]. 2017 [Erişim Tarihi 29.07.2019]. Erişim adresi: http://www.worldgastroenterology.org/UserFiles/file/guidelines/probiotics-and-prebiotics-english-2017.pdf

Yağcı, R. (2002). Prebiotics and probiotics. *Journal of Child Health and Diseases*, *45*(4), 337–344.

Yılmaz, M. (2004). Prebiotics and probiotics. *The Journal of Current Pediatrics*, *2*, 142–145.

Yüce, A. (2014) Probiotics and prebiotics in the treatment of constipation. In A. Kara & T. Coşkun (Eds.), Theory to Clinic Prebiotics, Probiotics (pp. 283-286). Istanbul: Academy Publishing.

Chapter 7
In Inflamation Dietary Inflammatory Index and the Role of Different Diet Types

Ramazan Mert Atan
https://orcid.org/0000-0003-4608-605X
University Bandırma Onyedi Eylül, Turkey

Uğur Günşen
https://orcid.org/0000-0001-9858-6019
Bandırma Onyedi Eylül University, Turkey

ABSTRACT

Inflammation usually occurs as a result of imbalances between pro-inflammatory and anti-inflammatory cytokines. Diet is one of the factors that play a role in their development and prevent them from developing. Therefore, it is important to determine the pro- and anti-inflammatory properties of foods. Diet is an important and modifiable determinant of chronic diseases. There is a lot of scientific evidence to support the fact that foods consumed have positive and negative effects on individuals' health. In addition to being effective whole of diet, it is seen that the food groups contained in the diet affect the inflammatory biomarkers separately. This section provides information about dietary inflammatory index (DII) and diets that are effective on inflammation.

DOI: 10.4018/978-1-7998-3594-3.ch007

BACKGROUND

Inflammation can be defined as both friend and enemy. The most important its tasks is the ability of the individual to defend himself / herself against microbial attacks and to heal the wounds that occur. It can also produce negative consequences. If the response to inflammation by the individual remains insufficient, inflammation may spread to organs and cause chronic diseases to occur (Sears, 2015). Chronic inflammatory response is characterized by abnormal cytokine production and activation of inflammatory signaling pathways (Ridker, Brown, Vaughan, Harrison, & Mehta, 2004; Wellen & Hotamisligil, 2003).

Inflammation usually occurs as a result of imbalances between pro-inflammatory and anti-inflammatory cytokines (Şentürk, 2013). Diet is one of the factors that play a role in their development and prevent them from developing. Therefore, it is important to determine the pro- and anti-inflammatory properties of foods (O'Neil et al., 2015). Diet is an important and modifiable determinant of chronic diseases. There is a lot of scientific evidence to support the fact that foods consumed have positive and negative effects on individuals' health (Philip C Calder et al., 2011). Various dietary components are known to alter important pathways leading to inflammation. For example, oxidants such as superoxide radicals and hydrogen peroxide are produced during metabolism in our bodies after consumption of nutrients. These substances can activate the Nuclear Factor Kappa B (NF-kB) pathway, which contributes to the formation of inflammation by increasing the production of pro-inflammatory cytokines (Kiecolt-Glaser, 2010). Therefore, prevention of oxidative stress may be effective to reduce the production of inflammatory mediators (Calder et al., 2009).

In addition to being effective whole of diet, it is seen that the food groups contained in the diet affect the inflammatory biomarkers separately. For example, higher consumption of both fruits and vegetables may result in lower levels of C reactive protein (CRP), Interleukin (IL) -6 and Tumor Necrosis Factor-α (TNF-a) which are inflammatory biomarkers and it is also associated with higher levels of antioxidant capacity indicators (Root et al., 2012). In addition, it is known that the diet affects the intestinal microbiota (Kjeldsen-Kragh, Haugen, Borchgrevink, & Førre, 1994; Soltani, Chitsazi, & Salehi-Abargouei, 2018), whereas the intestinal microbiota also is an interaction with the immune system. Changes in the gut microbiota cause a decrease in immune response and a deterioration of tolerance to microorganisms. This is thought to result in low-grade chronic inflammation (Ferreira et al., 2014; Telle-Hansen, Holven, & Ulven, 2018).

There are many diet patterns and eating habits around the world. When the literature is examined, especially the positive effect of Mediterranean diet and DASH diet on inflammation comes to the fore. In addition, vegetarian diet, Nordic diet are thought to be associated with inflammation. Furthermore, dietary inflammatory index (DII) was developed to measure the inflammatory potential of a diet. In this section, diets that are impact on inflammation are examined.

THE DIETARY INFLAMMATORY INDEX

Acute inflammation helps to heal any part of the body after injury, while chronic inflammation is associated with chronic disease states such as cancer, cardiovascular disease (CVD) and diabetes mellitus (DM). Plasma levels of inflammatory biomarkers such as CRP, IL-6 or TNF-α are independent predictors of primary and secondary coronary heart disease (Crimarco et al., 2018). According to a study, elevated CRP levels of individuals showed that they predicted the risk of developing chronic diseases such as DM and hypertension in the future more accurately than body mass index (BMI) (Galland, 2010).

Recent studies show that diet plays an important role in regulating chronic, systemic inflammation (Cavicchia et al., 2009; Chalkiadaki & Guarente, 2012; Esposito et al., 2004). The health impact of inflammation and the role of diet in inflammation have led to the development of dietary inflammatory index (DII). Accordingly, this index includes the scoring of an individual's diet by evaluating the results of peer-reviewed articles associated with inflammatory biomarkers IL-1, IL-4, IL-6, IL-10, TNF-α, CRP (Shivappa, Steck, Hurley, Hussey, & Hébert, 2014).

First, DII developed for forty-two nutrient values by Cavicchia et al. (2009), has benefited from epidemiological studies, laboratory animals and cell culture studies in the literature (Wood, Shivappa, Berthon, Gibson, & Hebert, 2015). This dietary index was updated by Shivappa et al. in 2014 (Shivappa, Steck, Hurley, Hussey, & Hébert, 2014). Accordingly, Shivappa et al. Starting from peer-reviewed research articles published from 2010, they developed a DII scoring system to compare the inflammatory potentials of diets in different populations using 11 different data sets of countries (Japan, Korea, America, Canada, Mexico, Taiwan, Australia, New Zealand, Bahrain, Denmark and India). A reference database representing a wider population including a total of forty-five nutrients, including whole grains, nutrients and nutrients including bioactive components, was created (Shivappa, Steck, Hurley, Hussey, & Hébert, 2014).

DII; based on the pro- and anti-inflammatory content of the general dietary composition, including macronutrients, vitamins and minerals, alcohol intake and flavonoids, it is an effective way to predict the inflammatory potential of the diet (Neufcourt et al., 2015). The nutrient parameters are not limited to micro- and macro-nutrients, but also include commonly consumed dietary components such as tea and spices (Shivappa, 2014). In addition, it has been suggested that this index may be a marker of serum CRP level (Wood et al., 2015). According to a study examining the relationship between DII score and plasma CRP level; There was a significant correlation between elevated plasma CRP (> 3 mg / L) levels in individuals with high DII scores determined by food consumption records (Shivappa, Steck, Hurley, Hussey, Ma, et al., 2014). According to another study in which DII was calculated by taking the food consumption frequency of individuals; While there was a significant positive correlation between DII and plasma IL-6 (> 1.6 pg / ml) levels, no significant correlation was found between DII and plasma CRP concentrations (Shivappa et al., 2015). Since the development of DII, it has been used to measure whether a pro-inflammatory diet in cancer, metabolic syndrom and CVD increases risk (Crimarco et al., 2018).

Improving and Scoring of DII

It is grouped according to the effects of nutrient components on inflammation parameters in the improvement of DII. According to this grouping, foods that significantly increased IL-1β, IL-6, TNF-α, CRP level and decreased IL-4 or IL-10 are accepted as pro-inflammatory and the effect value is ''+1''. Conversely, if IL-1β, IL-6, TNF-α, CRP levels were significantly decreased and IL-4 or IL-10 levels were increased, they were accepted as anti-inflammatory and the effect value was taken as ''-1''. If the nutritional parameter does not have a significant effect on inflammatory markers, it is accepted as ''0''. If the nutrient parameter increases both proinflammatory and anti-inflammatory markers, the mean effect score was calculated to eliminate this conflict (Shivappa, Steck, Hurley, Hussey, & Hébert, 2014).

In the calculation of dietary inflammatory index, the median value of the total effect scores of all articles used to represent an intact literature pool was determined as the cut-off point '236'. When calculating the total inflammatory effect score specific to the nutrient parameter, the total weight score of that nutrient parameter is divided into '236' if the total effect score is smaller than 236, which is the median value of the nutrient parameter. The value obtained as a result of the procedure was multiplied by the raw inflammatory effect score and the total inflammatory effect score specific to that food was obtained. If the total weight score of the nutrient parameter was greater than '236', the calculated inflammatory effect score was also determined as the total inflammatory effect score specific to that nutrient parameter. If the score for the nutrient parameter is negative, that nutrient shows anti-inflammatory effect and if it is positive, it shows pro-inflammatory effect (Shivappa, Steck, Hurley, Hussey, & Hébert, 2014).

While determining the contribution of each nutrient parameter to inflammation; The individual's nutrient consumption amount z score value is determined. Standard global consumption is subtracted from the average daily consumed amount of the individual's diet. It is divided by the standard deviation value specified for that nutrient. The determined values were converted to percentile scores to reduce skewness effect. In order to obtain a symmetrical distribution, the percentile score was calculated as the central value is zero and the limit values as ''-1'' (maximum anti-inflammatory) and ''+1'' (maximum pro-inflammatory). The percentile scores calculated for each nutrient were collected by multiplying that nutrient parameter with a specific inflammatory effect score for all nutrients. As a result, the inflammatory load of the diets of the individuals were determined. Then, the centered percentage value for each nutrient parameter is multiplied by the inflammatory effect score specific to the respective nutrient parameters in order to obtain the DII score specific to the nutrient parameters. Finally, all of the nutrient parameter-specific DII scores are summed to form the overall DII score for an individual (Shivappa, Steck, Hurley, Hussey, & Hébert, 2014).

According to the results obtained from the studies conducted with DII; Cavicchia et al. (2009), -20.9 to 24.7, Shivappa et al. (2014) -8.87 to 7.98, van Woudenbergh et al. (2013) calculated the DII in the range of -12.0 to 15.7. Shivappa et al. (2014), who recently created the updated version of DII, 's percentile values are given in the Table 1.

Table 1. The percentile values of DII

Rating	Score of DII
Max.	7.98
90-persantil	4.00
75-persantil	1.90
50-persantil (medyan)	0.23
25-persantil	-2.36
10-persantil	-3.37
Min.	-8.87

MEDITERRANEAN DIET

The Mediterranean diet is a nutrition model inspired by the traditional diet patterns of some countries in the Mediterranean basin. There are differences in Mediterranean diet among the countries in this basin and between the regions in the same country.

These differences are influenced by changes in culture, ethnicity, religion, economy and agricultural production. However, the Mediterranean diet has some common features. The main fat component of the diet should be olive oil. In addition, high amounts of fruit, vegetables, cereals (preferably whole grains), legumes, nuts and seeds must be included in the diet. It should also include moderately fish and shellfish, white meat, eggs and fermented dairy products (especially cheese and yogurt), as well as less red meat, processed meat and foods, contain added sugar. Small amounts of red wine are recommended, especially with meals. The Mediterranean diet contains low levels of saturated fatty acids and monounsaturated fatty acids especially from high amounts of olive oil. It is also rich in omega (n)-3 from fish and seafood (Casas, Sacanella, & Estruch, 2014).

Foods that should be consumed on a daily basis in the Mediterranean diet are: Bread, pasta, rice, couscous or other cereals should be consumed one or two servings at each meal. Vegetables should be consumed in 2 or more portions at each meal. At least one portion should be consumed raw to provide the necessary vitamins and minerals on a daily basis. Fruits should be 1 or 2 servings per meal. Taking fluid is important for water balance in the body. Therefore, 1.5-2 liters of water (8-10 glasses) must be consumed. Dairy products should be consumed at moderate levels (2 servings a day) and should be preferred in the form of low-fat yogurt, cheese or other fermented dairy products. Olive oil is at the center of the Mediterranean diet and should be particularly extra-virgin. Healthy snack options include a handful of olives and oil seeds. Wine consumption is recommended at moderate level (1 glass for women and 2 glasses for men) (Bach-Faig et al., 2011).

When the portions of foods that should be consumed on weekly basis are examined; 2 or more servings of fish and shellfish, 2 servings of white meat, 2-4 servings of eggs are recommended. Consumption of red meat (preferably from lean portions) should be less than 2 servings per week. The consumption of processed meats should not exceed 1 serving per week. It is recommended that dried legumes be consumed 2 servings or more per week. Potatoes are one of the foods included in meat and fish recipes and should be consumed 3 servings or less a week. Foods that are rarely recommended are; sugar and deserts which contain unhealthy fats. Sugar, confectionery, cakes, sugary fruit juices and sugary soft drinks can be consumed in small amounts.

In epidemiological and clinical studies, the Mediterranean diet was first found to have protective properties from CVD (Carter, Roberts, Salter, & Eaton, 2010; Fung et al., 2009; Martínez-González et al., 2011). Further studies have shown that the Mediterranean diet reduces the risk of type 2 DM, obesity and cancer (Kabaran et al., 2012; Pérez-López, Chedraui, Haya, & Cuadros, 2009; Romaguera, 2011) In addition, the Mediterranean diet is associated with prolonged survival and adherence to the Mediterranean diet has been found to be reduced death by 10-20% due to health problems such as CVD and cancer (Pérez-López et al., 2009). With all these features, the Mediterranean diet provides health protection and increases the quality of life (Willett et al., 1995)

In order to evaluate compliance with the Mediterranean diet, an assessment method called the Mediterranean diet adherence score was developed. It is also known that the Mediterranean diet adherence score has different forms of assessment in different countries. One of these methods was developed by Martinez-Gonzalez et al. (2012). In this scale, there are totally 14 questions, 12 of them are related to the frequency of food consumption and 2 of them are about food consumption habits. The score given for each question is 0 or 1 point. The scoring range of the Mediterranean Diet Compliance Scale was 0-14 points (Martinez-Gonzalez et al., 2012).

Another method of assessing compliance with the Mediterranean Diet was developed by Trichopoulou et al. (2003). A value of 0 or 1 was assigned to each of nine indicated components with the use of the sex-specific median as the cutoff. For beneficial components (vegetables, legumes, fruits and nuts, cereal, and fish), persons whose consumption was below the median were assigned a value of 0, and persons whose consumption was at or above the median were assigned a value of 1. For components presumed to be detrimental (meat, poultry, and dairy products, which are rarely nonfat or low-fat in Greece), persons whose consumption was below the median were assigned a value of 1, and persons whose consumption was at or above the median were assigned a value of 0. In addition, ''+1'' points are given in case of alcohol consumption of men 10-50 g / day and women 5-25 g / day. Finally, all the figures obtained are summed up and evaluated as the lowest adaptation to the Mediterranean diet, moderate adaptation and high adaptation (Trichopoulou, Costacou, Bamia, & Trichopoulos, 2003).

Serra-Majem et. al. (2004) developed the Mediterranean Diet Quality Index (KIDMED). This index is scored between 0 and 12. 12 of the questions included in the KIDMED index are positive and 4 are negative questions. Questions denoting a negative connotation with respect to the Mediterranean diet were assigned a value of ''-1'', and those with a positive aspect ''+1''. According to the total score obtained from the index, the quality of the diet is classified under 3 groups. If the total score is greater than 8, it is classified as an optimal Mediterranean type diet. If the total score is between 4 and 7, the quality of the diet should be improved and if the total score is less than 3, the quality of the diet is classified as very low (Serra-Majem et al., 2004).

The Effect of Mediterranean Diet on Inflamation

In general, western diet patterns with high red meat content, rich in whole-fat dairy products and refined sugars are considered pro-inflammatory. In addition, healthy diets (such as low-fat, vegetable-based or Mediterranean diets) are considered anti-inflammatory (Mayr et al., 2018). In the randomized controlled trials, the Mediterranean diet has the strongest evidence for a reduction in the levels of markers of inflammation (Neale, Batterham, & Tapsell, 2016; Schwingshackl & Hoffmann, 2014).

Nutrition according to the Mediterranean diet has been shown to be associated with decreases in systemic inflammation markers such as IL-6, TNF-α and CRP (Casas, Sacanella, Urpí-Sardà, et al., 2014; Richard et al., 2013; Viscogliosi et al. (2013). Regardless of weight loss, a significant decrease in serum CRP levels has been reported in individuals adherence to the Mediterranean diet (Chrysohoou, Panagiotakos, Pitsavos, Das, & Stefanadis, 2004; Esposito, Kastorini, Panagiotakos, & Giugliano, 2013; Richard et al., 2013). In the PREDIMED (Prevención con Dieta Mediterránea) study, a significant reduction in circulating CRP and IL-6 levels was detected after 12 months of intervention with Mediterranean diet (Casas, Sacanella, Urpí-Sardà, et al., 2014). In a study of approximately 22,000 adults from Greece, it was shown that there was an inverse relationship at individuals who adherence to a Mediterranean-style diet and showed greater mortality (Brownlee, 2001). In particular, an approximately 2/9 increase in the Mediterranean diet score was associated with a 25% reduction in total mortality and a 33% reduction in CVD mortality. In the ATTICA study in Greece, 1,514 males and 1,528 females were examined, and those who followed a Mediterranean diet were found to be associated with 20% low CRP and 17% low IL-6 levels (Chrysohoou et al., 2004).

Olive oil, the main component of the Mediterranean diet, regulates the expression of vascular cell adhesion molecule-1 (VCAM-1), intercellular adhesion molecule-1 (ICAM-1) and E-selectin in circulating lymphocytes and monocytes in clinical. It has shown that olive oil reduces plasma concentrations of soluble ICAM-1, soluble VCAM-1, soluble E-selectin, IL-6 and CRP in high-risk patients. In the Nurses Health Study, it was found to be associated with lower concentrations of inflammation and biological concentrations of endothelial dysfunction in individuals with high Mediterranean diet index score (CRP, IL6, ICAM-1 and VCAM-1) (Athyros et al., 2011). According to a meta-analysis study, 17 studies were examined and it was reported that nutrition suitable for the Mediterranean diet was associated with a significantly greater decrease in IL-6 and CRP compared to control groups by improving endothelial function of individuals (L Schwingshackl & Hoffmann, 2014). In addition, decreases in serum CRP, IL-6, IL-7 and IL-18 concentrations were found in patients with metabolic syndrome who were adherence to the Mediterranean diet.

In addition, the present study showed that the Mediterranean diet reduced insulin resistance and improved endothelial function (Esposito et al., 2004).

Mediterranean style nutrition model; It has a 2:1 ratio compared to the 14:1 omega 6 / omega 3 ratio seen in the western diet (Castro-Quezada, Román-Viñas, & Serra-Majem, 2014; Kris-Etherton, Eckel, Howard, St. Jeor, & Bazzarre, 2001). Omega-6 fatty acids such as arachidonic acid, prostoglandin-E2 and leukotriene-B4; increases the production of eicosanodies with pro-inflammatory properties. Omega-3 fatty acids such as eicosa pentaenoic acid (EPA), prostoglandin-E3 and leukotriene-B5 lead to the production of eicosanoids with less pro-inflammatory properties or more anti-inflammatory properties (Mena et al., 2009). Inflammatory markers influenced by the Mediterranean diet are shown in Table 2 (Casas, Sacanella, & Estruch, 2014).

Table 2. Inflammatory Markers Affected by Mediterranean Diet

IMMUNE FACTORS						
Interleukins & CRP	**Tumor Necrosis Factor & Receptors**	**Tumor Necrosis Factor & Receptors**	**Chemokines**	**Stability / Unstability of Atheromatic Plaque**	**Circulating Adhesion Molecules**	**Leukocyte Adhesion Molecules**
IL-1	TNF-α	TGF-β1	MCP-1	MMP-9	sICAM	CD11a
IL-6	TNFR60			TIMP-1	sVCAM-1	CD11b
IL-7	TNFR80			IL-10	sP-Seletin	CD49d
CRP				IL-18	sE-Selectin	CD40

There are high amounts of polyphenols in foods such as fruits, vegetables, cereals, legumes and wine in the Mediterranean Diet. Polyphenols are divided into two groups as flavonoids and phenolic acids. Flavonoids are effective in enzymatic modulations, inhibition of cellular proliferation; it is also known to have antioxidant and anti-inflammatory properties. Although the effects of polyphenolic compounds in the human body are not fully elucidated, it is assumed that they may prevent the development of Type 2 DM due to their antioxidant properties (Schröder, 2007). Red wine contains phenolic compounds (catechin, epicatechin, procyanidins) that have anti-inflammatory and antioxidant properties. Quercetin is one of the important flavonoids. Resveratrol is one of the antioxidants found in grape skin and seeds. It reduces the biosynthesis of pro-inflammatory such as prostaglandin-E2. Moderate alcohol consumption is recommended in the Mediterranean diet. Accordingly, consumption of 1 glass (140 ml) for women and 2 glasses of wine for men are defined as moderate. In summary, the polyphenols contained in the red wine recommended in the Mediterranean diet show anti-inflammatory properties (Kwan et al., 2017). In addition, due to the abundance of vegetables, fruits and whole grains in the Mediterranean diet, the amount of fiber is high. It is known that there is an inverse relationship between dietary fiber intake and inflammation indicators (Samur & Mercanlıgil, 2008).

DASH DIET

Dietary Approaches to Stop Hypertension (DASH) diet emerged in the 1990s. The National Institute of Health was planned in 1992 to determine the impact of medical nutrition on the treatment of hypertension. Accordingly, only dietary intervention was given to the individuals included in the study and no other lifestyle changes were recommended. As a result of this diet, systolic blood pressure of the individuals decreased approximately 6 to 11 mm Hg. This effect was seen in both hypertensive and normotensive individuals (Challa, Tadi, & Uppaluri, 2019). The DASH diet, when used in conjunction with other lifestyle changes, helps to control blood pressure and prevent elevation. If blood pressure is not too high, it may be possible to control hypertension with healthy lifestyle changes. Lifestyle changes include healthy weight management in overweight individuals, regular physical activity, and reduced alcohol consumption (NHLBI, 2006). Although this diet style was initially recommended to individuals to prevent or treat hypertension (Saneei, Salehi-Abargouei, Esmaillzadeh, & Azadbakht, 2014), this nutritional model also controls body weight (Blumenthal et al., 2010), improving lipid profile (Siervo et. al., 2015), the provision of glycemic control (Azadbakht, Surkan, Esmaillzadeh, & Willett, 2011; Shirani, Salehi-Abargouei, & Azadbakht, 2013) and has been found to reduce the risk of CVD (Salehi-Abargouei, Maghsoudi, Shirani, & Azad, 2013).

The DASH diet is a diet rich in fruits, vegetables, low-fat dairy products, dietary fiber, potassium, calcium and magnesium. It has a moderately high amount in terms of protein content. It is also a poor diet in terms of saturated fat, cholesterol and total fat. The DASH diet contains a high proportion of dietary fiber, especially seeds from nuts and low-fat dairy products. It also contains nutrients containing antioxidant vitamins such as vitamins A, C and E which are suggested to be beneficial to human health (Sakhaei et al., 2018). This nutritional model suggests sodium restriction on a daily basis. This diet recommends avoiding consumption of processed foods and consuming fresh foods (Challa et al., 2019). The portion amounts of the recommended food groups and nutrients in the DASH diet are as follows:

1. Vegetables: about 5 servings per day
2. Fruits: about 5 servings per day
3. Carbohydrates: about 7 servings per day
4. Low-fat dairy products: about 2 servings per day
5. Lean meat products: about 2 or less servings per day
6. Nuts and seeds: 2 or 3 servings per week (Challa et al., 2019).

According to NHLBI, the daily nutrient consumption targets of a 2100 kcal DASH diet are indicated in Table 3 (NHLBI, 2006).

Table 3. Objectives of DASH Diet

NUTRIENTS	DESTINATIONS
Total fat	27.0% of total energy
Saturated fat	6.0% of total energy
Protein	18.0% of total energy
Carbohydrate	55.0% of total energy
Cholesterol	150 mg
Sodium	2300 mg
Potassium	4700 mg
Calcium	1250 mg
Magnesium	500 mg
Fiber	30 g

DASH diet scoring was developed to assess compliance with DASH diet content (Mellen, Gao, Vitolins, & Goff, 2008). According to this scoring, when calculating the total DASH diet index score, a certain score was determined for each food group (0, 0.5 and 1 point) and 11 nutrients were collected. For example; The DASH diet recommends 4-5 servings of vegetables per day for individuals with a daily need of 2000 kcal. Accordingly, 4 or more servings of vegetables were given full score points (+1), while 2-3 servings of individuals consumed half (+0.5) score points, 2 servings or less of vegetables consumed daily individuals who score zero (0). For food groups whose consumption amount should be low, the opposite of normal scoring system is done. For example; individuals who consume 5 or less servings of sugar per week are given full score, whereas individuals who consume 6-7 servings of sugar per week are given half a score and individuals who consume 8 or more servings per week are given zero points (Folsom, Parker, & Harnack, 2007). At the end of the DASH scoring, total score <4.5 was considered to be low-fit and ^{3}4.5 points were considered as high-fit (Casanova, Medeiros, Oigman, & Neves, 2014).

The Effect of Dash Diet on Inflammation

When the content of DASH diet is examined, it is reported that it is rich in dietary fiber, whole grains, vegetables, fruits, legumes, low-fat dairy products, magnesium content and thus shows an anti-inflammatory feature. Furthermore, the DASH-style diet model is a type of diet with a low glycemic index / load ratio (Soltani et al., 2018). According to a systematic review, diets containing low glycemic index / load ratio have beneficial effects on decreasing serum CRP concentrations in obese individuals (L. Schwingshackl & Hoffmann, 2013). In addition, consumption of legume rich in dietary fiber results in a decrease in serum CRP levels of 0.21 mg / dl (Salehi-Abargouei, Saraf-Bank, Bellissimo, & Azadbakht, 2015). The anti-inflammatory properties of high-fiber and low-glycemic index nutrition models are due to the slowing of glucose absorption and consequently suppressing the production of inflammatory cytokines. In addition, such nutritional models increase the production of short-chain fatty acids, reducing circulating free fatty acid levels and thereby suppressing inflammation (Soltani et al., 2018). Another effect of dietary fiber on inflammation is the change in the microflora of individuals by fermentation by colonic bacteria. Thus, it provides the development of microbial species that produce anti-inflammatory cytokines (Poullis, Foster, Shetty, Fagerhol, & Mendall, 2004).

When the content of DASH nutrition model is examined, it is seen that there are significant amounts of low-fat dairy products. According to a systematic review, abundant consumption of dairy products has been shown to have a positive or neutral effect on inflammatory biomarkers than diets poor in dairy products (Labonté, Couture, Richard, Desroches, & Lamarche, 2013). Calcium in dairy products is involved in the regulation of inflammatory stress and suppresses angiotensin-converting enzyme and α1, 25-dihydroxycholecalciferol. In addition, bioactive peptides such as lactoferrin in dairy products have positive effects on inflammatory biomarkers through regulation and activation of cytokine-secreting immune cells (Soltani et al., 2018). Conjugated linoleic acid, riboflavin and high-quality protein, which are the other components of dairy products, are thought to have positive effects on systemic inflammation (Sakhaei et al., 2018).

The DASH diet is rich in magnesium minerals. According to a meta-analysis, 7 cross-sectional studies were examined and dietary magnesium levels were found to be inversely related to serum CRP levels (Dibaba, Xun, & He, 2014). It is known that free radical production increases as a result of magnesium deficiency in individuals and thus increases the release of pro-inflammatory cytokines (Soltani et al., 2018).

Restriction of sodium intake in the DASH diet is recommended. High sodium consumption appears to be associated with increased levels of inflammation (Fogarty, Lewis, McKeever, & Britton, 2009). Foods with a high sodium content generally have a high energy content (Zhu et al., 2014). High sodium consumption of individuals in the studies conducted has been associated with increased adipocyte tissue (Libuda, Kersting, & Alexy, 2012). In addition, high sodium consumption causes increased plasma leptin levels. Leptin is one of the most important adipokines secreted by fat cells. Control of metabolism has various physiological roles, such as the maintenance of energy homeostasis and body weight, inflammatory response, excretion of urine and sodium. Disorders such as hypertension and obesity occur as a result of changes in leptin (Fogarty et al., 2009).

It is known that inflammatory processes are closely related to pathological mechanisms such as glycotoxicity, lipotoxicity and oxidative stress. Dietary components may be affected by a number of factors including physical inactivity, smoking, alcohol consumption and other lifestyle changes. These stimuli increase the release of pro-inflammatory factors from various tissues, leading to chronic low-grade inflammation, defined as a risk factor for insulin resistance, cell dysfunction and ultimately development of Type 2 DM. This condition is defined as 2-3-fold increase in circulating inflammatory markers. Insulin resistance is also known to be a process triggered by oxidative stress, exacerbated by inflammatory mechanisms (Yalçın & Rakıcıoğlu, 2018). The DASH diet recommends the consumption of foods such as fish, soy, beans, lentils, whole grains, nuts, parsley and fresh basil. Therefore, this diet contains high amounts of arginine. The high arginine content of the DASH diet also has positive effects on insulin resistance. Arginine is thought to have positive effects on insulin resistance by increasing nitric oxide production in individuals and improving endothelial function. Another mechanism of action is the positive effects of high levels of magnesium and calcium contained in this diet (Asemi, Samimi, Tabassi, Sabihi, & Esmaillzadeh, 2013).

The high antioxidant content of the DASH diet may also explain the positive effects of this diet on inflammation. Antioxidants have been shown to reduce systemic inflammation (Aeberli et al., 2006). Dietary antioxidants are thought to have a positive effect on inflammation by affecting the expression of pro-inflammatory cytokines (Saneei et al., 2014). High levels of vitamin C in the DASH diet are a major component of plasma total antioxidant capacity. Vitamin C can reduce the activity of nicotinamide adenine dinucleotide phosphate-oxidase, a superoxide-producing enzyme (Asemi et al., 2013).

High amounts of vegetables and fruits contained in DASH diet prevent oxidative stress. Furthermore, the arginine content of the DASH diet contributes to the reduction of oxidative stress. Arginine has been shown to reduce serum angiotensin-II levels and oxidative stress measurements (Asemi et al., 2013).

VEGETARIAN DIET

Vegetarian nutrition is a form of nutrition that has been going on for centuries for religious and economic reasons or disliking the taste / texture of animal-derived foods. Especially as of the 20th century, animal rights and ethical considerations, ecological concerns and positive effects on health have led to an increase in the number of individuals who prefer this diet (Orlich et al., 2013). In this nutritional pattern, individuals partially or completely remove nutrients from animal diets. People who partially exclude animal-derived foods from their diet are defined under different groups according to the types of animal-derived foods they continue to consume. People who remove all nutrients of animal origin from their diets are called vegan. People who include all the nutrients of animal origin in their diet are defined as omnivores. Different types of vegetarian nutrition are described in Table 4 (Clarys et al., 2014).

Table 4. Vegetarian Nutrition Patterns

Vegetarian Nutrition Patterns	Definition
Semi-vejetaryen	From time to time red meat, poultry or fish and so on. consumes seafood.
Pesko-vejetaryen	Does not consume red meat and poultry, consumes seafood.
Lakto-ovo-vejetaryen	It removes all types of meat from its diet, consumes milk and dairy products and eggs.
Ovo-vejetaryen	It removes all types of meat and dairy products from its diet and consumes eggs.
Lakto-vejetaryen	It removes all types of meat and eggs from its diet and consumes milk and dairy products.
Vegan	Removes all nutrients of animal origin from the diet.

It is known that vegetarian diet has positive effects on health. This diet is positively effective for BMI, total cholesterol levels, ischemic heart disease risk, type 2 DM risk, constipation, diverticular diseases, gallstone and appendicitis disease and is associated with longer life expectancy (Crowe, Appleby, Allen, & Key, 2011; Key, Appleby, & Rosell, 2006). The reasons for these positive effects of vegetarian nutrition on health include the fact that individuals have a high amount of foods (vegetables, fruits, legumes etc.) that contain protective nutrients against diseases and do not consume nutrients (saturated fatty acids, cholesterol) that increase the risk of chronic diseases (Dewell, Weidner, Sumner, Chi, & Ornish, 2008). The nutrient content of vegetarian diets is rich in complex carbohydrates, carotenoids, fiber, vitamin C, vitamin E, folic acid and omega-6 fatty acids, magnesium, compared to mixed diets; protein, saturated fats, omega3 fatty acid, retinol, cholesterol, vitamin B_{12}, calcium and zinc content in terms of poorer (Davey et al., 2003).

In addition to the positive effect of vegetarian diets, a number of non-nutritional factors brought about by vegetarianism also have an impact on the increase quality of life and decrease in disease risks. These; adoption of a healthy lifestyle, a physically active life, low rate of smoking and alcohol use, and high educational levels of vegetarian individuals (Pilis, Stec, Zych, & Pilis, 2014).

The Effect of Vegetarian Diet on Inflammation

Although the definition of vegetarianism varies, it generally has a richer diet content than antioxidant micronutrients such as vitamins C and E, phytochemicals and fiber compared to the diets of omnivores. These healthy dietary components have a positive effect on inflammation processes. Accordingly, reducing circulating levels of inflammatory biomarkers, improving inflammation, and thus reducing the risk of age-related diseases may occur. Numerous studies have reported that vegetarian individuals have lower serum inflammatory biomarker concentrations than omnivores (Haghighatdoost, Bellissimo, Totosy De Zepetnek, & Rouhani, 2017). In addition, vegetarian diets have been shown to significantly alter fecal flora, which plays an important role in the inflammatory response (Glick-Bauer & Yeh, 2014).

In a recent clinical study, vegan and vegetarian individuals have been shown to have lower levels of inflammatory biomarkers than omnivores (Sutliffe, Wilson, de Heer, Foster, & Carnot, 2015). In a systematic review study, it was found out that 15 studies who examined the relationship between CRP levels and vegetarian and omnivor diets had lower CRP concentrations compared to omnivorous individuals. In addition, according to the results of 3 studies examining the relationship between IL-6 levels and these diets, it was found that IL-6 levels were higher in individuals who applied vegetarian diet than omnivores (Haghighatdoost et al., 2017). In a randomized controlled study, it was observed that vegan diet administered for 8 weeks in patients with coronary artery disease significantly reduced serum CRP levels compared to the American Heart Association recommended diet. However, no significant difference was observed in terms of weight loss, glycemic control, and improvement of lipid profile of individuals in both diet groups (Kim, Hwang, Park, & Bae, 2013). In another study, a long-term vegetarian diet was found to be associated with significantly lower CRP concentrations (Szeto, Kwok, & Benzie, 2004).

High inflammatory biomarkers, including TNFα and IL-6, are remarkable in overweight and obese subjects (Bastard et al., 2017). CRP, fibrinogen and total leukocyte concentrations are lower in individuals who are fed according to vegetarian diet patterns compared to omnivorous diets. It is thought that low BMIs observed in those fed in accordance with vegetarian diet patterns are effective in the formation of these low levels (Spencer, Appleby, Davey, & Key, 2003).

It is seen that uric acid level in vegetarian individuals is lower than those consuming meat and meat products. High levels of nucleic acid in meat, uric acid is formed in individuals consuming meat and meat products with higher purine content. Therefore, low uric acid concentration occurs in those who are vegetarian-style diet. High uric acid level has been reported to be directly associated with insulin resistance, hypertension and CVD risk. Therefore, vegetarian diets are thought to be effective in reducing mortality (Szeto et al., 2004).

In order to make a clearer comment on the efficacy of vegetarian dietary patterns on inflammation, a sufficient variety of inflammatory biomarkers has not been examined. However, it is especially noteworthy in studies that it has an impact on inflammation with changes in CRP levels. The lack of randomized controlled trials to determine the effectiveness of vegetarian diets on inflammation is striking (Craddock, Neale, Peoples, & Probst, 2019).

Diets rich in fruits and vegetables have a protective feature against chronic, degenerative diseases. These beneficial effects are thought to be due to the ability of plant-based antioxidant compounds such as ascorbic acid, carotenoids and flavonoids to protect important biological sites such as lipoproteins, membranes and DNA from oxidative damage. The World Cancer Research Fund recommends five or more portions of fruit and vegetables each day. In addition, the recently recommended daily intake of vitamin C in the US has been revised to 75 mg / day for women and 90 mg / day for men (Szeto et al., 2004). Although the identity of the preservative component or components in fruits and vegetables is not yet clear, vitamin C (ascorbic acid) intake and plasma concentrations have been reported to be inversely correlated with all-cause mortality rates (Khaw et al., 2001). In addition, vitamin E (mostly-tocopherol) is an important anti-atherogenic and anti-inflammatory agent. Due to the increase in the consumption of antioxidant components, dietary patterns of vegetarians are thought to improve the overall health status (Szeto et al., 2004). In addition, fruits and vegetables can regulate the intestinal microbiota through dietary fiber. *Faecalibacterium prausnitzii*, an anti-inflammatory bacterium, was found to be higher in vegetarian diets (Glick-Bauer & Yeh, 2014).

It is thought that nutrients and non-nutrient components contained in vegetarian diet patterns create levels of low inflammatory biomarkers (Craddock et al., 2019). Consumption of flavonoids such as quercetin, kaempferol, malvidin, peonidin, daidzein and genistein; is inversely related to serum CRP even after adjustment for covariants such as vitamin C vitamin E, carotenes, fruit and vegetable consumption (Chun, Chung, Claycombe, & Song, 2008). Flavonoids are important antioxidants that prevent LDL oxidation, an early inflammatory event in the development of atherosclerosis. Similarly, carotenoids are potent antioxidants embedded in the lipid bilayer, which reduces the harmful effect of free radicals and is inversely related to signs of inflammation (Craddock et al., 2019). Both flavonoids and carotenoids are found in higher concentrations in individuals who comply with vegetarian-based diet patterns and it provides anti-inflammatory effects of vegetarian-based diets (Craig, Mangels, & American Dietetic Association, 2009).

The type and amount of fat intake in the diet affects low-grade inflammation concentrations. Some studies have shown that increased serum CRP and fibrinogen levels are associated with dietary saturated fatty acids (Arya et al., 2006; Clarke, Shipley, Armitage, Collins, & Harris, 2009). Saturated fatty acid intake is higher in non-vegetarian diet models due to the increased consumption of animal-based products (Craig et al., 2009). This is thought to be the cause of high serum CRP and fibrinogen concentration observed in individuals. Individuals fed in accordance with vegetarian diet patterns consume higher amounts of unsaturated fatty acids than non-vegetarians (Craddock et al., 2019).

Nuts rich in monounsaturated fatty acids and polyunsaturated fatty acids and poor from free fatty acids reduce oxidation and provide a decrease in CRP, IL-6 and pro-inflammatory cytokines. Thus, they provide anti-inflammation effect and prevent cardiovascular health. One of the reasons for the low risk of CVD in vegetarian nutrition is the presence of nuts that are rich in protective nutrients in the diet (Ros, 2009). It has been reported that there is a positive effect on inflammation due to the high amount of magnesium, fiber, α-linolenic acid, L-arginine, antioxidants and monounsaturated fatty acids, especially in the nuts content of the nuts in the vegetarian diet patterns (Casas-Agustench, Bulló, & Salas-). Salvadó, 2010). However, since the composition of various nuts varies, the types of nuts consumed play an important role in the anti-inflammatory effect observed due to hazelnut consumption (Moodley, Kindness, & Jonnalagadda, 2007).

Dairy products in vegetarian diets have both positive and negative effects on inflammation. Although the fatty acid composition contained in dairy products is mostly saturated fatty acid, it is an important dietary source for the calcium intake of the individual. To minimize the adverse effects of dairy products on inflammation, it is recommended to replace dairy products with another calcium-containing food source (Haghighatdoost et al., 2017).

NORDIC DIET

It is a healthy diet characterized by high intake of traditional and locally sourced food in Scandinavian countries such as Norway, Denmark, Sweden and Finland. The Nordic diet consists of fruits and vegetables (especially cabbages and root vegetables), legumes, potatoes, fresh plants, weeds, nuts, whole grains, poultry and hunting meats, oily dairy products, wild-collected fungi, fish, shellfish and algae (Mithril et al., 2012). The Nordic diet varies according to different Scandinavian countries and regions. These changes include fruits, vegetables and bread types (Lankinen, Uusitupa, & Schwab, 2019). The Nordic diet has many similarities to the Mediterranean diet. Both dietary models emphasize the abundance of fruits and vegetables, whole grain products and fish and limit the consumption of saturated fat (milk fat), red and processed meat. The most important difference between the two diets is that the Mediterranean diet is the most important source of unsaturated fat for olive oil, while the Nordic diet is canola oil. In addition, the Nordic diet includes fruits such as blueberries and strawberries (Matti Uusitupa & Schwab, 2013). Both diets emphasize fish consumption. Although the fish species consumed are slightly different, the quality and quantity of fat is approximately the same. In the northern countries, fish species such as salmon, rainbow trout, herring, mackerel, saithe and cod are consumed (Lankinen et al., 2019).

The Effect of Nordic Diet on Inflammation

Studies have shown that the Nordic Diet has positive effects on weight loss (Fritzen et al., 2015) and insulin sensitivity (Adamsson et al., 2011). Furthermore, the Nordic Diet has been suggested to improve adipose tissue metabolism, lipid profile, and systemic inflammation (Brader, Uusitupa, Dragsted, & Hermansen, 2014; Vanessa D. F. De Mello et al., 2009; O'Connor et al., 2014). Randomized clinical trials have examined the effect of Nordic Diet on inflammatory markers, with different results. For example, one study found that the Nordic Diet had positive effects on low-grade inflammation (Fritzen et al., 2015). In addition, other studies have shown that the Nordic Diet has no effect on the levels of inflammatory markers (Adamsson et al., 2011; V. D. F. De Mello et al., 2011; M. Uusitupa et al., 2013). A systematic review of recent randomized controlled clinical trials and meta-analysis showed that Nordic Diet did not significantly affect inflammatory markers such as IL-6, TNF-α and CRP (Sakhaei, Ramezani-Jolfaie, Mohammadi, & Salehi-Abargouei, 2019). According to the results of another meta-analysis study, adherence to Nordic, Mediterranean, Tibetan and DASH dietary models has been shown to be associated with a significant reduction in CRP concentrations (Neale et al., 2016).

A questionnaire-based Anti-Infammatory Diet Index (AIDI) has been developed to predict systemic chronic inflammation in the Scandinavian population (Kaluza, Harris, Melhus, Michaëlsson, & Wolk, 2018). This index is based on food frequency surveys among 3503 women. Overall, 20 nutrients were found to be significantly correlated with CRP levels of individuals. Accordingly, foods with anti-inflammatory potential; fruit and vegetables, tea, coffee, whole grain bread, breakfast cereal, low fat cheese, chocolate, dried fruits, olive and canola oils, legumes, nuts, flax seeds, red wine and beer. Foods with high pro-inflammatory potential are raw and processed red meat, organ meats, chips and soft drinks. This study did not investigate the entire Nordic diet model. However, it is assumed that these nutrients may be associated with systemic chronic inflammation, especially in the Scandinavian population (Lankinen et al., 2019). In a study by Fritzen et al. (2015), it was found that adherence to Nordic Diet resulted in a significant decrease in CRP among female subjects only. Accordingly, it was interpreted that the nutrients contained in the Nordic diet decreased CRP levels due to their weight loss and low glycemic index.

The fruits of the Nordic Diet, such as blueberries, raspberries and cranberries, are thought to show anti-inflammatory effects because they contain high amounts of polyphenols. Polyphenols; There are studies that show anti-inflammatory effect by decreasing oxidative stress and inhibiting inflammatory gene expression (Sakhaei et al., 2019).

Fish and shellfish found in high amounts in the Nordic Diet are a good source of n-3 fatty acids (Mithril et al., 2012). According to the results of a meta-analysis, n-3 taken with seafood consumption has been shown to significantly reduce circulating levels of CRP, IL-6 and TNF-α (Li, Huang, Zheng, Wu, & Li, 2014).

The Nordic Diet seems to have a less beneficial effect on reducing inflammation compared to other healthy diet models such as the Mediterranean diet. Although the Nordic Diet is largely similar to the Mediterranean diet, the type of fat consumed (canola and olive oil) is the main difference between the two dietary models. Olive oil is the largest component of the Mediterranean diet and contains more monounsaturated fatty acids, lower saturated fatty acids and has an anti-inflammatory effect (Chrysohoou et al., 2004). According to the results of a meta-analysis, olive oil has a positive effect on the markers of inflammation (Lukas Schwingshackl, Christoph, & Hoffmann, 2015), while the effect of canola oil on inflammation is contradictory (Junker et al., 2001; Stricker, Duchini, Facchini, & Mombelli, 2008).). In addition, there are no studies comparing the effects of the Mediterranean diet and the Nordic Diet on inflammatory markers (Sakhaei et al., 2019).

CONCLUSION

Diet is an important and modifiable determinant of chronic diseases. In particular, the dietary groups and components contained in diets ensure that diets are pro or anti-inflammatory on inflammation. DII has an important role in measuring the inflammatory potential of a diet. Future studies will reveal more clearly the relationship between nutrition and inflammation. In particular, the number of studies investigating the relationship between inflammation-related diseases and DII should increase.

It is seen that Mediterranean diet and DASH diet are the most important anti-inflammatory diets. Although there are common features in both diets, there are some differences such as the presence of olive oil at the focal point of the Mediterranean diet and the presence of milk and products in the DASH diet. There are few studies evaluating the efficacy of these two diets on inflammation. Therefore, there is insufficient information as to which one is more effective on inflammation. The vegetarian diet, which is another form of nutrition, is thought to be anti-inflammatory because it is especially rich in micronutrients, phytochemicals and fiber. However, the variety of inflammatory biomarkers studied in studies is insufficient. Similarly, in order to interpret the efficacy of Nordic diet on inflammation, more studies need to be performed with various inflammatory biomarkers. As a result, the role of diet on inflammation is better understood at the present. The diet affects inflammation positively or negatively, both as a whole and with the effectiveness of the individual food groups.

REFERENCES

Adamsson, V., Reumark, A., Fredriksson, I. B., Hammarström, E., Vessby, B., Johansson, G., & Risérus, U. (2011). Effects of a healthy Nordic diet on cardiovascular risk factors in hypercholesterolaemic subjects: A randomized controlled trial (NORDIET). *Journal of Internal Medicine*, *269*(2), 150–159. doi:10.1111/j.1365-2796.2010.02290.x PMID:20964740

Aeberli, I., Molinari, L., Spinas, G., Lehmann, R., L'Allemand, D., & Zimmermann, M. B. (2006). Dietary intakes of fat and antioxidant vitamins are predictors of subclinical inflammation in overweight Swiss children. *The American Journal of Clinical Nutrition*, *84*(4), 748–755. doi:10.1093/ajcn/84.4.748 PMID:17023700

Arya, S., Isharwal, S., Misra, A., Pandey, R. M., Rastogi, K., Vikram, N. K., ... Luthra, K. (2006). C-reactive protein and dietary nutrients in urban Asian Indian adolescents and young adults. *Nutrition*, *22*(9), 865–871. doi:10.1016/j.nut.2006.05.002 PMID:16829027

Asemi, Z., Samimi, M., Tabassi, Z., Sabihi, S., & Esmaillzadeh, A. (2013). A randomized controlled clinical trial investigating the effect of DASH diet on insulin resistance, inflammation, and oxidative stress in gestational diabetes. *Nutrition (Burbank, Los Angeles County, Calif.)*, *29*(4), 619–624. doi:10.1016/j.nut.2012.11.020 PMID:23466048

Athyros, V. G., Kakafika, A. I., Papageorgiou, A. A., Tziomalos, K., Peletidou, A., Vosikis, C., ... Mikhailidis, D. P. (2011). Effect of a plant stanol ester-containing spread, placebo spread, or Mediterranean diet on estimated cardiovascular risk and lipid, inflammatory and haemostatic factors. *Nutrition, Metabolism, and Cardiovascular Diseases*, *21*(3), 213–221. doi:10.1016/j.numecd.2009.08.014 PMID:19939653

Azadbakht, L., Surkan, P. J., Esmaillzadeh, A., & Willett, W. C. (2011). The Dietary Approaches to Stop Hypertension Eating Plan Affects C-Reactive Protein, Coagulation Abnormalities, and Hepatic Function Tests among Type 2 Diabetic Patients. *The Journal of Nutrition*, *141*(6), 1083–1088. doi:10.3945/jn.110.136739 PMID:21525259

Bach-Faig, A., Berry, E. M., Lairon, D., Reguant, J., Trichopoulou, A., Dernini, S., ... Padulosi, S. (2011). Mediterranean diet pyramid today. Science and cultural updates. *Public Health Nutrition*, *14*(12A), 2274–2284. doi:10.1017/S1368980011002515 PMID:22166184

Bastard, J.-P., Maachi, M., Lagathu, C., Kim, M. J., Caron, M., Vidal, H., ... Bastard, J. P. (2017). Recent advances in the relationship between obesity, inflammation, and insulin resistance. *European Cytokine Network*, *17*(1), 4–12. PMID:16613757

Blumenthal, J. A., Babyak, M. A., Hinderliter, A., Watkins, L. L., Craighead, L., Lin, P. H., ... Sherwood, A. (2010). Effects of the DASH diet alone and in combination with exercise and weight loss on blood pressure and cardiovascular biomarkers in men and women with high blood pressure: The ENCORE study. *Archives of Internal Medicine*, *170*(2), 126–135. doi:10.1001/archinternmed.2009.470 PMID:20101007

Brader, L., Uusitupa, M., Dragsted, L. O., & Hermansen, K. (2014). Effects of an isocaloric healthy Nordic diet on ambulatory blood pressure in metabolic syndrome: A randomized SYSDIET sub-study. *European Journal of Clinical Nutrition*, *68*(1), 57–63. doi:10.1038/ejcn.2013.192 PMID:24129358

Brownlee, M. (2001, December 13). Biochemistry and molecular cell biology of diabetic complications. *Nature*, *414*(6865), 813–820. doi:10.1038/414813a PMID:11742414

Calder, P. C., Ahluwalia, N., Brouns, F., Buetler, T., Clement, K., Cunningham, K., ... Winklhofer-Roob, B. M. (2011). Dietary factors and low-grade inflammation in relation to overweight and obesity. *British Journal of Nutrition, 106*(S3), S5–S78. doi:10.1017/S0007114511005460 PMID:22133051

Calder, P. C., Albers, R., Antoine, J.-M., Blum, S., Bourdet-Sicard, R., Ferns, G. A., ... Zhao, J. (2009). Inflammatory disease processes and interactions with nutrition. *British Journal of Nutrition, 101*(S1), S1–S45. doi:10.1017/S0007114509377867 PMID:19586558

Carter, S. J., Roberts, M. B., Salter, J., & Eaton, C. B. (2010). Relationship between Mediterranean Diet Score and atherothrombotic risk: Findings from the Third National Health and Nutrition Examination Survey (NHANES III), 1988-1994. *Atherosclerosis, 210*(2), 630–636. doi:10.1016/j.atherosclerosis.2009.12.035 PMID:20138282

Casanova, M. A., Medeiros, F., Oigman, W., & Neves, M. F. (2014). Low Concordance with the DASH Plan Is Associated with Higher Cardiovascular Risk in Treated Hypertensive Patients. *ISRN Hypertension, 2014*, 1–8. doi:10.1155/2014/618710

Casas, R., Sacanella, E., & Estruch, R. (2014). The Immune Protective Effect of the Mediterranean Diet against Chronic Low-grade Inflammatory Diseases. *Endocrine, Metabolic & Immune Disorders Drug Targets, 14*(4), 245–254. doi:10.2174/1871530314666140922153350 PMID:25244229

Casas, R., Sacanella, E., Urpí-Sardà, M., Chiva-Blanch, G., Ros, E., Martínez-González, M. A., ... Estruch, R. (2014). The effects of the Mediterranean diet on biomarkers of vascular wall inflammation and plaque vulnerability in subjects with high risk for cardiovascular disease. A randomized trial. *PLoS One, 9*(6), e100084. doi:10.1371/journal.pone.0100084 PMID:24925270

Casas-Agustench, P., Bulló, M., & Salas-Salvadó, J. (2010). Nuts, inflammation and insulin resistance. *Asia Pacific Journal of Clinical Nutrition, 19*(1), 124–130. PMID:20199997

Castro-Quezada, I., Román-Viñas, B., & Serra-Majem, L. (2014, January 3). The mediterranean diet and nutritional adequacy: A review. *Nutrients.*

Cavicchia, P. P., Steck, S. E., Hurley, T. G., Hussey, J. R., Ma, Y., Ockene, I. S., & Hébert, J. R. (2009). A New Dietary Inflammatory Index Predicts Interval Changes in Serum High-Sensitivity C-Reactive Protein. *The Journal of Nutrition, 139*(12), 2365–2372. doi:10.3945/jn.109.114025 PMID:19864399

Chalkiadaki, A., & Guarente, L. (2012). High-fat diet triggers inflammation-induced cleavage of SIRT1 in adipose tissue to promote metabolic dysfunction. *Cell Metabolism*, *16*(2), 180–188. doi:10.1016/j.cmet.2012.07.003 PMID:22883230

Challa, H. J., Tadi, P., & Uppaluri, K. R. (2019). *DASH Diet (Dietary Approaches to Stop Hypertension)*. StatPearls.

Chrysohoou, C., Panagiotakos, D. B., Pitsavos, C., Das, U. N., & Stefanadis, C. (2004). Adherence to the Mediterranean diet attenuates inflammation and coagulation process in healthy adults: The ATTICA study. *Journal of the American College of Cardiology*, *44*(1), 152–158. doi:10.1016/j.jacc.2004.03.039 PMID:15234425

Chun, O. K., Chung, S.-J., Claycombe, K. J., & Song, W. O. (2008). Serum C-Reactive Protein Concentrations Are Inversely Associated with Dietary Flavonoid Intake in U.S. Adults. *The Journal of Nutrition*, *138*(4), 753–760. doi:10.1093/jn/138.4.753 PMID:18356331

Clarke, R., Shipley, M., Armitage, J., Collins, R., & Harris, W. (2009). Plasma phospholipid fatty acids and CHD in older men: Whitehall study of London civil servants. *British Journal of Nutrition*, *102*(2), 279–284. doi:10.1017/S0007114508143562 PMID:19105853

Clarys, P., Deliens, T., Huybrechts, I., Deriemaeker, P., Vanaelst, B., De Keyzer, W., ... Mullie, P. (2014). Comparison of nutritional quality of the vegan, vegetarian, semi-vegetarian, pesco-vegetarian and omnivorous diet. *Nutrients*, *6*(3), 1318–1332. doi:10.3390/nu6031318 PMID:24667136

Craddock, J. C., Neale, E. P., Peoples, G. E., & Probst, Y. C. (2019, May 1). Vegetarian-Based Dietary Patterns and their Relation with Inflammatory and Immune Biomarkers: A Systematic Review and Meta-Analysis. In *Advances in Nutrition*. Oxford University Press. doi:10.1093/advances/nmy103

Craig, W. J., & Mangels, A. R. (2009). Position of the American Dietetic Association: Vegetarian diets. *Journal of the American Dietetic Association*, *109*(7), 1266–1282. doi:10.1016/j.jada.2009.05.027 PMID:19562864

Crimarco, A., Turner-McGrievy, G. M., Wirth, M. D., Shivappa, N., Dunn, C., Vyas, S., ... Hébert, J. R. (2018). Baseline markers of inflammation, lipids, glucose, and Dietary Inflammatory Index scores do not differ between adults willing to participate in an intensive inflammation reduction intervention and those who do not. *Nutrition and Health (Berkhamsted, Hertfordshire)*. PMID:30229691

Crowe, F. L., Appleby, P. N., Allen, N. E., & Key, T. J. (2011). Diet and risk of diverticular disease in Oxford cohort of European Prospective Investigation into Cancer and Nutrition (EPIC): Prospective study of British vegetarians and non-vegetarians. *BMJ (Online), 343*(7817).

Davey, G. K., Spencer, E. A., Appleby, P. N., Allen, N. E., Knox, K. H., & Key, T. J. (2003). EPIC–Oxford:lifestyle characteristics and nutrient intakes in a cohort of 33 883 meat-eaters and 31 546 non meat-eaters in the UK. *Public Health Nutrition, 6*(3), 259–268. doi:10.1079/PHN2002430 PMID:12740075

De Mello, V. D. F., Erkkilä, A. T., Schwab, U. S., Pulkkinen, L., Kolehmainen, M., Atalay, M., ... Uusitupa, M. (2009). The effect of fatty or lean fish intake on inflammatory gene expression in peripheral blood mononuclear cells of patients with coronary heart disease. *European Journal of Nutrition, 48*(8), 447–455. doi:10.100700394-009-0033-y PMID:19506932

De Mello, V. D. F., Schwab, U., Kolehmainen, M., Koenig, W., Siloaho, M., Poutanen, K., ... Uusitupa, M. (2011). A diet high in fatty fish, bilberries and wholegrain products improves markers of endothelial function and inflammation in individuals with impaired glucose metabolism in a randomised controlled trial: The Sysdimet study. *Diabetologia, 54*(11), 2755–2767. doi:10.100700125-011-2285-3 PMID:21870174

Dewell, A., Weidner, G., Sumner, M. D., Chi, C. S., & Ornish, D. (2008). A Very-Low-Fat Vegan Diet Increases Intake of Protective Dietary Factors and Decreases Intake of Pathogenic Dietary Factors. *Journal of the American Dietetic Association, 108*(2), 347–356. doi:10.1016/j.jada.2007.10.044 PMID:18237581

Dibaba, D. T., Xun, P., & He, K. (2014). Dietary magnesium intake is inversely associated with serum C-reactive protein levels: Meta-analysis and systematic review. *European Journal of Clinical Nutrition, 68*(4), 510–516. doi:10.1038/ejcn.2014.7 PMID:24518747

Esposito, K., Kastorini, C. M., Panagiotakos, D. B., & Giugliano, D. (2013). Mediterranean diet and metabolic syndrome: An updated systematic review. *Reviews in Endocrine & Metabolic Disorders, 14*(3), 255–263. doi:10.100711154-013-9253-9 PMID:23982678

Esposito, K., Marfella, R., Ciotola, M., Di Palo, C., Giugliano, F., Giugliano, G., ... Giugliano, D. (2004). Effect of a Mediterranean-style diet on endothelial dysfunction and markers of vascular inflammation in the metabolic syndrome: A randomized trial. *Journal of the American Medical Association, 292*(12), 1440–1446. doi:10.1001/jama.292.12.1440 PMID:15383514

Ferreira, C. M., Vieira, A. T., Vinolo, M. A. R., Oliveira, F. A., Curi, R., & Martins, F. dos S. (2014). The central role of the gut microbiota in chronic inflammatory diseases. *Journal of Immunology Research, 2014*, 689492. doi:10.1155/2014/689492 PMID:25309932

Fogarty, A. W., Lewis, S. A., McKeever, T. M., & Britton, J. R. (2009). Is higher sodium intake associated with elevated systemic inflammation? A population-based study. *The American Journal of Clinical Nutrition*, *89*(6), 1901–1904. doi:10.3945/ajcn.2008.27006 PMID:19386745

Folsom, A. R., Parker, E. D., & Harnack, L. J. (2007). Degree of Concordance With DASH Diet Guidelines and Incidence of Hypertension and Fatal Cardiovascular Disease. *American Journal of Hypertension*, *20*(3), 225–232. doi:10.1016/j.amjhyper.2006.09.003 PMID:17324731

Fritzen, A. M. H., Lundsgaard, A. M., Jordy, A. B., Poulsen, S. K., Stender, S., Pilegaard, H., ... Kiens, B. (2015). New nordic diet-induced weight loss is accompanied by changes in metabolism and AMPK signaling in adipose tissue. *The Journal of Clinical Endocrinology and Metabolism*, *100*(9), 3509–3519. doi:10.1210/jc.2015-2079 PMID:26126206

Fung, T. T., Rexrode, K. M., Mantzoros, C. S., Manson, J. E., Willett, W. C., & Hu, F. B. (2009). Mediterranean diet and incidence of and mortality from coronary heart disease and stroke in women. *Circulation*, *119*(8), 1093–1100. doi:10.1161/CIRCULATIONAHA.108.816736 PMID:19221219

Galland, L. (2010, December). Diet and inflammation. *Nutrition in Clinical Practice*, *25*(6), 634–640. doi:10.1177/0884533610385703 PMID:21139128

Glick-Bauer, M., & Yeh, M. C. (2014). *The health advantage of a vegan diet: Exploring the gut microbiota connection. Nutrients*. MDPI AG.

Haghighatdoost, F., Bellissimo, N., Totosy De Zepetnek, J. O., & Rouhani, M. H. (2017). *Association of vegetarian diet with inflammatory biomarkers: A systematic review and meta-analysis of observational studies. Public Health Nutrition*. Cambridge University Press.

Junker, R., Kratz, M., Neufeld, M., Erren, M., Nofer, J.-R., Schulte, H., ... Wahrburg, U. (2001). Effects of Diets Containing Olive Oil, Sunflower Oil, or Rapeseed Oil on the Hemostatic System. *Thrombosis and Haemostasis*, *85*(02), 280–286. doi:10.1055-0037-1615680 PMID:11246548

Kabaran, S., Gezer, C., Üniversitesi, D. A., Fakültesi, S. B., Ve, B., Bölümü, D., ... Lefkoşa, K. (2012). Kuzey Kıbrıs Türk Cumhuriyeti'ndeki Çocuk ve Adolesanlarda Akdeniz Diyetine Uyum ile Obezitenin Belirlenmesi. *Turkish Journal of Pediatric Disease*, *1*, 11–20.

Kaluza, J., Harris, H., Melhus, H., Michaëlsson, K., & Wolk, A. (2018). *Questionnaire-Based Anti-Inflammatory Diet Index as a Predictor of Low-Grade Systemic Inflammation. Antioxidants and Redox Signaling*. Mary Ann Liebert Inc.

Key, T. J., Appleby, P. N., & Rosell, M. S. (2006). Health effects of vegetarian and vegan diets. *The Proceedings of the Nutrition Society*, *65*(1), 35–41. doi:10.1079/PNS2005481 PMID:16441942

Khaw, K. T., Bingham, S., Welch, A., Luben, R., Wareham, N., Oakes, S., & Day, N. (2001). Relation between plasma ascorbic acid and mortality in men and women in EPIC-Norfolk prospective study: A prospective population study. *Lancet*, *357*(9257), 657–663. doi:10.1016/S0140-6736(00)04128-3 PMID:11247548

Kiecolt-Glaser, J. K. (2010). Stress, food, and inflammation: Psychoneuroimmunology and nutrition at the cutting edge. *Psychosomatic Medicine*, *72*(4), 365–369. doi:10.1097/PSY.0b013e3181dbf489 PMID:20410248

Kim, M. S., Hwang, S. S., Park, E. J., & Bae, J. W. (2013). Strict vegetarian diet improves the risk factors associated with metabolic diseases by modulating gut microbiota and reducing intestinal inflammation. *Environmental Microbiology Reports*, *5*(5), 765–775. PMID:24115628

Kjeldsen-Kragh, J., Haugen, M., Borchgrevink, C. F., & Førre, Ø. (1994). Vegetarian diet for patients with rheumatoid arthritis - Status: Two years after introduction of the diet. *Clinical Rheumatology*, *13*(3), 475–482. doi:10.1007/BF02242946 PMID:7835013

Kris-Etherton, P., Eckel, R. H., Howard, B. V., St. Jeor, S., & Bazzarre, T. L. (2001). Lyon diet heart study: Benefits of a Mediterranean-style, National Cholesterol Education Program/American Heart Association Step I dietary pattern on cardiovascular disease. *Circulation*, *103*(13), 1823–1825. doi:10.1161/01.CIR.103.13.1823 PMID:11282918

Kwan, H. Y., Chao, X., Su, T., Fu, X., Tse, A. K. W., Fong, W., & Yu, Z.-L. (2017). The anticancer and antiobesity effects of Mediterranean diet. *Critical Reviews in Food Science and Nutrition*, *57*(1), 82–94. doi:10.1080/10408398.2013.852510 PMID:25831235

Labonté, M. È., Couture, P., Richard, C., Desroches, S., & Lamarche, B. (2013). Impact of dairy products on biomarkers of inflammation: A systematic review of randomized controlled nutritional intervention studies in overweight and obese adults. *The American Journal of Clinical Nutrition*, *97*(4), 706–717. doi:10.3945/ajcn.112.052217 PMID:23446894

Lankinen, M., Uusitupa, M., & Schwab, U. (2019). *Nordic Diet and Inflammation-A Review of Observational and Intervention Studies. Nutrients. NLM*. Medline.

Li, K., Huang, T., Zheng, J., Wu, K., & Li, D. (2014). Effect of marine-derived n-3 polyunsaturated fatty acids on C-reactive protein, interleukin 6 and tumor necrosis factor α: A meta-analysis. *PLoS One*, *9*(2). PMID:24505395

Libuda, L., Kersting, M., & Alexy, U. (2012). Consumption of dietary salt measured by urinary sodium excretion and its association with body weight status in healthy children and adolescents. *Public Health Nutrition*, *15*(3), 433–441. doi:10.1017/S1368980011002138 PMID:21929845

Martínez-González, M. A., García-Arellano, A., Toledo, E., Salas-Salvado, J., Buil-Cosiales, P., Corella, D., ... Fiol, M. (2012). A 14-item Mediterranean diet assessment tool and obesity indexes among high-risk subjects: The PREDIMED trial. *PLoS One*, *7*(8), e43134. doi:10.1371/journal.pone.0043134 PMID:22905215

Martínez-González, M. A., García-López, M., Bes-Rastrollo, M., Toledo, E., Martínez-Lapiscina, E. H., Delgado-Rodriguez, M., ... Beunza, J. J. (2011). Mediterranean diet and the incidence of cardiovascular disease: A Spanish cohort. *Nutrition, Metabolism, and Cardiovascular Diseases*, *21*(4), 237–244. PMID:20096543

Mayr, H. L., Tierney, A. C., Thomas, C. J., Ruiz-Canela, M., Radcliffe, J., & Itsiopoulos, C. (2018). Mediterranean-type diets and inflammatory markers in patients with coronary heart disease: A systematic review and meta-analysis. *Nutrition Research (New York, N.Y.)*, *50*, 10–24. doi:10.1016/j.nutres.2017.10.014 PMID:29540268

Mellen, P. B., Gao, S. K., Vitolins, M. Z., & Goff, D. C. (2008). Deteriorating dietary habits among adults with hypertension: Dash dietary accordance, NHANES 1988-1994 and 1999-2004. *Archives of Internal Medicine*, *168*(3), 308–314. doi:10.1001/archinternmed.2007.119 PMID:18268173

Mena, M. P., Sacanella, E., Vazquez-Agell, M., Morales, M., Fitó, M., Escoda, R., ... Estruch, R. (2009). Inhibition of circulating immune cell activation: A molecular antiinflammatory effect of the Mediterranean diet. *The American Journal of Clinical Nutrition*, *89*(1), 248–256. doi:10.3945/ajcn.2008.26094 PMID:19056596

Mithril, C., Dragsted, L. O., Meyer, C., Blauert, E., Holt, M. K., & Astrup, A. (2012). Guidelines for the New Nordic Diet. *Public Health Nutrition, 15*(10), 1941–1947. doi:10.1017/S136898001100351X PMID:22251407

Moodley, R., Kindness, A., & Jonnalagadda, S. B. (2007). Elemental composition and chemical characteristics of five edible nuts (almond, Brazil, pecan, macadamia and walnut) consumed in Southern Africa. *Journal of Environmental Science and Health. Part. B, Pesticides, Food Contaminants, and Agricultural Wastes, 42*(5), 585–591. doi:10.1080/03601230701391591 PMID:17562467

Neale, E. P., Batterham, M. J., & Tapsell, L. C. (2016). *Consumption of a healthy dietary pattern results in significant reductions in C-reactive protein levels in adults: A meta-analysis. Nutrition Research.* Elsevier Inc. doi:10.1016/j.nutres.2016.02.009

Neufcourt, L., Assmann, K. E., Fezeu, L. K., Touvier, M., Graffouillère, L., Shivappa, N., ... Kesse-Guyot, E. (2015). Prospective association between the dietary inflammatory index and metabolic syndrome: Findings from the SU.VI. MAX study. *Nutrition, Metabolism, and Cardiovascular Diseases, 25*(11), 988–996. doi:10.1016/j.numecd.2015.09.002 PMID:26482566

O'Connor, L. M., Lentjes, M. A. H., Luben, R. N., Khaw, K. T., Wareham, N. J., & Forouhi, N. G. (2014). Dietary dairy product intake and incident type 2 diabetes: A prospective study using dietary data from a 7-day food diary. *Diabetologia, 57*(5), 909–917. doi:10.100700125-014-3176-1 PMID:24510203

O'Neil, A., Shivappa, N., Jacka, F. N., Kotowicz, M. A., Kibbey, K., Hebert, J. R., & Pasco, J. A. (2015). Pro-inflammatory dietary intake as a risk factor for CVD in men: A 5-year longitudinal study. *British Journal of Nutrition, 114*(12), 2074–2082. doi:10.1017/S0007114515003815 PMID:26450630

Orlich, M. J., Singh, P. N., Sabaté, J., Jaceldo-Siegl, K., Fan, J., Knutsen, S., ... Fraser, G. E. (2013). Vegetarian dietary patterns and mortality in adventist health study 2. *JAMA Internal Medicine, 173*(13), 1230–1238. doi:10.1001/jamainternmed.2013.6473 PMID:23836264

Pérez-López, F. R., Chedraui, P., Haya, J., & Cuadros, J. L. (2009). *Effects of the Mediterranean diet on longevity and age-related morbid conditions. Maturitas.* Elsevier Ireland Ltd.

Pilis, W., Stec, K., Zych, M., & Pilis, A. (2014). Health benefits and risk associated with adopting a vegetarian diet. *Roczniki Panstwowego Zakladu Higieny, 65*(1), 9–14. PMID:24964573

Poullis, A., Foster, R., Shetty, A., Fagerhol, M. K., & Mendall, M. A. (2004). Bowel Inflammation as Measured by Fecal Calprotectin: A Link between Lifestyle Factors and Colorectal Cancer Risk. *Cancer Epidemiology, Biomarkers & Prevention, 13*(2), 279–284. doi:10.1158/1055-9965.EPI-03-0160 PMID:14973103

Richard, C., Royer, M.-M., Couture, P., Cianflone, K., Rezvani, R., Desroches, S., & Lamarche, B. (2013). Effect of the Mediterranean diet on plasma adipokine concentrations in men with metabolic syndrome. *Metabolism: Clinical and Experimental, 62*(12), 1803–1810. doi:10.1016/j.metabol.2013.07.012 PMID:23993420

Ridker, P. M., Brown, N. J., Vaughan, D. E., Harrison, D. G., & Mehta, J. L. (2004). Established and Emerging Plasma Biomarkers in the Prediction of First Atherothrombotic Events. *Circulation, 109*(25 suppl. 1), IV-6-IV–19.

Romaguera, D. (2011). Mediterranean diet and type 2 diabetes risk in the European prospective investigation into cancer and nutrition (EPIC) study: The interAct project. *Diabetes Care, 34*(9), 1913–1918. doi:10.2337/dc11-0891 PMID:21788627

Root, M. M., McGinn, M. C., Nieman, D. C., Henson, D. A., Heinz, S. A., Shanely, R. A., ... Jin, F. (2012). Combined fruit and vegetable intake is correlated with improved inflammatory and oxidant status from a cross-sectional study in a community setting. *Nutrients, 4*(1), 29–41. doi:10.3390/nu4010029 PMID:22347616

Ros, E. (2009). Nuts and novel biomarkers of cardiovascular disease. *The American Journal of Clinical Nutrition, 89*(5), 1649–1656. doi:10.3945/ajcn.2009.26736R PMID:19321561

Sakhaei, R., Ramezani-Jolfaie, N., Mohammadi, M., & Salehi-Abargouei, A. (2019, February 1). The healthy Nordic dietary pattern has no effect on inflammatory markers: A systematic review and meta-analysis of randomized controlled clinical trials. *Nutrition.*

Sakhaei, R., Shahvazi, S., Mozaffari-Khosravi, H., Samadi, M., Khatibi, N., Nadjarzadeh, A., ... Salehi-Abargouei, A. (2018). The Dietary Approaches to Stop Hypertension (DASH)-Style Diet and an Alternative Mediterranean Diet are Differently Associated with Serum Inflammatory Markers in Female Adults. *Food and Nutrition Bulletin, 39*(3), 361–376. doi:10.1177/0379572118783950 PMID:29969908

Salehi-Abargouei, A., Maghsoudi, Z., Shirani, F., & Azadbakht, L. (2013). Effects of Dietary Approaches to Stop Hypertension (DASH)-style diet on fatal or nonfatal cardiovascular diseases-Incidence: A systematic review and meta-analysis on observational prospective studies. *Nutrition (Burbank, Los Angeles County, Calif.)*, *29*(4), 611–618. doi:10.1016/j.nut.2012.12.018 PMID:23466047

Salehi-Abargouei, A., Saraf-Bank, S., Bellissimo, N., & Azadbakht, L. (2015). Effects of non-soy legume consumption on C-reactive protein: A systematic review and meta-analysis. *Nutrition (Burbank, Los Angeles County, Calif.)*, *31*(5), 631–639. doi:10.1016/j.nut.2014.10.018 PMID:25837205

Samur, G., & Mercanlıgil, S. (2008). *Diyet Posası ve Beslenme (1st ed.)*. Ankara: Klasmat Matbaacılık.

Saneei, P., Salehi-Abargouei, A., Esmaillzadeh, A., & Azadbakht, L. (2014). Influence of Dietary Approaches to Stop Hypertension (DASH) diet on blood pressure: A systematic review and meta-analysis on randomized controlled trials. *Nutrition, Metabolism, and Cardiovascular Diseases*, *24*(12), 1253–1261. doi:10.1016/j.numecd.2014.06.008 PMID:25149893

Schröder, H. (2007). Protective mechanisms of the Mediterranean diet in obesity and type 2 diabetes. *The Journal of Nutritional Biochemistry*, *18*(3), 149–160. doi:10.1016/j.jnutbio.2006.05.006 PMID:16963247

Schwingshackl, L., Christoph, M., & Hoffmann, G. (2015). Effects of olive oil on markers of inflammation and endothelial function—A systematic review and meta-analysis. *Nutrients*, *7*(9), 7651–7675. doi:10.3390/nu7095356 PMID:26378571

Schwingshackl, L., & Hoffmann, G. (2013). Long-term effects of low glycemic index/load vs. high glycemic index/load diets on parameters of obesity and obesity-associated risks: A systematic review and meta-analysis. *Nutrition, Metabolism, and Cardiovascular Diseases*, *23*(8), 699–706. doi:10.1016/j.numecd.2013.04.008 PMID:23786819

Schwingshackl, L., & Hoffmann, G. (2014). Mediterranean dietary pattern, inflammation and endothelial function: A systematic review and meta-analysis of intervention trials. *Nutrition, Metabolism, and Cardiovascular Diseases*, *24*(9), 929–939. doi:10.1016/j.numecd.2014.03.003 PMID:24787907

Şentürk, N. (2013). Kütanöz inflamasyon. *Turkderm Deri Hastaliklari ve Frengi Arsivi*, *47*(Suppl. 1), 28–36.

Serra-Majem, L., Ribas, L., Ngo, J., Ortega, R. M., García, A., Pérez-Rodrigo, C., & Aranceta, J. (2004). Food, youth and the Mediterranean diet in Spain. Development of KIDMED, Mediterranean Diet Quality Index in children and adolescents. *Public Health Nutrition*, *7*(7), 931–935. doi:10.1079/PHN2004556 PMID:15482620

Shirani, F., Salehi-Abargouei, A., & Azadbakht, L. (2013). Effects of Dietary Approaches to Stop Hypertension (DASH) diet on some risk for developing type 2 diabetes: A systematic review and meta-analysis on controlled clinical trials. *Nutrition (Burbank, Los Angeles County, Calif.)*, *29*(7–8), 939–947. doi:10.1016/j.nut.2012.12.021 PMID:23473733

Shivappa, N. (2014). *Dietary Inflammatory Index and its relationship with inflammation, metabolic biomarkers and mortality*. University of South Carolina - Columbia.

Shivappa, N., Hébert, J. R., Rietzschel, E. R., De Buyzere, M. L., Langlois, M., Debruyne, E., ... Huybrechts, I. (2015). Associations between dietary inflammatory index and inflammatory markers in the Asklepios Study. *British Journal of Nutrition*, *113*(4), 665–671. doi:10.1017/S000711451400395X PMID:25639781

Shivappa, N., Steck, S. E., Hurley, T. G., Hussey, J. R., & Hébert, J. R. (2014). Designing and developing a literature-derived, population-based dietary inflammatory index. *Public Health Nutrition*, *17*(8), 1689–1696. doi:10.1017/S1368980013002115 PMID:23941862

Shivappa, N., Steck, S. E., Hurley, T. G., Hussey, J. R., Ma, Y., Ockene, I. S., ... Hébert, J. R. (2014). A population-based dietary inflammatory index predicts levels of C-reactive protein in the Seasonal Variation of Blood Cholesterol Study (SEASONS). *Public Health Nutrition*, *17*(8), 1825–1833. doi:10.1017/S1368980013002565 PMID:24107546

Siervo, M., Lara, J., Chowdhury, S., Ashor, A., Oggioni, C., & Mathers, J. C. (2015). Effects of the dietary approach to stop hypertension (DASH) diet on cardiovascular risk factors: A systematic review and meta-analysis. *British Journal of Nutrition*, *113*(1), 1–15. doi:10.1017/S0007114514003341 PMID:25430608

Soltani, S., Chitsazi, M. J., & Salehi-Abargouei, A. (2018). The effect of dietary approaches to stop hypertension (DASH) on serum inflammatory markers: A systematic review and meta-analysis of randomized trials. *Clinical Nutrition (Edinburgh, Scotland)*, *37*(2), 542–550. doi:10.1016/j.clnu.2017.02.018 PMID:28302405

Spencer, E. A., Appleby, P. N., Davey, G. K., & Key, T. J. (2003). Diet and body mass index in 38000 EPIC-Oxford meat-eaters, fish-eaters, vegetarians and vegans. *International Journal of Obesity and Related Metabolic Disorders*, *27*(6), 728–734. doi:10.1038j.ijo.0802300 PMID:12833118

Stricker, H., Duchini, F., Facchini, M., & Mombelli, G. (2008). Canola oil decreases cholesterol and improves endothelial function in patients with peripheral arterial occlusive disease - a pilot study. *Artery Research*, *2*(2), 67–73. doi:10.1016/j.artres.2008.02.001

Sutliffe, J. T., Wilson, L. D., de Heer, H. D., Foster, R. L., & Carnot, M. J. (2015). C-reactive protein response to a vegan lifestyle intervention. *Complementary Therapies in Medicine*, *23*(1), 32–37. doi:10.1016/j.ctim.2014.11.001 PMID:25637150

Szeto, Y. T., Kwok, T. C. Y., & Benzie, I. F. F. (2004). Effects of a long-term vegetarian diet on biomarkers of antioxidant status and cardiovascular disease risk. *Nutrition*, *20*(10), 863–866. doi:10.1016/j.nut.2004.06.006 PMID:15474873

Telle-Hansen, V. H., Holven, K. B., & Ulven, S. M. (2018). Impact of a Healthy Dietary Pattern on Gut Microbiota and Systemic Inflammation in Humans. *Nutrients*, *10*(11), 1783. doi:10.3390/nu10111783 PMID:30453534

Trichopoulou, A., Costacou, T., Bamia, C., & Trichopoulos, D. (2003). Adherence to a Mediterranean diet and survival in a Greek population. *The New England Journal of Medicine*, *348*(26), 2599–2608. doi:10.1056/NEJMoa025039 PMID:12826634

Uusitupa, M., Hermansen, K., Savolainen, M. J., Schwab, U., Kolehmainen, M., Brader, L., ... Åkesson, B. (2013). Effects of an isocaloric healthy Nordic diet on insulin sensitivity, lipid profile and inflammation markers in metabolic syndrome - a randomized study (SYSDIET). *Journal of Internal Medicine*, *274*(1), 52–66. doi:10.1111/joim.12044 PMID:23398528

Uusitupa, M., & Schwab, U. (2013). Diet, Inflammation and Prediabetes-Impact of Quality of Diet. *Canadian Journal of Diabetes*, *37*(5), 327–331. doi:10.1016/j.jcjd.2013.07.029 PMID:24500560

van Woudenbergh, G. J., Theofylaktopoulou, D., Kuijsten, A., Ferreira, I., van Greevenbroek, M. M., van der Kallen, C. J., ... Feskens, E. J. M. (2013). Adapted dietary inflammatory index and its association with a summary score for low-grade inflammation and markers of glucose metabolism: The Cohort study on Diabetes and Atherosclerosis Maastricht (CODAM) and the Hoorn study. *The American Journal of Clinical Nutrition*, *98*(6), 1533–1542. doi:10.3945/ajcn.112.056333 PMID:24153342

Viscogliosi, G., Cipriani, E., Liguori, M. L., Marigliano, B., Saliola, M., Ettorre, E., & Andreozzi, P. (2013). Mediterranean dietary pattern adherence: Associations with prediabetes, metabolic syndrome, and related microinflammation. *Metabolic Syndrome and Related Disorders*, *11*(3), 210–216. doi:10.1089/met.2012.0168 PMID:23451814

Wellen, K. E., & Hotamisligil, G. S. (2003). Obesity-induced inflammatory changes in adipose tissue. *The Journal of Clinical Investigation*, *112*(12), 1785–1788. doi:10.1172/JCI20514 PMID:14679172

Willett, W. C., Sacks, F., Trichopoulou, A., Drescher, G., Ferro-Luzzi, A., Helsing, E., & Trichopoulos, D. (1995). Mediterranean diet pyramid: A cultural model for healthy eating. *The American Journal of Clinical Nutrition*, *61*(6 Suppl.), 1402–1406. doi:10.1093/ajcn/61.6.1402S PMID:7754995

Wood, L. G., Shivappa, N., Berthon, B. S., Gibson, P. G., & Hebert, J. R. (2015). Dietary inflammatory index is related to asthma risk, lung function and systemic inflammation in asthma. *Clinical and Experimental Allergy*, *45*(1), 177–183. doi:10.1111/cea.12323 PMID:24708388

Yalçın, T., & Rakıcıoğlu, N. (2018). Dietary Factors, Type 2 Diabetes and Inflammation. *Sakarya Tıp Dergisi*, *8*(4), 686–694.

Zhu, H., Pollock, N. K., Kotak, I., Gutin, B., Wang, X., Bhagatwala, J., ... Dong, Y. (2014). Dietary sodium, adiposity, and inflammation in healthy adolescents. *Pediatrics*, *133*(3), e635–e642. doi:10.1542/peds.2013-1794 PMID:24488738

Related Readings

To continue IGI Global's long-standing tradition of advancing innovation through emerging research, please find below a compiled list of recommended IGI Global book chapters and journal articles in the areas of nutrition, inflammation, and food science. These related readings will provide additional information and guidance to further enrich your knowledge and assist you with your own research.

Ababio, G. K. (2018). Nutraceuticals: The Dose Makes the Difference – It's All in the Dose. In A. Verma, K. Srivastava, S. Singh, & H. Singh (Eds.), *Nutraceuticals and Innovative Food Products for Healthy Living and Preventive Care* (pp. 24–47). Hershey, PA: IGI Global. doi:10.4018/978-1-5225-2970-5.ch002

Agrawal, R. P., Agrawal, R., Faris, M. A., & Ghazzawi, H. A. (2020). Potential Anti-Diabetic Effect of Camel Milk. In O. Alhaj, B. Faye, & R. Agrawal (Eds.), *Handbook of Research on Health and Environmental Benefits of Camel Products* (pp. 185–196). Hershey, PA: IGI Global. doi:10.4018/978-1-7998-1604-1.ch009

Al-Sayyed, H. F. (2020). Historical Background and Population of Camels. In O. Alhaj, B. Faye, & R. Agrawal (Eds.), *Handbook of Research on Health and Environmental Benefits of Camel Products* (pp. 1–14). Hershey, PA: IGI Global. doi:10.4018/978-1-7998-1604-1.ch001

Alhaj, O. A. (2017). Functional Properties of Camel Milk. In H. Shekhar, Z. Howlader, & Y. Kabir (Eds.), *Exploring the Nutrition and Health Benefits of Functional Foods* (pp. 147–164). Hershey, PA: IGI Global. doi:10.4018/978-1-5225-0591-4.ch007

Alhaj, O. A. (2020). Exploring Potential Therapeutic Properties of Camel Milk. In O. Alhaj, B. Faye, & R. Agrawal (Eds.), *Handbook of Research on Health and Environmental Benefits of Camel Products* (pp. 123–154). Hershey, PA: IGI Global. doi:10.4018/978-1-7998-1604-1.ch007

Andreea, I. R. (2018). Beyond Macroeconomics of Food and Nutrition Security. *International Journal of Sustainable Economies Management, 7*(1), 13–22. doi:10.4018/IJSEM.2018010102

Asirvatham, J. (2018). Does Impulsive Response to Internal and External Food Cues Lead to Higher Calorie Intake?: Self-Control and Food Intake. *International Journal of Applied Behavioral Economics*, *7*(1), 14–34. doi:10.4018/IJABE.2018010102

Bajaj, S., & Manchanda, S. (2019). Nutraceutical and Functional Foods in Cancer Management and Therapy. In R. Keservani, A. Sharma, & R. Kesharwani (Eds.), *Nutraceutical and Functional Foods in Disease Prevention* (pp. 341–390). Hershey, PA: IGI Global. doi:10.4018/978-1-5225-3267-5.ch012

Basu, A., Sarkar, A., & Basak, P. (2018). Nutraceuticals for Human Health and Hypersensitivity Reaction. In A. Verma, K. Srivastava, S. Singh, & H. Singh (Eds.), *Nutraceuticals and Innovative Food Products for Healthy Living and Preventive Care* (pp. 323–341). Hershey, PA: IGI Global. doi:10.4018/978-1-5225-2970-5.ch015

Bohra, M., & Visen, A. (2018). Nutraceutical Properties in Flowers. In A. Verma, K. Srivastava, S. Singh, & H. Singh (Eds.), *Nutraceuticals and Innovative Food Products for Healthy Living and Preventive Care* (pp. 217–235). Hershey, PA: IGI Global. doi:10.4018/978-1-5225-2970-5.ch010

Buffo, R. (2017). Yerba Mate: Chemistry, Technology, and Biological Properties. In H. Shekhar, Z. Howlader, & Y. Kabir (Eds.), *Exploring the Nutrition and Health Benefits of Functional Foods* (pp. 185–194). Hershey, PA: IGI Global. doi:10.4018/978-1-5225-0591-4.ch009

Cascella, M., Muzio, M. R., Bimonte, S., & Cuomo, A. (2018). Nutraceuticals for Prevention of Chemotherapy-Induced Peripheral Neuropathy. In A. Verma, K. Srivastava, S. Singh, & H. Singh (Eds.), *Nutraceuticals and Innovative Food Products for Healthy Living and Preventive Care* (pp. 236–259). Hershey, PA: IGI Global. doi:10.4018/978-1-5225-2970-5.ch011

Choudhary, M., Tripathi, S., & Kesharwani, R. K. (2019). Nutraceuticals Role in Stress, Aging, and Neurodegenerative Disorders. In R. Keservani, A. Sharma, & R. Kesharwani (Eds.), *Nutraceutical and Functional Foods in Disease Prevention* (pp. 288–306). Hershey, PA: IGI Global. doi:10.4018/978-1-5225-3267-5.ch010

Dahiya, K., & Dhankhar, R. (2018). Role of Nutraceuticals in Cancer. In A. Verma, K. Srivastava, S. Singh, & H. Singh (Eds.), *Nutraceuticals and Innovative Food Products for Healthy Living and Preventive Care* (pp. 176–194). Hershey, PA: IGI Global. doi:10.4018/978-1-5225-2970-5.ch008

Dimitriou, M., Giazitzi, K., Stavridi, E., Palisidis, G., Karathanos, V., & Boskou, G. (2017). Evaluation of an Electronic Application for Nutritional Information in Food Service Outlets: A Pilot mHealth Application. *International Journal of Reliable and Quality E-Healthcare*, *6*(1), 46–58. doi:10.4018/IJRQEH.2017010104

Disouza, J. I., Patil, K. S., Kakade, P. S., & Patravale, V. B. (2019). Dietary Fibers and Nutraceuticals in Prevention of Hypertension. In R. Keservani, A. Sharma, & R. Kesharwani (Eds.), *Nutraceutical and Functional Foods in Disease Prevention* (pp. 192–232). Hershey, PA: IGI Global. doi:10.4018/978-1-5225-3267-5.ch007

Elsahoryi, N. A., & Al-Sayyed, H. F. (2020). Manufacture of Dairy and Non-Dairy Camel Milk Products. In O. Alhaj, B. Faye, & R. Agrawal (Eds.), *Handbook of Research on Health and Environmental Benefits of Camel Products* (pp. 75–109). Hershey, PA: IGI Global. doi:10.4018/978-1-7998-1604-1.ch005

Eshiet, E. R., & Smith, E. E. (2017). Herbal Benefits of Tea. In H. Shekhar, Z. Howlader, & Y. Kabir (Eds.), *Exploring the Nutrition and Health Benefits of Functional Foods* (pp. 117–146). Hershey, PA: IGI Global. doi:10.4018/978-1-5225-0591-4.ch006

Faris, M. A., & Attlee, A. (2017). Lentils (Lens culinaris, L.): A Novel Functional Food. In H. Shekhar, Z. Howlader, & Y. Kabir (Eds.), *Exploring the Nutrition and Health Benefits of Functional Foods* (pp. 42–72). Hershey, PA: IGI Global. doi:10.4018/978-1-5225-0591-4.ch003

Faris, M. A., & Ghazzawi, H. (2020). Health-Improving and Disease-Preventing Potential of Camel Milk Against Chronic Diseases and Autism: Camel Milk and Chronic Diseases. In O. Alhaj, B. Faye, & R. Agrawal (Eds.), *Handbook of Research on Health and Environmental Benefits of Camel Products* (pp. 155–184). Hershey, PA: IGI Global. doi:10.4018/978-1-7998-1604-1.ch008

Faye, B. (2020). Interaction Between Camel Farming and Environment. In O. Alhaj, B. Faye, & R. Agrawal (Eds.), *Handbook of Research on Health and Environmental Benefits of Camel Products* (pp. 363–378). Hershey, PA: IGI Global. doi:10.4018/978-1-7998-1604-1.ch017

Goswami, S., Mitra, S., Paul, P., Dey, D., & Das, S. (2019). Biochemic System of Medicine: Oldest Form of Nutraceutical Therapy. In R. Keservani, A. Sharma, & R. Kesharwani (Eds.), *Nutraceutical and Functional Foods in Disease Prevention* (pp. 403–431). Hershey, PA: IGI Global. doi:10.4018/978-1-5225-3267-5.ch014

Gupta, A. (2017). Functional Foods in Hypertension: Functional Foods in Cardiovascular Diseases. In H. Shekhar, Z. Howlader, & Y. Kabir (Eds.), *Exploring the Nutrition and Health Benefits of Functional Foods* (pp. 376–396). Hershey, PA: IGI Global. doi:10.4018/978-1-5225-0591-4.ch017

Gupta, C., Pacheco, C., & Prakash, D. (2018). Anti-Inflammatory Functional Foods. In A. Verma, K. Srivastava, S. Singh, & H. Singh (Eds.), *Nutraceuticals and Innovative Food Products for Healthy Living and Preventive Care* (pp. 48–78). Hershey, PA: IGI Global. doi:10.4018/978-1-5225-2970-5.ch003

Gupta, C., Pacheco, C., & Prakash, D. (2019). Lactoserum: As a Complete Nutraceutical. In R. Keservani, A. Sharma, & R. Kesharwani (Eds.), *Nutraceutical and Functional Foods in Disease Prevention* (pp. 432–456). Hershey, PA: IGI Global. doi:10.4018/978-1-5225-3267-5.ch015

Gupta, C., Prakash, D., & Gupta, S. (2019). Nutraceutical Intervention of Phytosterols in Cardiovascular Aging. In R. Keservani, A. Sharma, & R. Kesharwani (Eds.), *Nutraceutical and Functional Foods in Disease Prevention* (pp. 166–190). Hershey, PA: IGI Global. doi:10.4018/978-1-5225-3267-5.ch006

Hamid, S. B., & Hamid, A. F. (2019). Roles of Nutraceuticals and Functional Food in Prevention of Cardiovascular Disease: Sustaining Health. In R. Keservani, A. Sharma, & R. Kesharwani (Eds.), *Nutraceutical and Functional Foods in Disease Prevention* (pp. 126–165). Hershey, PA: IGI Global. doi:10.4018/978-1-5225-3267-5.ch005

Hasi, S., Amu, G., & Zhang, W. (2020). Camel Hair Structure, Properties, and Commercial Products. In O. Alhaj, B. Faye, & R. Agrawal (Eds.), *Handbook of Research on Health and Environmental Benefits of Camel Products* (pp. 328–347). Hershey, PA: IGI Global. doi:10.4018/978-1-7998-1604-1.ch015

Hemansi, V. R. K., Shukla, R., Gupta, R., & Saini, J. K. (2018). Food Grade Microorganisms for Nutraceutical Production for Industrial Applications. In A. Verma, K. Srivastava, S. Singh, & H. Singh (Eds.), Nutraceuticals and Innovative Food Products for Healthy Living and Preventive Care (pp. 342-367). Hershey, PA: IGI Global. doi:10.4018/978-1-5225-2970-5.ch016

Hosni, H., Periklis, D., & Baourakis, G. (2017). Consumers Attitude Towards Healthy Food: "Organic and Functional Foods. *International Journal of Food and Beverage Manufacturing and Business Models*, *2*(2), 85–99. doi:10.4018/IJFBMBM.2017070105

Howlader, M. Z., & Shekhar, H. U. (2017). Health Benefits and Risks of Rice. In H. Shekhar, Z. Howlader, & Y. Kabir (Eds.), *Exploring the Nutrition and Health Benefits of Functional Foods* (pp. 195–222). Hershey, PA: IGI Global. doi:10.4018/978-1-5225-0591-4.ch010

Ismail, T., Akhtar, S., & Riaz, M. (2017). Pomegranate Peel and Fruit Extracts: A Novel Approach to Avert Degenerative Disorders – Pomegranate and Degenerative Diseases. In H. Shekhar, Z. Howlader, & Y. Kabir (Eds.), *Exploring the Nutrition and Health Benefits of Functional Foods* (pp. 165–184). Hershey, PA: IGI Global. doi:10.4018/978-1-5225-0591-4.ch008

Jain, A., & Rani, V. (2017). Food and Cardiac Health: Protective Effects of Food on Cardiovascular System. In H. Shekhar, Z. Howlader, & Y. Kabir (Eds.), *Exploring the Nutrition and Health Benefits of Functional Foods* (pp. 1–15). Hershey, PA: IGI Global. doi:10.4018/978-1-5225-0591-4.ch001

Jaswir, I., Al-Kahtani, H. A., Octavianti, F., Lestari, W., & Yusof, N. (2020). Camel Gelatin Composition, Properties, Production, and Applications. In O. Alhaj, B. Faye, & R. Agrawal (Eds.), *Handbook of Research on Health and Environmental Benefits of Camel Products* (pp. 306–327). Hershey, PA: IGI Global. doi:10.4018/978-1-7998-1604-1.ch014

Jrad, Z., Oussaief, O., Khorchani, T., & El-Hatmi, H. (2020). Camel Colostrum Composition, Nutritional Value, and Nutraceuticals. In O. Alhaj, B. Faye, & R. Agrawal (Eds.), *Handbook of Research on Health and Environmental Benefits of Camel Products* (pp. 240–262). Hershey, PA: IGI Global. doi:10.4018/978-1-7998-1604-1.ch011

Ju, K. H., & Eung-Soo, H. (2017). Health Promoting Effects of Kimchi. In H. Shekhar, Z. Howlader, & Y. Kabir (Eds.), *Exploring the Nutrition and Health Benefits of Functional Foods* (pp. 73–98). Hershey, PA: IGI Global. doi:10.4018/978-1-5225-0591-4.ch004

Kadim, I. T., Mbaga, M., Ibrahim, G. A., & Nour, I. A. (2020). Camel Meat Production, Structure, and Quality. In O. Alhaj, B. Faye, & R. Agrawal (Eds.), *Handbook of Research on Health and Environmental Benefits of Camel Products* (pp. 263–284). Hershey, PA: IGI Global. doi:10.4018/978-1-7998-1604-1.ch012

Kadim, I. T., Purchas, R., Al-Amri, I., Alkindi, A., & Abbas, G. (2020). Camel Meat Nutrient Content and Potential Health Benefits. In O. Alhaj, B. Faye, & R. Agrawal (Eds.), *Handbook of Research on Health and Environmental Benefits of Camel Products* (pp. 285–305). Hershey, PA: IGI Global. doi:10.4018/978-1-7998-1604-1.ch013

Kaindi, D. W., & Njage, P. M. (2020). Microbial Aspect of Lactic Acid Bacteria Isolated From Camel Milk. In O. Alhaj, B. Faye, & R. Agrawal (Eds.), *Handbook of Research on Health and Environmental Benefits of Camel Products* (pp. 54–74). Hershey, PA: IGI Global. doi:10.4018/978-1-7998-1604-1.ch004

Konuspayeva, G. S. (2020). Camel Milk Composition and Nutritional Value. In O. Alhaj, B. Faye, & R. Agrawal (Eds.), *Handbook of Research on Health and Environmental Benefits of Camel Products* (pp. 15–40). Hershey, PA: IGI Global. doi:10.4018/978-1-7998-1604-1.ch002

Konuspayeva, G. S. (2020). Manufacture and Challenges of Camel Milk Cheese. In O. Alhaj, B. Faye, & R. Agrawal (Eds.), *Handbook of Research on Health and Environmental Benefits of Camel Products* (pp. 110–122). Hershey, PA: IGI Global. doi:10.4018/978-1-7998-1604-1.ch006

Krbez, J. M., & Shaout, A. (2019). Interval Type-2 Fuzzy Application for Diet Journaling. *International Journal of Fuzzy System Applications, 8*(2), 34–67. doi:10.4018/IJFSA.2019040103

Kumar, B., Singh, S., Srivastava, K., & Wani, K. A. (2018). New Product Development and Regulatory Challenges in Nutraceutical Industry. In A. Verma, K. Srivastava, S. Singh, & H. Singh (Eds.), *Nutraceuticals and Innovative Food Products for Healthy Living and Preventive Care* (pp. 280–303). Hershey, PA: IGI Global. doi:10.4018/978-1-5225-2970-5.ch013

Kumar, R., & Rizvi, S. I. (2019). The Protective Role of Nutraceuticals and Functional Food in Hyperlipidemia. In R. Keservani, A. Sharma, & R. Kesharwani (Eds.), *Nutraceutical and Functional Foods in Disease Prevention* (pp. 233–254). Hershey, PA: IGI Global. doi:10.4018/978-1-5225-3267-5.ch008

Lee, C. (2017). Application of the Dietary Processed Sulfur Supplementation for Enhancing Nutritional and Functional Properties of Meat Products. In H. Shekhar, Z. Howlader, & Y. Kabir (Eds.), *Exploring the Nutrition and Health Benefits of Functional Foods* (pp. 254–264). Hershey, PA: IGI Global. doi:10.4018/978-1-5225-0591-4.ch012

Luiz, O. J., Weber, V. A., Cagnin, M. I., Raposo de Medeiros, S., Gomes, R. D., Cristine de Souza, L., & Paiva, D. M. (2018). Computational System to Support Bovine Nutritional Behavior. *International Journal of Agricultural and Environmental Information Systems, 9*(3), 22–37. doi:10.4018/IJAEIS.2018070102

Mayo, B., Guadamuro, L., Flórez, A. B., & Delgado, S. (2017). Soy and Soy Products, Isoflavones, Equol, and Health. In H. Shekhar, Z. Howlader, & Y. Kabir (Eds.), *Exploring the Nutrition and Health Benefits of Functional Foods* (pp. 223–253). Hershey, PA: IGI Global. doi:10.4018/978-1-5225-0591-4.ch011

Mboya, R. M. (2019). The Nutritional and Health Potential of Blackjack (Bidens pilosa l.): A Review – Promoting the Use of Blackjack for Food. *International Journal of Applied Research on Public Health Management, 4*(1), 47–66. doi:10.4018/IJARPHM.2019010104

Mehta, R. D., & Agrawal, R. (2020). Camel Milk Disguised Cosmeceutical. In O. Alhaj, B. Faye, & R. Agrawal (Eds.), *Handbook of Research on Health and Environmental Benefits of Camel Products* (pp. 348–362). Hershey, PA: IGI Global. doi:10.4018/978-1-7998-1604-1.ch016

Mentado, M. N., & Pérez, E. S. (2019). Low Glycemic Index Diets for Subjects With Diabetes by Minimizing Glycemic Load of Individual Foods. *International Journal of Privacy and Health Information Management, 7*(1), 1–17. doi:10.4018/IJPHIM.2019010101

Metwalli, A. A., & Hailu, Y. (2020). Effects of Industrial Processing Methods on Camel Milk Composition, Nutritional Value, and Health Properties. In O. Alhaj, B. Faye, & R. Agrawal (Eds.), *Handbook of Research on Health and Environmental Benefits of Camel Products* (pp. 197–239). Hershey, PA: IGI Global. doi:10.4018/978-1-7998-1604-1.ch010

Mishra, A., Chaudhari, D. D., Patel, H. K., & Patel, B. D. (2018). Nutraceutical Properties of Important Weeds in India. In A. Verma, K. Srivastava, S. Singh, & H. Singh (Eds.), *Nutraceuticals and Innovative Food Products for Healthy Living and Preventive Care* (pp. 304–322). Hershey, PA: IGI Global. doi:10.4018/978-1-5225-2970-5.ch014

Mitra, S., & Khandelwal, S. (2017). Health Benefits of Tea: Beneficial Effects of Tea on Human Health. In H. Shekhar, Z. Howlader, & Y. Kabir (Eds.), *Exploring the Nutrition and Health Benefits of Functional Foods* (pp. 99–116). Hershey, PA: IGI Global. doi:10.4018/978-1-5225-0591-4.ch005

Mudila, H., Prasher, P., Khati, B., Kumar, S., & Punetha, H. (2018). Nutraceuticals for Healthy Sporting. In A. Verma, K. Srivastava, S. Singh, & H. Singh (Eds.), *Nutraceuticals and Innovative Food Products for Healthy Living and Preventive Care* (pp. 79–107). Hershey, PA: IGI Global. doi:10.4018/978-1-5225-2970-5.ch004

Muyonga, J. H., Nansereko, S., Steenkamp, I., Manley, M., & Okoth, J. K. (2017). Traditional African Foods and Their Potential to Contribute to Health and Nutrition: Traditional African Foods. In H. Shekhar, Z. Howlader, & Y. Kabir (Eds.), *Exploring the Nutrition and Health Benefits of Functional Foods* (pp. 320–346). Hershey, PA: IGI Global. doi:10.4018/978-1-5225-0591-4.ch015

Oussaief, O., Jrad, Z., Khorchani, T., & El-Hatmi, H. (2020). Strategies and Technologies for Camel Milk Preservation. In O. Alhaj, B. Faye, & R. Agrawal (Eds.), *Handbook of Research on Health and Environmental Benefits of Camel Products* (pp. 41–53). Hershey, PA: IGI Global. doi:10.4018/978-1-7998-1604-1.ch003

Parsad, C., Chandra, C. P., & Suman, S. (2019). A Product Feature Prioritization-Based Segmentation Model of Consumer Market for Health Drinks. *International Journal of Strategic Decision Sciences, 10*(2), 70–83. doi:10.4018/IJSDS.2019040104

Passi, S. J. (2017). Functional Foods and Cardiac Health. In H. Shekhar, Z. Howlader, & Y. Kabir (Eds.), *Exploring the Nutrition and Health Benefits of Functional Foods* (pp. 16–41). Hershey, PA: IGI Global. doi:10.4018/978-1-5225-0591-4.ch002

Patravale, V. B., & Joshi, A. K. (2019). An Overview of the Therapeutic Aspect of Living Drugs Probiotics. In R. Keservani, A. Sharma, & R. Kesharwani (Eds.), *Nutraceutical and Functional Foods in Disease Prevention* (pp. 1–34). Hershey, PA: IGI Global. doi:10.4018/978-1-5225-3267-5.ch001

Patravale, V. B., Kadwadkar, N. A., Patki, S. R., & Disouza, J. I. (2019). Nutraceutical and Functional Foods in Treatment of Anemia. In R. Keservani, A. Sharma, & R. Kesharwani (Eds.), *Nutraceutical and Functional Foods in Disease Prevention* (pp. 308–339). Hershey, PA: IGI Global. doi:10.4018/978-1-5225-3267-5.ch011

Patravale, V. B., Naik, S. V., & Dhage, S. N. (2019). Role of Diet, Functional Foods, and Nutraceuticals in Brain Disorders. In R. Keservani, A. Sharma, & R. Kesharwani (Eds.), *Nutraceutical and Functional Foods in Disease Prevention* (pp. 256–287). Hershey, PA: IGI Global. doi:10.4018/978-1-5225-3267-5.ch009

Poonia, A. (2017). Antimicrobial Edible Films and Coatings for Fruits and Vegetables. In H. Shekhar, Z. Howlader, & Y. Kabir (Eds.), *Exploring the Nutrition and Health Benefits of Functional Foods* (pp. 301–319). Hershey, PA: IGI Global. doi:10.4018/978-1-5225-0591-4.ch014

Poonia, A. (2019). Recent Trends in Functional Foods for Obesity Management. In R. Keservani, A. Sharma, & R. Kesharwani (Eds.), *Nutraceutical and Functional Foods in Disease Prevention* (pp. 69–92). Hershey, PA: IGI Global. doi:10.4018/978-1-5225-3267-5.ch003

Punetha, H., Kumar, S., Mudila, H., & Prakash, O. (2018). Brassica Meal as Source of Health Protecting Neuraceutical and Its Antioxidative Properties. In A. Verma, K. Srivastava, S. Singh, & H. Singh (Eds.), *Nutraceuticals and Innovative Food Products for Healthy Living and Preventive Care* (pp. 108–131). Hershey, PA: IGI Global. doi:10.4018/978-1-5225-2970-5.ch005

Rani, K. (2019). Clinical Role of Antioxidants in the Treatment of Diseases. In R. Keservani, A. Sharma, & R. Kesharwani (Eds.), *Nutraceutical and Functional Foods in Disease Prevention* (pp. 392–401). Hershey, PA: IGI Global. doi:10.4018/978-1-5225-3267-5.ch013

Saeed, N., Khan, S. K., Raheed, H. M., & Hussain, M. Z. (2018). Empirical Analysis of Socio-economic Factors Effecting Nutritional Status of Children (1-5) of Age. *International Journal of Civic Engagement and Social Change*, *5*(4), 1–18. doi:10.4018/IJCESC.2018100101

Sen, S., & Chakraborty, R. (2017). Food in Health Preservation and Promotion: A Special Focus on the Interplay between Oxidative Stress and Pro-Oxidant/Antioxidant. In H. Shekhar, Z. Howlader, & Y. Kabir (Eds.), *Exploring the Nutrition and Health Benefits of Functional Foods* (pp. 265–300). Hershey, PA: IGI Global. doi:10.4018/978-1-5225-0591-4.ch013

Sidhu, J. S., & Zafar, T. A. (2017). Functional Foods of the Indian Subcontinent. In H. Shekhar, Z. Howlader, & Y. Kabir (Eds.), *Exploring the Nutrition and Health Benefits of Functional Foods* (pp. 347–375). Hershey, PA: IGI Global. doi:10.4018/978-1-5225-0591-4.ch016

Thakur, K., Zhang, J. G., Wei, Z., Kumar, N., Tomar, S. K., & Pophaly, S. D. (2018). Cross Talk Between Functional Foods and Gut Health. In A. Verma, K. Srivastava, S. Singh, & H. Singh (Eds.), *Nutraceuticals and Innovative Food Products for Healthy Living and Preventive Care* (pp. 195–216). Hershey, PA: IGI Global. doi:10.4018/978-1-5225-2970-5.ch009

Tingirikari, J. M. (2019). Functional Foods for Treatment and Prevention of Obesity and Its Associated Disorders. In R. Keservani, A. Sharma, & R. Kesharwani (Eds.), *Nutraceutical and Functional Foods in Disease Prevention* (pp. 93–124). Hershey, PA: IGI Global. doi:10.4018/978-1-5225-3267-5.ch004

Tingirikari, J. M., Sarathy, M. V., & Karthigarani, A. K. (2019). Impact of Probiotics in Human Health and Disease Treatment. In R. Keservani, A. Sharma, & R. Kesharwani (Eds.), *Nutraceutical and Functional Foods in Disease Prevention* (pp. 35–67). Hershey, PA: IGI Global. doi:10.4018/978-1-5225-3267-5.ch002

Uvanesh, K., Nayak, S. K., Sagiri, S. S., Banerjee, I., Ray, S. S., & Pal, K. (2018). Effect of Non-Ionic Hydrophilic and Hydrophobic Surfactants on the Properties on the Stearate Oleogels: A Comparative Study. In A. Verma, K. Srivastava, S. Singh, & H. Singh (Eds.), *Nutraceuticals and Innovative Food Products for Healthy Living and Preventive Care* (pp. 260–279). Hershey, PA: IGI Global. doi:10.4018/978-1-5225-2970-5.ch012

Verma, A. K., Singh, A., & Negi, M. S. (2018). Nutriproteomics: An Advance Methodology of Nutrichemical Analysis. In A. Verma, K. Srivastava, S. Singh, & H. Singh (Eds.), *Nutraceuticals and Innovative Food Products for Healthy Living and Preventive Care* (pp. 1–23). Hershey, PA: IGI Global. doi:10.4018/978-1-5225-2970-5.ch001

Wani, K. A., Manzoor, J., Anjum, J., Bashir, M., & Mamta,. (2018). Pesticides in Vegetables: Their Impact on Nutritional Quality and Human Health. In A. Verma, K. Srivastava, S. Singh, & H. Singh (Eds.), *Nutraceuticals and Innovative Food Products for Healthy Living and Preventive Care* (pp. 132-157). Hershey, PA: IGI Global. doi:10.4018/978-1-5225-2970-5.ch006

About the Contributors

Uğur Günşen was born in Bandirma on October 22, 1965. He completed my undergraduate education at the Faculty of Veterinary, University of Uludağ. He has completed two different doctorate degrees, one in Biochemistry and another in Food Science and Technology, in University of Uludag. Since 2008, he has been working as a full Professor at the University of Bandirma Onyedi Eylul, Faculty of Health Sciences, Department of Nutrition and Dietetics. So far, he has presented 20 papers at international scientific congresses. He has twenty articles in international scientific journals, twenty articles in national journals, and two national books and books chapters.

Ramazan Mert Atan was born in Istanbul on February 21, 1995. He completed his undergraduate education in the Department of Nutrition and Dietetics, School of Health, Kırklareli University. He completed his master's degree with a thesis in the field of Nutrition and Dietetics from the Institute of Health Sciences of Tekirdağ Namık Kemal University. He is currently a PhD student in Nutrition and Dietetics at Istanbul Medipol University. Since 2018, he has been working as a research assistant at Bandırma Onyedi Eylül University, Faculty of Health Sciences, Department of Nutrition and Dietetics. So far, he has had 14 papers in international scientific congresses. He has two articles in international scientific journals, one article in a national journal, and one international book chapter.

Sedat Demir was born in Istanbul in 1960. He completed his undergraduate education in the Faculty of Medicine, University of İstanbul Cerrahpaşa. He specialized in General Internal Medicine at University of Fırat, Faculty of Medicine, Department of Internal Medicine. He became an Associate Professor of Internal Diseases in 1996 while he was a faculty member at the Department of Cardiology at University of Celal Bayar School of Medicine. In 2016, he was appointed as a professor to the Department of Internal Medicine, Faculty of Medicine, Istanbul Aydın University. He still works as a freelance physician in his own clinic. He has many research, scientific articles and studies.

Hüseyin Eseceli was born in 1968 in Kırıkkale, Turkey. He graduated from Istanbul University Veterinary Faculty in 1992. In 2003, he received his doctorate degree in Animal Nutrition and Nutritional Diseases, then in 2013 he became an associate professor and in 2017 he became a professor. Since 2017, he has been working as a Professor in the Department of Nutrition Sciences, Department of Nutrition and Dietetics, Faculty of Health Sciences, Bandırma Onyedi Eylül University and Professor Eseceli has 33 national and international research articles, 6 book chapters, 62 scientific papers, and 21 projects. These studies include research articles on the effects of probiotics and prebiotics in animals. He is a member of the Animal Nutrition Science Association and the Veterinary Poultry Association. He has 6 awards from the Scientific Publication Incentive (TÜBİTAK) and his scientific studies.

Fatma Esra Güneş was born in Istanbul, graduated from Hacettepe University Department of Nutrition and Dietetics in 1991. In 1994, she got a master's degree from Selcuk University, Faculty of Medicine, Department of Public Health. In 2007, she completed her PhD at Selcuk University, Faculty of Veterinary Medicine, Department of Food Hygiene and Technology. She received the title of Associate Professor in 2016 and since 2016, she has been working as the Head of the Nutrition and Dietetic Department at Health Sciences Faculty of Marmara University. She has more than 50 articles and papers published in SCI and other international journals and congresses. Her research interests include nutrition sciences, dietetics, community nutrition and epidemiology, and food technology.

Kevser Tarı Selçuk, Dr., was born in İzmir in 1981 and completed his primary, secondary, high school, and undergraduate education in Balıkesir. In 2010, she received her master's degree from Celal Bayar University, Institute of Health Sciences, Department of Public Health. In 2013, she received her PhD degree from Dokuz Eylül University Institute of Health Sciences, Department of Public Health. Kevser Tarı Selçuk worked in different health institutions as a midwife between 2001-2013, entered the academic life as a lecturer doctor in 2014. She is currently a faculty member in the Department of Nutrition and Dietetics, Faculty of Health Sciences at Bandırma Onyedi Eylül University and continues her studies in the field of public health.

Leyla Tevfikoğlu Pehlivan, Dr. Leyla, was originally from Targovishte, Bulgaria, and moved to Turkey in 1989. She works in the field of nutrition and dietetics. Her research interests include nutrition, medical nutrition therapies in diseases, and community nutrition. She is a member of Turkey Dietitians Association.

Index

L

M

N

O

P

R

V

www.ingramcontent.com/pod-product-compliance
Lightning Source LLC
LaVergne TN
LVHW081322300926
849161LV00008B/1856